# Foundations of Physical Therapy

## A 21st Century-Focused View of the Profession

# Foundations of Physical Therapy

## A 21st Century-Focused View of the Profession

Ron Scott, OCS, MSPT, JD

Associate Professor and Chair
Physical Therapy Dcpartment
Lebanon Valley College
Annville, Pennsylvania



**McGraw Hill**

Medical Publishing Division

New York Chicago San Francisco Lisbon London Madrid Mexico City Milan New Delhi
San Juan Seoul Singapore Sydney Toronto

**McGraw-Hill**

*A Division of The* ***McGraw-Hill*** *Companies*

**Foundations of Physical Therapy: A 21st Century-Focused View of the Profession**



1234567890 DOCDOC 0987654321

ISBN: 0-07-135590-1

**NOTICE**

Medicine is an ever-changing science. As new research and clinical experience broaden our knowledge, changes in treatment and drug therapy are required. The author and the publisher of this work have checked with sources believed to be reliable in their efforts to provide information that is complete and generally in accord with the standards accepted at the time of publication. However, in view of the possibility of human error or changes in medical sciences, neither the author nor the publisher nor any other party who has been involved in the preparation or publication of this work warrants that the information contained herein is in every respect accurate or complete, and they disclaim all responsibility for any errors or omissions or for the results obtained from use of the information contained in this work. Readers are encouraged to confirm the information contained herein with other sources. For example and in particular, readers are advised to check the product information sheet included in the package of each drug they plan to administer to be certain that the information contained in this work is accurate and that changes have not been made in the recommended dose or the contraindications for administration. This recommendation is of particular importance in connection with new or infrequently used drugs.

The book was set in Palatino by Circle Graphics.
The editors were Julie Scardiglia and Karen Davis.
The production supervisor was Lisa T. Mendez.
The text design was by José Fonfrias.
The cover designer was Aimée Nordin.
The index was prepared by Marilyn Rowland.
R. R. Donnelley & Sons, Crawfordsville, was printer and binder.

This book was printed on acid-free paper.

**Library of Congress Cataloging-in-Publication Data**

Scott, Ronald W.
Foundations of physical therapy : a 21st century-focused view of the profession / author, Ron Scott.
p. ; cm.
Includes bibliographical references and index.
ISBN 0-07-135590-1
1. Physical Therapy. I. Title.
[DNLM: 1. Physical Therapy. WB 460 S428f 2001]
RM700.S375 2001
615.8′2--dc21 2001044041

*I dedicate this book with love to my wonderful wife of 28 years*

*Maria Josefa Scott*

*who has consistently encouraged, inspired, and supported me.*

*I also dedicate the book to all of*

*the physical therapy (PT and PTA) professionals and their support staffs*

*who make this vocation such a rewarding and enjoyable one.*

*Thank you for your superlative service to patients,*

*the profession, and society.*

*Our deepest sympathy goes out*

*to the families of the victims*

*of the September 11, 2001, terrorist attack*

*on the United States.*

# Contributors

Dolores Bertoti, MS, PT, PCS
*Dean of Allied Health*
*Alvernia College*
*Reading, Pennsylvania*

Jennifer M. Bottomley, MS, PT, PhD
*President, Geriatric Section*
*American Physical Therapy Association*
*Alexandria, Virginia*

Ron Scott, OCS, MSPT, JD
*Associate Professor and Chair*
*Physical Therapy Department*
*Lebanon Valley College*
*Annville, Pennsylvania*

Penny Samuelson, MS, PT
*Lebanon Orthopedic Associates*
*Lebanon, Pennsylvania*

Kristin Zwemer, PT, MSPT
*HealthSouth*
*Mechanicsburg, Pennsylvania*

# Contents

# *Preface*

At the advent of the 21st century, the physical therapy profession is at a crossroads, as it has been at several points throughout its history. In its inaugural in the 20th century, physical therapy was formed and formalized; its initial scope of practice defined and developed; and its educational and scholarly roots cultivated. In the 21st century, physical therapy faces new problems, issues, and dilemmas, including, among myriad others, reconfiguration of the discipline of physical therapy as a doctorally prepared one; expanded scope of practice and concomitant competency and encroachment issues; the technological revolution directly and indirectly affecting all aspects of physical therapy practice (clinical, educational, and research); and globalization and resource allocation as they impact the profession and the patients and clients we serve.

Whatever the changes be that affect physical therapy, it will always remain an altruistically focused, patient/client-centered health professional service discipline, whose physical therapist and assistant professionals and their support professionals are committed to optimizing patient/client physical function and mental well being through their interventions. Political and economic realities, including the cost-focused managed care health care delivery paradigm, seemingly make this formidable responsibility more challenging, if not more difficult. But while political and economic theories and practices may come and go, fundamental health disciplines like physical therapy continue to thrive, in part because of the profession's human resources who continue to lead and follow in positive, new practice and service directions.

This text offers a vista of the physical therapy profession and its milieu. Chapter 1, The Physical Therapy Profession, explores with a historical perspective the profession at the commencement of the new millennium. The chapter addresses fundamental and current issues, including the nature of a profession and professionalism, and intra- and interdisciplinary health professional relations. Chapter 2, Education, addresses physical therapy education and vitally important accreditation processes; learning domains; curricular models; and postprofessional education generally. The most recent accreditation Evaluative Criteria of the Commission on Accreditation in Physical Therapy Education (CAPTE) are included (with permission) as an appendix to Chapter 2 primarily as a resource to facilitate student and clinician education program assessment and discussion.

Chapter 3 addresses physical therapy clinical practice in general and overviews, among other topics, clinical practice settings and specialties, direct access and evidence-based practice, the evolving *Guide to Physical Therapist Practice,* and the mentoring process as applied to physical therapy. Chapters 4 through 7 offer focused vignettes by clinical experts on neurologic, orthopaedic, geriatric, and pediatric clinical physical therapy practice, respectively.

Chapter 8 addresses legal and ethical standards as they affect physical therapy, and overviews the newly revised *Code of Ethics* and *Guide for Professional Conduct,* which govern the official conduct of physical therapist members of the American Physical Therapy Association (APTA); licensure, certification and credentialing; the Model Practice Act; patient bills of rights and responsibilities; civil rights, clinical affiliations contracts; physical therapy malpractice; the law and ethics of patient informed consent to care; and disciplinary processes and procedures of the APTA. The most recent edition of the Model Practice Act is included in its entirety (with grateful permission of the Federation of State Boards of Physical Therapy) to facilitate student/professor discussion on the comparative analyses of state and foreign practice acts.

Chapter 9, Professional Associations and Responsibility, overviews the APTA, World Confederation for Physical Therapy, and the Tri-Alliance of Health and Rehabilitation Professionals. Chapter 10, Salient Issues, addresses some, but not all, of the current issues affecting the profession at the time of the writing of the book. The broad brush of current issues offers discussion of managed care and physical therapy-specific education and practice issues, including the Vector Workforce Study and its aftermath.

Many chapters feature the following sections: Key Words and Phrases, a chapter abstract including objectives; a summary section; activities, cases, and questions; and additional readings. Focus on a Leader and Clinical Practice chapters draw in the special expertise and perspectives of selected leaders in the profession, including: Dolores Bertoti, Jennifer Bottomley, Beth Domholdt, Mary Jane Harris, Jonathan Cooperman, Rick Ritter, Penny Samuelson, Jayne Leigh Snyder, Mary Ann Wharton, Ted Yanchuleff, and Kris Zwemer. Select appendices, photographs, and figures augment the written text for clarification and/or illustration.

I hope that this text serves to foster discussion and debate within the physical therapy profession, and acts as a catalyst for continued positive evolution of the profession and self-actualization of its members, who are the foundation of physical therapy.

Ron Scott
December 2001

CHAPTER 1

# The Physical Therapy Profession

RON SCOTT

## Key Words and Phrases

Allied Health Professions
American Occupational Therapy Association
American Physical Therapy Association
Army Medical Specialist Corps
Certified Occupational Therapy Assistants
Classic Professions
Code of Ethics
Direct Access Practice
Extender Personnel
Federation of State Boards of Physical Therapy
*Guide for Conduct of the Affiliate Member*
*Guide for Professional Conduct*
*Guide to Physical Therapist Practice*
Gymnast
Infantile Paralysis
Interdisciplinary
Keens Chophouse
Managed Care
Mary McMillan
Multidisciplinary
National Board for Certification in Occupational Therapy
Occupational Therapists
Occupational Therapy
Occupational Therapy Code of Ethics
Orthotists
Physical Therapist Assistants
Physical Therapists
Physical Therapy
*Pro bono publico*
Profession
Professional
Prosthetists
Reconstruction Aide
Reed College
Reimbursement Policies
Standards of Ethical Conduct for the Physical Therapist Assistant
Support Professionals

*Physical therapy is a primary health profession composed of two interdependent disciplines: licensed physical therapists and physical therapist assistants. Physical therapist assistants carry out therapeutic interventions for patients under the supervision of physical therapists, who bear ultimate responsibility for patient care, safety, and welfare. Additional participants in physical therapy clinical activities include extender, support, administrative, and clerical professionals. Every physical therapy professional must develop an accurate, concise, and easily comprehensible personal definition of physical therapy to communicate to patients and relevant others. Managed care has made the role of fiduciary more difficult to fulfill for physical therapy professionals. Historically, physical therapy developed at the advent of the 20th century in response to infantile paralysis (polio) and in support of military servicemen in World War I. Mary McMillan, along with other women and men, formed wartime Reconstruction Aides, dedicated to physical rehabilitation and the mental well-being of injured military service personnel. From this genesis, the interrelated professions of physical and occupational therapy emerged. The precursor to the American Physical Therapy Association (see Appendix I) was formed in 1921 at Keens Chophouse in New York City. The Association today serves over 67,000 professional and affiliate members. Irrespective of whether physical therapists and physical therapist assistants are "classic professionals" (like attorneys, physicians, and clergy), physical therapy professionals clearly possess the attributes that characterize a true profession: a defined body of knowledge, relative autonomy, formal education, clinical research to validate practice, a code of professional ethics, recognition of advanced competencies, and public service. Physical therapy professionals, like* all *other health professionals, are allied health professionals, working in support of the patients they serve.*

## THE PROFESSION AT ADVENT OF THE 21st CENTURY

At the advent of the new millennium, the physical therapy profession stands, as it has several times in the 20th century, at a crossroads. As the principal work product of this primary clinical health care profession, physical therapy service delivery is vital to the health and well-being of patients and the public at large. The promise of optimal quality health care service delivery is the most significant expectation of the public, and of politicians and health care professionals in society. That expectation has been dampened somewhat by macro-level political events, especially resulting from the growth and predominance of managed care, the health care delivery and financing paradigm under which optimal quality health care service delivery has seemingly been displaced as the preeminent goal of the health care system by the desire for health care cost containment. Physical therapists and assistants and their support professionals have borne substantial hardship because of managed care, both in terms of their relative financial positions and in their abilities to serve patients and clients to the degree to which they have traditionally been accustomed to serve. Managed care will be examined in greater detail in Chapter 10, "Salient Issues."

Managed care is not the only external force adversely affecting the profession of physical therapy, and the ability of physical therapy professionals to fully serve their clientele. Federal (and resultant or complementary state and local) reimbursement public policy over the past decade has adversely affected all health professional disciplines, but particularly the rehabilitation professions, including, but not limited to, physical, occupational, and speech therapy. From restrictive numbers of patient care visits to arbitrary aggregate caps on service reimbursement, rehabilitation professionals have been forced to pare health care service delivery (in many or most cases) to subjectively suboptimal levels and to provide services for substantially less compensation. Although innovative measures, for example, clinical research to validate interventions, clinical practice guidelines, and the implementation of *pro bono publico* (free or reduced cost) care, have blunted somewhat the adverse effects of reimbursement reductions, virtually every physical therapy professional is "feeling the pinch." And, sadly, so are many physical therapy patients.

Not all problems affecting the profession of physical therapy are external ones. Some problems, although certainly not applicable to all or even a majority of professionals, emanate from within. These include, but are not limited to, apathy or lethargy, manifested in noninvolvement in professional association and other professional activities or in the political process; abuse of the reimbursement system; and the failure to maintain state-of-the-art clinical and practice competencies.

Physical therapy is representative of a primary health care discipline that, in many respects, can and will exercise substantial control over its own destiny in the 21st century through individual and collective political action. The assertion that physical therapy is a vital primary health care discipline may seem to be a truism; however, physical therapy professionals must assert their positions and political influence at all levels of government in order to remain prominent professionals on the American health care scene.

## PHYSICAL THERAPY DEFINED

The physical therapy profession is commonly thought of as a rehabilitation discipline; however, from its inception, it has always encompassed health care activities that fall outside the scope of physical rehabilitation, such as wound care, cardiopulmonary intervention, preventive interventions, and patient/client education, among many other activities. As such, "physical therapy" is difficult to define.

Every physical therapist and physical therapist assistant (including professional students) must formulate in his or her mind, and be ready to articulate to others, a personal definition of physical therapy. Nothing is more disconcerting than to encounter a physical therapist or physical therapist assistant who cannot clearly, completely, and concisely define and describe his or her own profession.

As an individual physical therapist or physical therapist assistant grows personally and professionally toward self-determination and self-actualization, that person's definition of physical therapy will become refined as it is augmented, perhaps hundreds of times over a career or lifetime. One of the exercises at the end of this chapter addresses the concept of formulating and recording one's own personal definition of, and place within, the profession.

A Model Definition of Physical Therapy, developed by the Federation of State Boards of Physical Therapy, and adopted by the Board of Directors of the American Physical Therapy Association in 1993, defined physical therapy as follows:

> Physical therapy means the assessment, evaluation, and treatment and prevention of physical disability, movement dysfunction and pain resulting from injury, disease, disability, or other health-related conditions. Physical therapy includes: (1) the performance and interpretation of tests and measurements to assess pathophysiological, pathomechanical, electrophysiologic, ergonomic, and developmental deficits of bodily systems to determine diagnosis, treatment, prognosis and prevention; (2) the planning, administration, and modification of therapeutic interventions that focus on posture, locomotion, strength, endurance, cardiopulmonary function, balance, coordination, joint mobility, flexibility, pain, healing and repair, and functional abilities in daily living skills, including work; and (3) the provision of consultative, educational, research, and other advisory services.
>
> The therapeutic interventions may include, but are not limited to, the use of therapeutic exercise with or without assistive devices, physical agents, electricity, manual procedures such as joint and soft tissue mobilization, neuromuscular reeducation, bronchopulmonary hygiene, and ambulation/gait training.

To some, within and external to the profession, this definition might appear either overbroad or incomplete, or simply not to the point. There are as many opinions and viewpoints as there are individuals. That is why it is critical to for each physical therapy professional to develop his or her own definition of what it is that he or she does, and can do, as a physical therapy professional.

The Model Definition above has become dated, in part, because of the publication by the American Physical Therapy Association in November 1997 of the *Guide to Physical Therapist Practice* (hereafter known as the *Guide*), within which words like "assessment" and "treatment" have been supplanted by broader inclusive terminology such as "examination" and "intervention," within which the former terms are components. The *Guide*, although not intended to represent a clinical practice guideline or the legal standard of care, has established common terminology and recommended standards for patient/client examination, evaluation, diagnosis, prognosis, and intervention, which will form, or at least evidence, the legal standard of care for physical therapy practice.

The *Guide* does a commendable job of explaining the relative roles of physical therapy professionals and the scope and breadth of physical therapist and physical therapist assistant practice because it does so using, to the extent feasible, lay-person terminology, which is also critically important for physical therapists and assistants to use in their communications with patients and clients and with relevant others. For example, in the "Introduction," the *Guide* describes the professional participants and practices as follows:

> As essential participants in the health care delivery system, physical therapists assume leadership roles in rehabilitation services, prevention and health maintenance programs, and professional and community organizations. They also play important roles in developing health care policy and appropriate standards for the various elements of physical therapist practice to ensure availability, accessibility, and excellence in the delivery of physical therapy services. The positive impact of physical therapists' rehabilitation, prevention, and health promotion services on health-related quality of life is well accepted. Physical therapy is covered by almost all federal, state, and private insurance plans.
>
> As clinicians, physical therapists engage in an examination process that includes taking the history, conducting a systems review, and administering tests and measures to identify potential and existing problems. To establish *diagnoses* and *prognoses,* physical therapists perform *evaluations* that synthesize the examination data. Physical therapists provide *interventions* (the interactions and procedures used in treating and instructing patients/clients), conduct reexaminations, modify interventions as necessary to achieve anticipated goals and desired outcomes, and develop and implement discharge plans. Physical therapy includes not only the services provided by physical therapists but those rendered under physical therapist direction and supervision.

## HISTORY OF PHYSICAL THERAPY IN THE UNITED STATES

Although the application of physical therapy to illnesses and injuries may be generically as old as humankind, the history of physical therapy as an organized profession in the United States is of relative recent vintage. And while this book may focus on the present and, particularly, on the future, it is critical to be familiar with historical developments in physical therapy in order to grow individually and collectively and to learn from past successes and mistakes.

A single pathologic condition was the primary genesis of the physical therapy profession in the late 1800s and early 1900s. That condition was the recurrent worldwide epidemic of infantile paralysis, or poliomyelitis, which seriously affected children in the United States for the first time (regionalized to New England) in 1894. Subsequent polio epidemics affected children in the same geographic region in 1914 and 1916.

Physicians and surgeons, including Dr Robert Lovett, a prominent New England-based orthopedist, began to recruit European-educated gymnasts and American physical educators to assist doctors and nurses in meeting the physical rehabilitation needs of polio patients and their families in the United States. One of the first such professionals to be formally recognized as a "physical therapist" was Mary McMillan (Fig. 1-1). Mary ("Mollie") McMillan was born in Hyde Park, Massachusetts, in 1880 and was educated in Liverpool, England, after her family sent her to live with Scottish relatives following the death from consumption (tuberculosis) of her mother and older sister in 1885. After graduating from Liverpool University and Liverpool Gymnasium College, Mollie studied corrective exercise science on the job under prominent European physicians and surgeons. She returned to Liverpool and worked primarily with children with poliomyelitis and scoliosis and other developmental conditions.

World War I was the next impetus for growth for physical therapy. Mary McMillan served first in the British and then in the American army during World War I as a physical rehabilitation specialist and a reconstruction aide. She, along with professional colleagues like Marguerite Sanderson, promoted the concept of physiotherapy as a profession to American military commanders and civilian leaders, particularly to Surgeon General William Gorgas. Gorgas authorized the establishment of a division of special hospitals and physical reconstruction.

Along with occupational therapists and dieticians (which later would form the core of the Army Medical Specialist Corps), physical therapy reconstruction aides were recruited and educated to serve the physical and vocational rehabilitation needs of military service personnel. Physical therapy reconstruction aides were educated at one of seven War Emergency Training Centers, including Walter Reed Medical Center in Silver Spring, Maryland; four centers located in Boston and New Haven, Connecticut; Columbia University, New York; the Kellogg Normal School, Michigan; and Reed College, Portland, Oregon.

As a representative example, the Reed College program was a 3-month program that became the model for early post-war physical therapy education. Its curriculum consisted of 457 hours of classroom instruction in human dissection anatomy, physiology, kinesiology, therapeutic exercise, massage, hydrotherapy, and ethics. The 800 students—all women, and referred to as the "Reed girls"—also received 163 contact hours in clinical internship experiences. Students could also take French as a humanities elective.

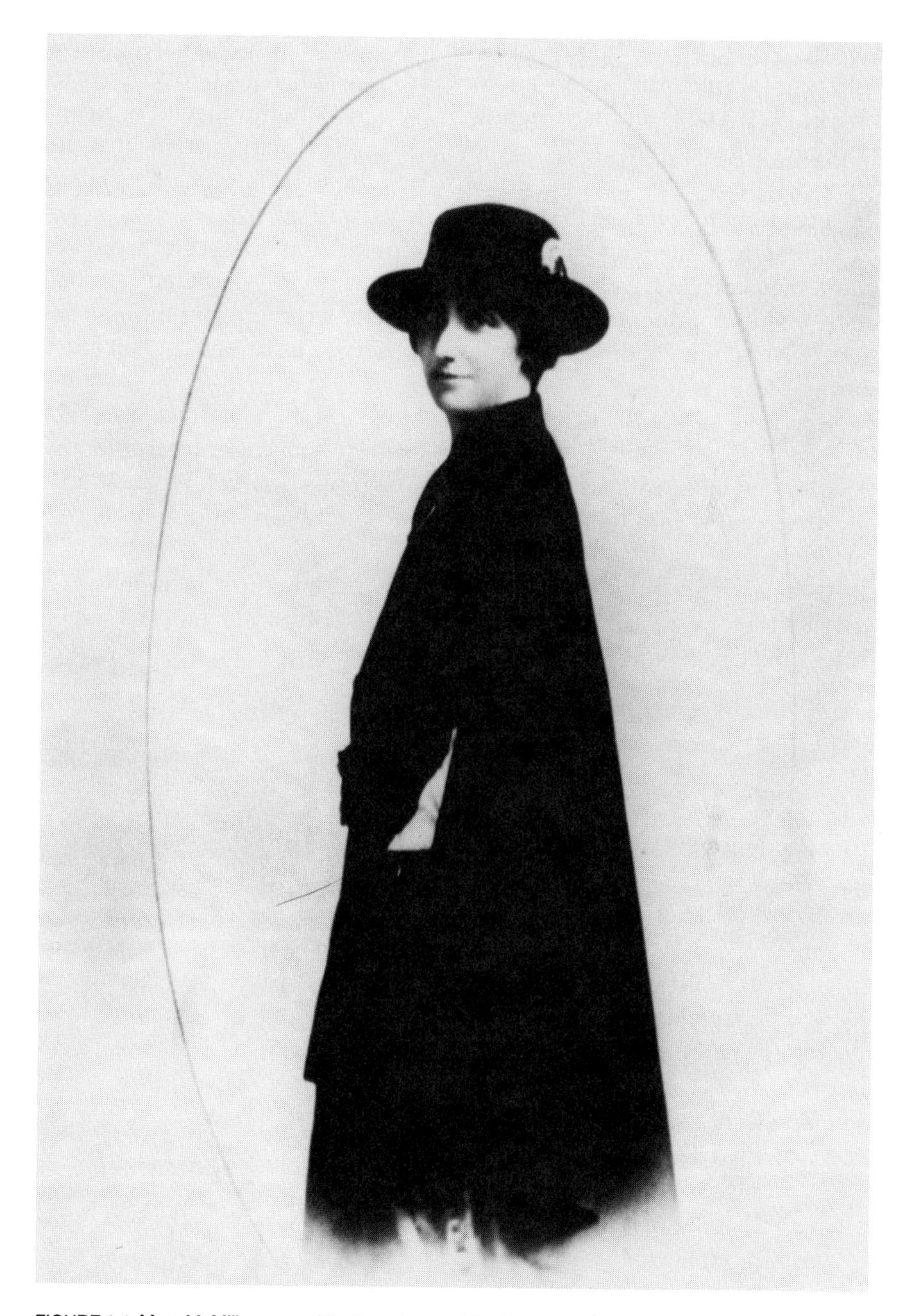

FIGURE 1-1 Mary McMillan, one of the founders and the first president of the American Physical Therapy Association, is shown here wearing her Reconstruction Aide uniform (WWI era, 1918–1919).

After World War I, Mary McMillan and 244 of her reconstruction aide colleagues formed the American Women's Physical Therapeutic Association in 1921. The founding meeting of the association was held at Keens Chophouse Restaurant at 72 West 36th St, New York City, a venue that did not welcome women until the British actress Lillie Langtry sued and won the legal right for women to be served there.

The charter American physical therapy professional association did not admit men. Its name was changed to the American Physiotherapy Association, and its charter amended in 1922, so that men could join the association. (Several men had been educated and served as reconstruction aides during World War I.)

According to McMillan, the domain of physical therapy practice in 1921 included four specialties: therapeutic exercise, massage, hydrotherapy (Fig. 1-2), and electrotherapy. Education programs between World Wars I and II were few in number and largely hospital-based and non-degree-awarding.

At the advent of World War II, there ensued emergent reemphasis on physical therapy education (Fig. 1-3). Some 1632 physical therapists served during the Great War. Post-World War II, the number and quality of pro-

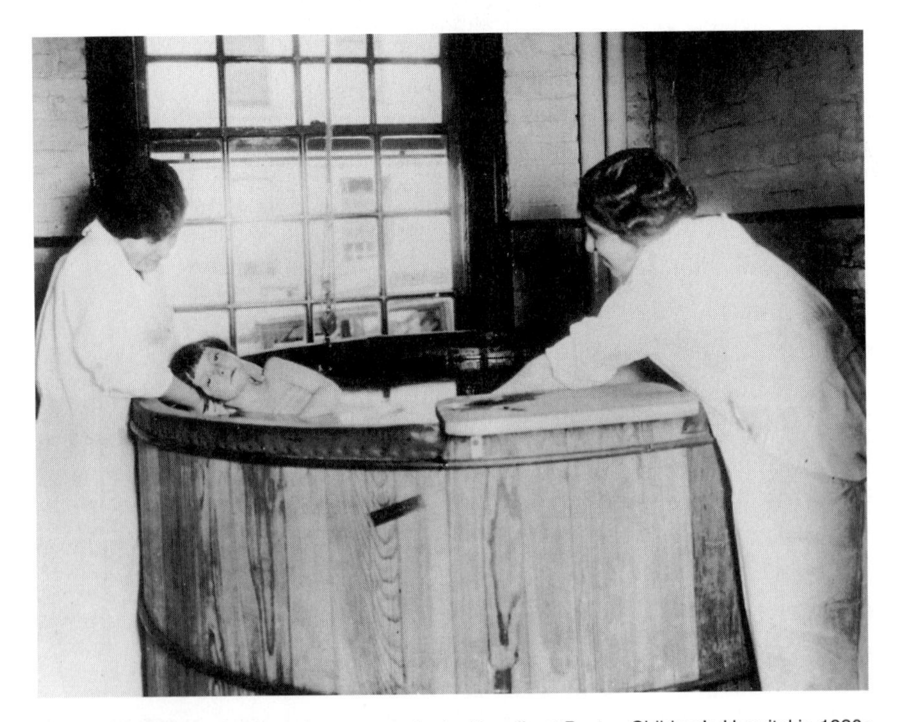

FIGURE 1-2 Early pool therapy for young patient with polio at Boston Children's Hospital in 1920s and 1930s (1920–1939 era).

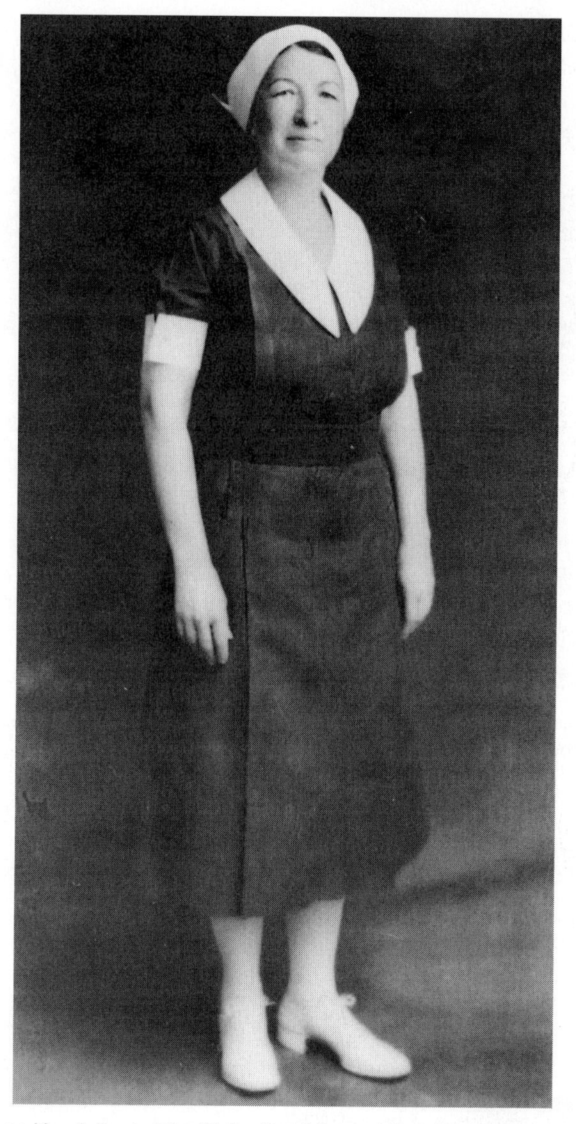

FIGURE 1-3 Emma Vogel directed the Walter Reed General Hospital program for physical therapists. After the outbreak of World War II, Vogel was deployed to direct the War Emergency Training courses at 10 Army hospitals (post–WWI through WWII era).

fessional education programs proliferated to approximately 200 by April 2000. This growth was fostered again by the recurrence of poliomyelitis epidemics after World War II (Fig. 1-4) and the relative dearth of physicians and concomitant need for physician surrogates.

Today, the domain of physical therapy clinical practice ranges from general to highly specialized practice, covering the human life span from

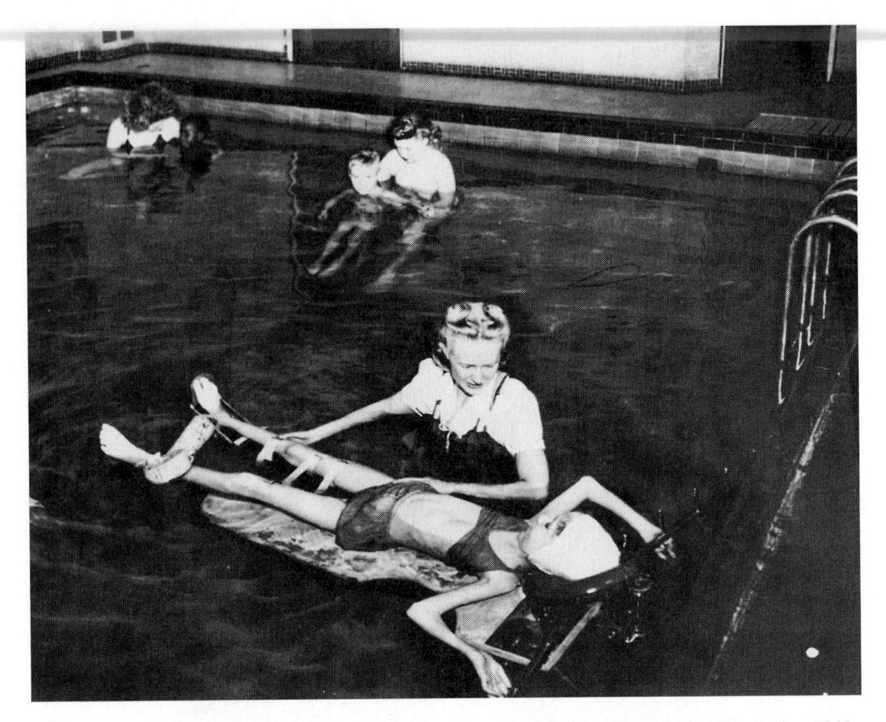

FIGURE 1-4 Physical therapists use pool therapy to treat children with poliomyelitis in the 1940s and 1950s (1946–1959 era).

neonates to geriatric clientele. In 32 states, physical therapists may examine and intervene for patients without physician or other provider referral or consultation. Such primary practice is referred to as direct access practice.

## REPRESENTATIVE PROFESSIONS AND SUPPORT PROFESSIONALS

Although it may seem self-evident that licensed physical therapists are the alter ego of the profession of physical therapy, in fact, the discipline *physical therapy* is composed of two distinct classes of professionals: physical therapists and physical therapist assistants. Let us examine whether these two classes of professionals constitute, by classic definition, a "profession."

The classic definition of a profession is that its members: (1) possess a defined body of knowledge or expertise; (2) exercise a degree of autonomy, or self-determination, over matters pertinent to their discipline; (3) undergo formal education processes to acquire practice competencies; (4) conduct research activities to validate and refine their professional practice; (5) recognize advanced member competency through certification or other activities; and (6) promote public welfare through their service.

Historically, only three classic professions were recognized: the practices of law, medicine, and the ministry. Today, however, many more classes of professionals exist in society, including physical therapists and physical therapist assistants. Although physical therapy professionals exercise only limited autonomy over their practice (either because, as physical therapists, they interact with patients pursuant to physician or other-entity referral or, as physical therapist assistants, they are supervised by licensed physical therapists), they nonetheless exercise practice autonomy over activities within their legal scope of practice and individual domain of personal competency. (Chapter 4 discusses how the representative codes of ethics for physical therapists and assistants give each of these classes of professionals professional status, based on distinct rights and duties.)

Members of a defined profession can be characterized by certain attributes. Members

- possess a defined body of knowledge or expertise
- exercise a degree of autonomy, or self-determination, over matters pertinent to their discipline
- undergo formal education processes to acquire practice competencies
- conduct research activities to validate and refine their professional practice
- recognize advanced member competency through certification or other activities
- promote public welfare through their service.

In addition to licensed physical therapists and physical therapist assistants, physical therapy is carried out by extenders working under the direction of licensed physical therapists, including, but not limited to, certified athletic trainers and exercise physiologists. Physical therapy aides augment the professional physical therapy team by providing patient support services, such as preparing patients and equipment for service delivery by physical therapists and/or assistants, assisting in interventions as allowed by law and customary practice, and sanitizing equipment and facilities, among others.

A salient political issue involving the term *physical therapy* is whether health professionals other than physical therapists and assistants may lawfully and ethically carry out physical therapy activities with patients and clients. This issue resulted in litigation with chiropractors in several states recently, and is not finally resolved in the courts. The issue turns in large part on whether the term physical therapy is generic in nature or exists for exclusive utilization by licensed physical therapists and their professional assistants.

## INTERDISCIPLINARY CO-PRIMARY HEALTH CARE DISCIPLINES

This section explores in brief two representative co-primary rehabilitation disciplines whose members interact in a substantial way in interdisciplinary processes with physical therapy professionals: occupational therapy and orthotics and prosthetics. The section begins with basic definitions for, and distinctions between, *interdisciplinary* and *multidisciplinary* processes.

*Interdisciplinary* health care professional activities include those that involve workers in multiple health care disciplines who cooperate and closely coordinate their efforts to achieve common goals or outcomes for the patients they serve. Examples of interdisciplinary health care teams include surgical teams working in operating room suites and physical rehabilitation teams caring for patients with significant physical impairments and disabilities, as patients with diagnoses of cerebrovascular accidents (strokes) and spinal cord injuries. A *multidisciplinary* health care group, on the other hand, exists largely for the convenience of patients it serves. Members of various disciplines may provide patient/client services in a common geographic site but do not necessarily work in concert toward common patient goals or outcomes.

The nonphysician primary health care disciplines, including physical and occupational therapists, speech–language–hearing professionals, orthotists and prosthetists, clinical laboratory scientists, and others, have been traditionally collectively called "allied health professionals." Many physical therapists chose to distance themselves from that label in the 1980s, in an attempt to exert their professional autonomy. That approach has had mixed results; some nonphysical therapy colleagues have come to view physical therapists executing that approach as aloof and noncollegial. If the intent of the strategy was to distance physical therapy from the perception of being physician dominated, then a better approach may be to broaden the definition of allied health to mean "health professionals allied in support of the patient." Under this open definition, all health care primary and support professionals (especially including physicians and physical therapists) are "allied health professionals."

Although traditionally physicians have been the de jure leaders of interdisciplinary health care teams, the best approach is to recognize the patient (or in the case of the patient lacking mental and/or legal capacity, the patient's surrogate decision maker) as the true head of any health care team. Medicine and health care generally have yet to fully embrace this approach, which most respects patient autonomy or self-determination.

Occupational therapy shares a common historical origin in the United States with physical therapy, in that both disciplines had their modern genesis in the form of reconstruction aides recruited as rehabilitation professionals serving military servicemen during World War I. Although the curricula for these reconstruction aide professionals were similar, the divergent directions that the two professionals took were distinct. Whereas physical therapy had as its professional core the basic physical rehabilitation (including wound and burn management) of war-injured personnel, occupational therapy developed a holistic occupational and psychosocial core that concentrated its physical dimension on optimizing patient/client abilities to perform occupational and avocational activities of daily living with maximum independence.

Both disciplines grew after the world wars to become coequal, critically important primary health care clinical disciplines. Each discipline refined and expanded its scope of professional practice, and developed specialty clinical practice domains that, to some degree, overlap with each other.

Like physical therapy, occupational therapy has two distinct professions within its purview of professional responsibility: licensed and/or registered occupational therapists and certified occupational therapy assistants. These professionals share attributes of classic professionals in the same manner as physical therapists and physical therapist assistants. Again, as in physical therapy, occupational therapy also employs extender personnel as support professionals in the form of occupational therapy aides and others.

The professional association for the 45,000 occupational therapists and certified occupational therapy assistants is the American Occupational Therapy Association (AOTA). Educational program accreditation and licensure is within the domain of the National Board for Certification in Occupational Therapy (NBCOT). The AOTA-administered Occupational Therapy Code of Ethics is similar to the American Physical Therapy Association's Code of Ethics, Standards of Ethical Conduct for the Physical Therapist Assistant, and implementing *Guide for Professional Conduct* and *Guide for Conduct of the Affiliate Member*. One important difference between the ethics documents of the two disciplines, however, is that the Occupational Therapy Code of Ethics is all inclusive of occupational therapy professional and support personnel in its express subject-matter jurisdiction instead of being bifurcated, as are the physical therapy ethical standards.

Although there have been over time moves to reconsolidate the professions, especially over the past few decades, such attempts have always failed because of political, practice domain, philosophical, or other rationale. In the managed care and postmodernist, postmanaged care eras, characterized by maximally cost-conservative, efficient and proficient interdisciplinary patient-focused health care delivery, renewed interest and initiatives in this direction may, and perhaps should, ensue.

## SUMMARY

As a primary clinical health care profession, physical therapy stands at the advent of the 21st century at a crossroads, from which the future of the profession and the welfare of patients it serves are held in the balance. Factors such as managed care, a health care delivery paradigm under which cost containment seemingly takes precedence over all other factors, and increased competition from complementary health care professions make evolutionary refinement of the profession a requisite to its survival.

Physical therapy is composed of two distinct disciplines: licensed physical therapists and physical therapist assistants. Although physical therapist assistants customarily carry out interventions delineated by supervisory physical therapists, they possess a defined scope of professional practice and have a distinct code of ethics, which creates for them at least limited independent duties and autonomy. Supporting clinical physical therapists and assistants are extender and support professionals, as well as critically important administrative, clerical, and other professionals. One obvious focus of this book is on recognition of each and every member of the interdisciplinary health care team as a professional, worthy of dignity and respect by all others on the team. Similarly, all health care professionals collectively should be viewed as "allied health professionals," since all work in support of patient care, safety, and welfare, and are fiduciaries charged by law to place patient welfare above all competing and subordinate interests.

Although historically there were only three "classic" professions requiring postsecondary education—law, medicine, and religion—modernly physical therapy is clearly a "profession," possessing the professional attributes of a defined body of knowledge, relative professional autonomy (if autonomous practice were a strict condition of professional status, only attorneys would, by definition, be professionals), formal education, research activities, ethical guidelines, recognition of advanced competencies, and a public service focus.

The historical genesis of contemporary physical therapy has two origins, both emerging at the advent of the last century: infantile paralysis (poliomyelitis) and World War I, with its emergent need for physical rehabilitation of war-wounded service members. Mary McMillan, Marguerite Sanderson, and others established reconstruction aides, civilian health care professionals recruited by US and British military commanders during World War I to take primary responsibility for optimal restoration of the physical and mental health of injured military service personnel. (The term *reconstruction aide* possibly derives from the term *reconstruction,* coined post-Civil War to describe the reintegration of seceded Confederate states into the United States.) From reconstruction aides post-World War I, the interrelated professions of physical and occupational therapy developed (along quite similar tracks).

The precursor to the American Physical Therapy Association was formed by Mary McMillan and her colleagues in 1922 with a historic founding meeting at Keens Chophouse in New York City. The American Physical Therapy Association, headquartered in Alexandria, Virginia (Fig. 1-5), currently serves the professional needs of its more than 70,000 professional (physical therapist), affiliate (physical therapist assistant), and professional and affiliate student members.

## Activities, Cases, and Questions

1. **Activity:** As a physical therapist or physical therapist assistant student or professional, initiate a professional diary in which you record in detail your personal definition of the profession and practice of physical therapy. Revisit the diary approximately every 3 years to rewrite and refine your definition of the profession and practice. Maintain this diary throughout your professional career.
2. **Case:** The physical rehabilitation service at ABC Medical Center, Anytown, USA, has been directed by the system's administration to develop a written plan to better coordinate professional service delivery by physical therapy, occupational therapy, speech–language–hearing professionals, orthotists and prosthetists, and rehabilitation nurses, so as to maximize efficiency and efficacy of service delivery, and to minimize unnecessary

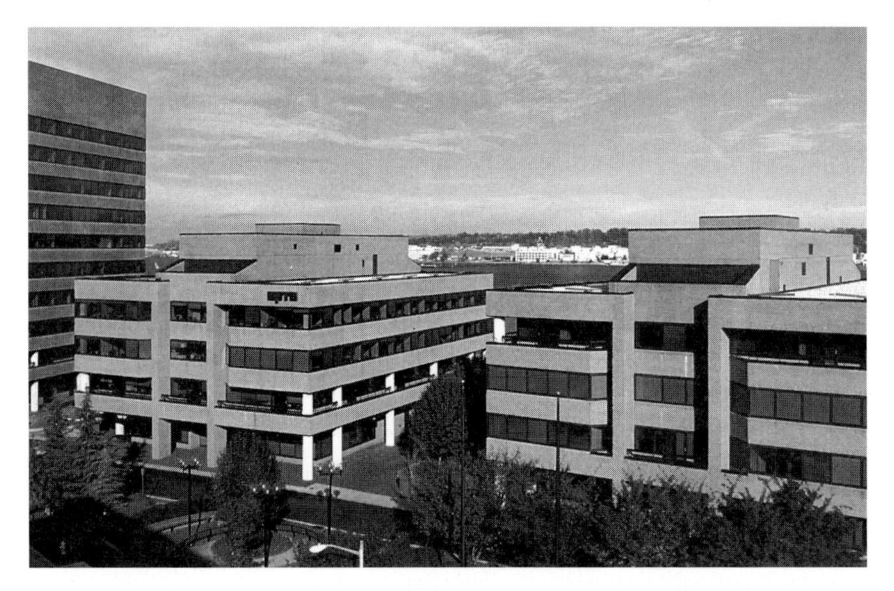

FIGURE 1-5 American Physical Therapy Association headquarters, Alexandria, VA.

cost outlays. What kinds of professional activities of these disciplines could form the basis of a quantitative "time-and-motion study" to effect closer coordination and enhance patient comfort and satisfaction?

3. **Question:** What is your personal opinion about being labeled an "allied health professional"?

## ADDITIONAL READINGS

APTA celebrates 75 years. *PT: Magazine of Physical Therapy.* 1996; 4(1).

Bicentennial Issue. *Physical Therapy.* 1976; 56(1):1–146.

Cleather J. *Head, Heart and Hands: The Story of Physiotherapy in Canada.* Toronto: Canadian Physiotherapy Association; 1995.

*Commonalities and Differences Between the Professions of Physical Therapy and Occupational Therapy: An American Physical Therapy Association White Paper.* Alexandria, VA: American Physical Therapy Association; 1994.

Courses for reconstruction aides at Reed College. *School and Society.* 1918; 7 (Apr 27): 494–495.

How the salvage of polio cases proceeds. *Survey.* 1916; 37 (Oct 21): 58–66.

Murphy W. *Healing the Generations: A History of Physical Therapy and the American Physical Therapy Association.* Alexandria, VA: American Physical Therapy Association; 1995.

Myers RS. *Saunders Manual of Physical Therapy Practice.* Philadelphia: WB Saunders Company; 1995.

Pagliarulo MA. *Introduction to Physical Therapy.* St. Louis: Mosby–Year Book; 1996.

Ritchie-Hartwick AM. *The Army Medical Specialist Corps: The 45th Anniversary.* Washington, DC: Center of Military History; 1993.

Scully RM, Barnes MR. *Physical Therapy.* Philadelphia: JB Lippincott; 1989.

The study of physical therapy advanced by the war. *School and Society.* 1946; 62 (Jan 26): 63.

## Focus on a Leader

**ELIZABETH DOMHOLDT, EDD, PT**
**PROFESSOR AND DEAN, KRANNERT SCHOOL OF PHYSICAL THERAPY**
**UNIVERSITY OF INDIANAPOLIS, INDIANAPOLIS, INDIANA**

*1. Beth, please briefly capsulize for readers your credentials, professional chronology, and current and recent professional activities.*
I received a BS in physical therapy from the University of Michigan in 1979. I then practiced full-time for 4 years at Wishard Memorial Hospital in Indianapolis. Patients included acute care and trauma of all types and acute and long-term rehabilitation for patients after burn, spinal cord injury, and amputation.

I was a member of the American Physical Therapy Association (APTA) as a student and as a clinician and was mentored to begin contributing to the profession through presentation of special interest papers at national conferences. I also began teaching part-time as an adjunct instructor in local physical therapy programs.

While working full-time in the clinic, I earned a Master of Science degree in health occupations education from Indiana University. I accepted a full-time academic position at the University of Indianapolis in 1983, after completing the MS degree. I began working on the Doctor of Education degree in Higher Education Administration soon after beginning the academic position. I taught full-time for 4 years, combining the teaching with clinical practice approximately 1 day per week and with scholarly publication and presentation activities.

I became Dean of the Krannert School of Physical Therapy at the University of Indianapolis in 1987 after completing the EdD degree from Indiana University the same year. This is a combined administrative and teaching role, and I have maintained a scholarly focus as well during the last 12 years. My textbook, *Physical Therapy Research: Principles and Applications, 2nd ed* (Philadelphia: W.B. Saunders; 2000) has been a major project, as have journal articles related to support personnel utilization and direct access.

*2. What is the "state of the physical therapy profession"?*
In 2000 the profession is experiencing the first of what I believe will be a cycle of ongoing sine waves. Most professions cycle through relatively

short bouts of shortage and oversupply, with opportunities for practitioners peaking during shortage periods and waning during the oversupply. In physical therapy we have been in a shortage situation for so long that the current oversupply seems like the end of an age. In my opinion, this is simply the first oversupply cycle we have ever experienced, and we will again experience shortages and then oversupply again. These ongoing fluctuations in the market will sometimes be related to the numbers of practitioners and will at other times be related to health care policy changes that alter demand for physical therapy services.

In 2000 we have more autonomy in our practice than ever before, but we are still striving to be recognized as first-contract practitioners within our scope of practice. Direct access laws often include many stipulations that limit practitioner autonomy, and reimbursers frequently require a referral even when one may not be required from a legal perspective.

In 2000 we have defined our scope of practice better than ever before, in the *Guide to Physical Therapist Practice*, but find it necessary to defend that scope of practice in a variety of arenas—with other health professionals, in the state legislatures, and with payers.

In 2000 we are in the midst of a health care system that seems to be emphasizing the chemical basis of health to a greater and greater extent, with pharmaceutical treatments for many conditions including depression, obesity, hair loss, high cholesterol, and inflammation. Physical therapy's unique contribution to this chemical soup is an anatomical/functional/activity basis for health.

3. *Where do you believe physical therapy will be in the year 2050? What needs to be accomplished to get the profession where you envision it being in 2050?*
For starters, I'll be 92 and retired, and observing my predictions from the sidelines! Entry-level education for physical therapists will be at the doctoral level. Physical therapists will have meaningful direct access, meaning that they will be able to see individuals without physician referrals and without the numerous stipulations that currently limit practice without referral in those states in which it exists. In addition, physical therapists will use this autonomy to a much greater extent than they do now.

Even though physical therapists will practice more autonomously than today, this "level playing field" for practice will also result in more collaborative practice with physicians and nurse practitioners, with PTs managing much of the routine musculoskeletal complaints that are brought to a primary care setting.

PTs will be more entrepreneurial in their approach to their practice. This entrepreneurship will be in the form of seeking new markets for care and capitalizing on the public's interest in fitness and wellness.

PTs will be influenced greatly by technology and will use high-tech ways of communicating with patients. However, one of the strengths of PT lies in the "high touch" aspect of what we do. We will somehow find a balance that permits us to be both "high tech" and "high touch."

The aging of America will result in more opportunities for PTs to deal with chronic disease and long-term disability and PTs will play a major role in enabling the US population to grow old in more functional ways than ever before.

How do we get to this future? We look for ways to partner with other providers, with community organizations, with other disciplines. We seek autonomy, but then use it to practice collaboratively, rather than in isolation. So why do we need the autonomy? So that we can collaborate on a level playing field with the other players. For example, at present, when we collaborate with physicians, most of the referrals go one way—from physician to physical therapist. With meaningful autonomy, there could be a balance of referrals from physician to physical therapist and from physical therapist to physician. When this balance in possible, the elements of a true partnership are in place.

CHAPTER 2

# Education

RON SCOTT

## Key Words and Phrases

Accreditation
Affect
Affective Learning Domain
Analysis
Andragogical Model
Application
Auditory Learner
Bloom's Taxonomy of Learning
Candidacy for Accreditation
Case-based Model
Clinical Education
Cognitive Learning Domain
Collaborative Learning
Commission on Accreditation in Physical Therapy Education (CAPTE)
Comprehension
Cooperative Learning
Curriculum
Declaration of Intent
Didactic Education
Evaluation
*Evaluative Criteria*
Generic (Professional) Abilities/Attributes
Guide-based Model
*Guide to Physical Therapist Practice*
Knowledge
Learning Disabilities
Lifespan-based Model
Mentor
Pedagogical Model
Problem-based Learning Model
Protégée
Psychomotor Learning Domain
Renaissance Person
Self-Study
Student-Led Teaching/Learning
Synthesis
Tactical Learner
Traditional Model
Visual Learner

*The goal of entry-level physical therapy professional education is the preparation of physical therapists and physical therapist assistants who can function independently and safely in basic professional clinical practice. Approximately 492 educational institutions worldwide, housing 530 physical therapy programs, carry out that task. The chapter explores in detail the structure and operations of the Commission on Accreditation in Physical Therapy Education (CAPTE), a private regulatory body and component of the American Physical Therapy Association. The CAPTE is responsible for education program accreditation under the direction of three accreditation panels and 26 appointed commissioners. Developing education programs must achieve Candidacy for Accreditation status before embarking on professional-phase physical therapy education of students. CAPTE evaluates physical therapy education programs using* Evaluative Criteria *based on the* Normative Models for Physical Therapist and Physical Therapist Assistant Education. *Education programs for physical therapists must award postbaccalaureate entry-level degrees in order to remain CAPTE-accredited after January 1, 2002. Also discussed in this chapter are physical therapy professional education processes, which include pedagogy, andragogy, and the three learning domains: the cognitive (knowledge-based) domain, psychomotor (skills-based) domain, and affective (behavioral) domain. Curricular models are explained, from traditional through case- and problem-based learning models. The progression of learning from base to higher order learning through comprehension, application, analysis, synthesis, and evaluation is also discussed. This chapter contains two* Focus on a Leader *vignettes, one from Mary Jane Harris, CAPTE Director, and the other from Professor Mary Ann Wharton, Physical Therapy Program, Saint Francis University.*

## BACKGROUND

As of April 1, 2000, 492 educational institutions worldwide support 530 professional entry-level physical therapist and physical therapist assistant education programs accredited by the Commission on Accreditation in Physical Therapy Education. Of that number, 203 US-based education institutions support 214 programs dedicated to the education of physical therapists: 183 master's degree-level (MPT/MS) programs, 11 doctoral degree-level (DPT) programs, and 20 baccalaureate programs. Twenty-one foreign educational institutions support 24 physical therapist entry-level education programs (13 Canadian, 11 other), all at the baccalaureate degree level. Two hundred sixty-eight US-based educational institutions support 292 physical therapist assistant (associate degree level) education programs.

Of 557 postbaccalaureate physical therapy education program faculty surveyed in 1995, 63% were women and 37% were men. Forty-one percent of them had PhD degrees, and 6.6% possessed professional doctoral degrees.

## HISTORY OF PHYSICAL THERAPY EDUCATION PROGRAM ACCREDITATION

The American Physiotherapy Association initially had autonomous accreditation responsibility for physical therapist professional education programs from 1923 to 1933. From 1934 to 1956, the Council on Medical Education and Hospitals of the American Medical Association (AMA) accredited physical therapist professional education programs (as it did for most allied health education programs) at the request of the American Physical Therapy Association (APTA). From 1957 to 1963, the APTA and the AMA informally jointly accredited physical therapy education programs. This arrangement was formalized in 1964 and continued through 1976. In 1977, the Commission on Accreditation in Education was formed by the APTA, and it alone accredited physical therapy education programs from that time on. Its current name is the Commission on Accreditation in Physical Therapy Education (CAPTE). The Commission is recognized as an independent educational accrediting body by the US Department of Education and the Council on Higher Education Accreditation.

## CAPTE AND ACCREDITATION ACTIVITIES

CAPTE is an autonomous division of the APTA that accredits and reaccredits entry-level physical therapist professional and physical therapist assistant education programs. Its current accreditation standards for physical therapy education programs are known as the *Evaluative Criteria* (see Appendix 2-1).

Twenty-six appointed commissioners make up CAPTE. These include experienced physical therapy education professionals (who possess substantial experience as on-site program evaluators, among other qualifications), higher education administrators, and consumers of physical therapy accreditation services. CAPTE consists of three panels: the physical therapist education program panel, the physical therapist assistant educational program panel, and the central (appellate and policy) panel.

Before admitting students to the professional phase of study, developing (newly formed) physical therapist professional education programs are required to obtain candidate status from CAPTE, and must be approved by the Commission for initial accreditation before graduates are eligible to take the national licensure examination, a requisite for professional practice.

The *Evaluative Criteria* for program accreditation are specific and detailed. They are divided into four sections:

- Section 1: Organization
- Section 2: Resources and Services

- Section 3: Curriculum Development and Content, and
- Section 4: Program Assessment

Section 1 sets out the legal, administrative, and financial duties of sponsoring institutions of higher education and the rights and duties of the institution, faculty, and students. Section 2 addresses the qualifications for program core and adjunct faculty, fiscal planning and management, administrative and support services, learning/library resources, and equipment and materials. Section 3 delineates the requisites of curriculum planning and acceptable curriculum content in terms of didactic, clinical, and research educational content areas.

As of January 1, 2000, CAPTE no longer conducts accreditation activities for baccalaureate physical therapy education programs. This controversial policy decision took two decades to achieve consensus, in part because of its antitrust implications and in part because it spells the demise of a substantial minority of programs that educate physical therapists at the baccalaureate level and all of the foreign education programs under the jurisdiction of CAPTE (unless they are willing and able to convert to graduate programs by 2002).

This policy decision was based on multiple criteria, but particularly on the fact that the professional scope and depth of clinical physical therapy practice has developed to the point that public safety demands expanded, graduate-level preparation for licensed physical therapists. Standard 3.9 of the *Evaluative Criteria* reads: "The first professional degree for physical therapists is awarded at the postbaccalaureate level at the completion of the physical therapy program."

Section 4 of the *Evaluative Criteria* details the requisites for systematic, formal program assessment, from mission, philosophy, and goals to admissions to resourcing to postgraduate placement and activities of graduates.

Accreditation is both evaluative and educative in nature (for the educational institution/program accredited) and protective of public and societal interests and the reputation of the profession. It is a process that occurs along a continuum from inception to dissolution of an educational program. The steps involved in physical therapy education program accreditation include: development of evaluative standards, institution/program self-appraisal, external evaluation, dissemination of evaluative findings and recommendations, and systematic, ongoing review.

To achieve candidacy (pre-accreditation) status, allowing a developing education program to proceed to the professional phase of teaching/learning, an educational institution planning to implement a physical therapist professional education program must: (1) have hired a full-time qualified physical therapy program director for program development; (2) have in place at least one additional full-time physical therapy faculty member; (3) meet 30 additional detailed achievement objectives outlined in the *CAPTE Accreditation Manual*; and (4) submit to CAPTE an Application for Candidacy (AFC). Similar standards apply to developing physical therapist assistant programs.

Once an AFC is received and the developing program is billed for its administrative processing by CAPTE, CAPTE staff screen the report for completeness and assign a reader/consultant to thoroughly evaluate the AFC and the developing program. This assessment process includes: (1) the formulation of a report sent by the reader/consultant to the developing program director for review and revisions; (2) submission of a revised AFC by the developing program director to CAPTE; and (3) a 2-day candidacy visit by the reader/consultant to assess the developing program in person. On the basis of the reader/consultant's final report, the appropriate CAPTE panel makes a decision, subject to specified reconsideration and appeal processes, to award candidacy or not.

Once pre-accreditation candidacy status is granted to a developing physical therapy education program, students in the charter class may be admitted to the professional phase of study. During this phase of the application, the developing program director, faculty, and institutional administration officials complete the Self-Study Report. After the submission of this report, an on-site CAPTE-appointed team (three members for physical therapist education programs; two for physical therapist assistant programs) visits the developing program and sponsoring institution and reports to CAPTE on the evaluative findings; and CAPTE decides to grant initial (5-year maximal) accreditation status to the developing program, subject to reconsideration and appellate procedures outlined in the *CAPTE Accreditation Manual*.

Renewal of accreditation normally occurs thereafter every 8 years. All physical therapy education programs, developing to accredited, must submit biennial accreditation (update) reports (now computerized) to CAPTE for recordation, analysis, and support of educational research activities. (See Fig. 2-1.)

## PROFESSIONAL (ENTRY-LEVEL) EDUCATION: PHILOSOPHY AND PROCESSES

Physical therapy professional or entry-level education involves didactic classroom instruction and educational experiences in clinical settings. The teaching–learning process in the classroom, laboratory, and clinic typically progresses along a continuum from a relative pedagogical (structured and directive) model to an andragogical (self-directed) one as students gain competence, autonomy, and responsibility.

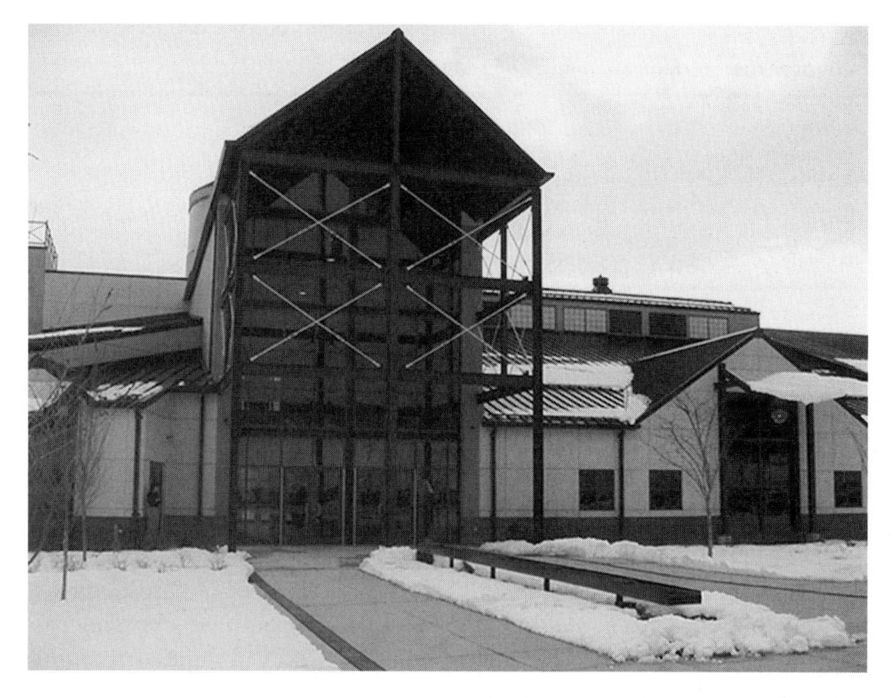

FIGURE 2-1 Lebanon Valley College, Annville, Pennsylvania (Developing Master of Physical Therapy Program, Heilman Center).

Professors and other instructors must be cognizant of the fact that all students have distinct optimal learning styles and preferences—visual, auditory, tactile—and must adjust teaching methods accordingly. Similarly, educators must accommodate learning and related physical and psychological disabilities in students as part of their fiduciary duty owed to them.

## Curricular Models

Classroom instruction may follow a traditional curricular model, within which basic science precedes clinical science instruction, followed by physical therapy–specific science instruction. Nontraditional progressive curricular methods include, among possible others, (1) the case-based model, within which patient/client case scenarios augment traditional instruction; (2) lifespan-based (prenatal through geriatric age groupings) and reference-based (*Guide to Physical Therapist Practice*) models; (3) systems-based, within which curricular content is centered on physiologic organ systems; and (4) problem-based, within which students independently assess, resolve, present, and defend hypothetical and real patient/client comprehensive case presentations (Table 2-1).

TABLE 2-1

**Physical Therapy Education Curricular Models**

- Traditional
- Case-based
- Reference-based (*Guide to Physical Therapist Practice*)
- Lifespan-based
- Problem-based
- Systems-based

Instructional delivery models range from traditional (live) lecture to small group dynamic teaching/learning processes to self-directed textual programmed learning to distance and Internet-based computerized delivery systems. One small group teaching/learning process—cooperative learning—is described in greater detail below

Small group activities, such as case studies, problem-based learning exemplars, and negotiations exercises, are collaborative in nature, meaning that students work together in a collegial, noncompetitive manner to identify and solve the problem(s) presented therein. Cooperative learning is a form of collaborative andragogical (self-directed) learning that focuses dually on positive interdependence of group members and on individual member accountability for the group's work product.

Cooperative learning activities are typically more structured than traditional collaborative group activities. Procedures common to all cooperative learning activities include the following:

- The class is divided into small heterogeneous groups of between three and eight students. The term *heterogeneous* indicates that group members may have ethnic, language, and lifestyle diversity; may be male or female; and may possess different learning abilities and styles, among other attributes.
- The groups work cooperatively on various academic tasks, at any and all levels of intellectual complexity, including skills, concepts, principles, problem identification and resolution, and creative thinking. A formal presentation by an instructor may or may not precede group activities.
- The instructor provides guidance to promote optimal cooperation and interdependence, and serves as a process observer for follow-on reporting and analysis of perceived positive and negative aspects of the experience. (The instructor serves as a "guide on the side," instead of a "sage on the stage" (Millis, 1988)).

What distinguishes cooperative learning methods from other collaborative group learning activities? In addition to *positive interdependence,* wherein students teach and learn from each other during the exercises, *individual accountability* characterizes cooperative learning. Because activities and assignments are carefully structured, and grading is reflective of individual, not group effort, each student learner has a vested interest in contributing to the success of the project and helping his or her colleagues to succeed. Group performance grades and peer evaluation may also constitute small parts of the final grade mix under cooperative learning models.

### Cooperative Learning Formats

Cooperative learning formats include, among others: think–pair–share, three-step interview, numbered heads together, roundtable, structured controversy, and group investigation. *Think–pair–share* entails the presentation of a problem by the instructor, followed by individual student analysis of its solution(s), then paired analysis of possible solutions, and later the sharing of ideas within a larger group or with the entire class. *Three-step interview* involves pairs of students interviewing each other on a specific topic or question, and the presentation and discussion of each other's answers to another pair within a 4-person small group. *Numbered heads together* starts with students counting off, i.e., 1, 2, 3. . . . After the instructor presents a problem, students with the same numbers come together to solve the problem. After a set amount of time, the instructor reconvenes the class and calls on a numbered group for its answer and analysis, which is presented through a spokesperson selected by the instructor. *Roundtable* is another name for brainstorming, in which all potential solutions to a given problem are identified and discussed. *Structured controversy* requires that group members take opposing positions on controversial topics and defend them in role-playing exercises. *Group investigation* involves shared responsibilities in researching and presenting on topics of mutual interest.

Cooperative learning strategies are particularly useful in administration and management, professional ethics, and legal issues courses. Students could be asked to divide into small groups of between three and eight students each, to brainstorm and report on the significant issues presented in real or hypothetical cases (using numbered heads, roundtable, or think–pair–share cooperative learning techniques). Groups might be asked to take opposing positions on well-defined management, professional ethical, or legal issues, and role-play the defense of their positions (structured controversy). Student groups might also sign up for, research, and report on salient practice-related problems, issues, and dilemmas of mutual interest (group investigation). All these techniques, and variations thereof, are excellent ways to utilize cooperative learning to facilitate learning of physical therapy malpractice and related concepts.

There are significant potential benefits to augmenting existing teaching/learning activities with cooperative learning group activities. Cooperative learning promotes higher order thinking, i.e., analysis, synthesis, and evaluation. It facilitates critical reflective thinking, creative problem identification and resolution strategies, active versus passive learning, and independent, self-directed learning. Cooperative learning advances the development of critical social skills, especially tolerance of diverse opinions and perspectives. It makes apparent boundaries between instruction and research less distinct. Finally, it serves as an easy means to break the tedium of the straight lecture teaching format.

Cooperative learning has been found to be an effective adjunct to traditional teaching/learning strategies from kindergarten through graduate and professional school. Faculty in physical therapy professional education programs are urged to augment their teaching methods with some or all of the cooperative learning techniques described herein. Clinical educators and continuing education providers are similarly encouraged to try cooperative learning techniques in their programs to enhance self-directed learning and retention of vital material.

Student learning is assessed through evaluation in physical therapy education in all three learning domains (Table 2-2) described by Bloom: the cognitive (factual knowledge-based) domain, the psychomotor (skills) domain, and the affective (behavioral) domain. Universal or generic attributes (abilities) generally expected of physical therapy professional education program graduates include, but are not limited to, interpersonal and communicative life skills; a sense of professional responsibility, including compliance with, and enforcement of, legal and ethical standards; reflective profession-related problem-solving skills; effective personal life-management skills; the ability to accept and act on constructive criticism; and a life-long commitment to continued professional and personal learning and growth. These attributes, inherent in the balanced, liberal education espoused in CAPTE Accreditation Criterion 3.7, are what make up the Renaissance man or woman.

Learning objectives for curricular content are centered on Bloom's hierarchal taxonomy of learning levels (Table 2-3). These include, in ascending order, base comprehension, application of concepts and principles, analysis

**TABLE 2-2**

**The Three Classic Learning Domains**

- Cognitive
- Psychomotor
- Affective

TABLE 2-3

| Taxonomy of Learning Levels (in ascending order) |
|---|
| ■ Comprehension<br>■ Application<br>■ Analysis<br>■ Synthesis<br>■ Evaluation |

of content, synthesis of segmented learning into the whole, and evaluation of content and learning. Instructor assessment of student learning in all there domains may derive from written, oral, and practical examinations, with or without formal prior or concomitant student self-assessment (i.e., 180° assessment). A broader (270° and 360°) assessment may include input from peers, patients/clients, and relevant others. In clinical settings, assessments commonly are made through standardized clinical competency-assessment instruments, such as the American Physical Therapy Association's *Clinical Performance Instrument* and Texas Consortium's *Blue MACS,* among others.

## POSTPROFESSIONAL EDUCATION

Focused postprofessional education of physical therapists and physical therapist assistants involves augmentation of entry-level cognitive, psychomotor, and affective domain skills with advanced-level knowledge, skills, and behaviors that enhance the external value and promote the self-determination and self-actualization of the physical therapy professional. Informal training, education, and development programs range from short continuing education courses to intermediate-range certificate programs to longer residencies in specific clinical practice areas (e.g., orthopedics and sports physical therapy). Formal postprofessional degree programs may lead to the earning and award of Master of Science, academic and professional, e.g., advanced-standing Doctor of Physical Therapy (DPT), and other degrees. (See Fig. 2-2.)

## SUMMARY

Physical therapy education is designed to prepare professional-phase physical therapist and physical therapist assistant students to perform entry-level clinical practices safely and independently. CAPTE is a private regulatory body of 26 commissioners responsible for accrediting over 500 physical therapy education programs worldwide.

Health professional education takes place progressively in pedagogical (early directed teaching-learning) and andragogical (mature, self-directed

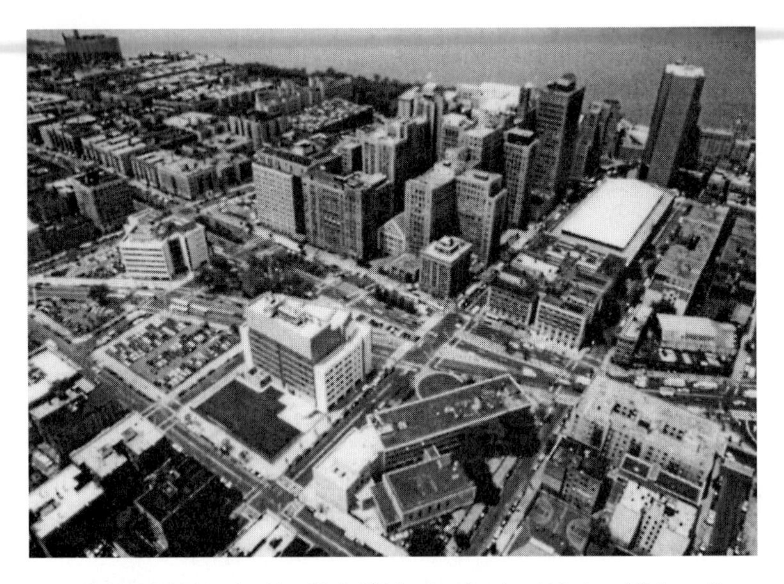

FIGURE 2-2 Columbia University, New York, NY (postprofessional Master of Science Degree program; only physical therapy program housed within an Ivy League college/university).

teaching-learning) modes, and in various curricular models from traditional to case-based to problem-based. Learning objectives impart, in hierarchal fashion, comprehension, application, and higher order: analysis, synthesis, and evaluation. Students are evaluated by academic and clinical faculty in all three learning domains: the cognitive (knowledge-based) domain, the psychomotor (skills-based) domain, and the affective (behavioral) domain.

For physical therapist professional students, entry-level degrees are uniformly graduate degrees in CAPTE-accredited programs after January 1, 2002. Postprofessional education may be focused on training, education, and/or development (refinement) of existing cognitive and psychomotor skill sets.

## Activities, Cases, and Questions

1. **Activity:** Obtain curriculum outlines from local or regional physical therapist and physical therapist assistant education programs. Evaluate them in terms of sequencing, clinical education component, and comprehensiveness. Recommend improvements to the respective program directors and/or curriculum coordinators.
2. **Case:** X., a senior student physical therapist, is on her final clinical affiliation at XYZ Medical Center, Anytown, USA. X. has failed to report for work on time on three occasions over a 2-week period, in contravention of specific direction by her clinical instructor and CCCE. What can and

should be done to remediate X.'s deficient behavior? Which one(s) of Bloom's three learning domains is/are involved in this behavioral manifestation?

3. **Question.** What is the appropriate level for professional educational preparation for the physical therapist in your opinion? For the physical therapist assistant?

## ADDITIONAL READINGS

Accreditation Update [current and past issues]. Alexandria, VA: American Physical Therapy Association, Department of Accreditation.

*A Future in Physical Therapy: A Hands-On Health Care Profession. Education Programs Accredited by the Commission on Accreditation in Physical Therapy Education 2000.* Alexandria, VA: American Physical Therapy Association.

Aleamoni LM. *Techniques for Evaluating and Improving Instruction.* San Francisco: Jossey-Bass; 1987.

*A Normative Model of Physical Therapist Professional Education: Version 97.* Alexandria, VA: American Physical Therapy Association; 1997.

*CAPTE Accreditation Manual* [current edition]. Alexandria, VA: American Physical Therapy Association, Department of Accreditation.

Cooper J. Cooperative learning: Why does it work? *Coop Learn College Teach* 1990; 1(1):3.

DeYoung S. *Teaching Nursing.* Redwood City, CA: Addison-Wesley Nursing, 1990.

Domholdt E. *Professional Education and the Liberal Arts: Physical Therapy Programs at Liberal Arts Institutions* [dissertation]. Bloomington, IN: Indiana University; 1987.

Faculty Development Course Books. San Antonio, TX: The University of Texas Health Sciences Center at San Antonio, Office of Educational Resources, Division of Instructional Development; 1994.

Gronlund NE. *Stating Objectives for Classroom Instruction,* 3rd ed. New York: Macmillan; 1985.

*Guidelines and Self-Assessments for Clinical Education.* Rev ed. Alexandria, VA: American Physical Therapy Association, Department of Education; 1999.

Higgs J, Edwards H. *Educating Beginning Practitioners: Challenges for Health Professional Education.* Oxford, England: Butterworth-Heinemann; 1999.

Hrachovy J et al. Use of the Blue MACS: Acceptance by clinical instructors and self-reports of adherence. *Phys Ther.* 2000;80:652–661.

*Journal of Physical Therapy Education* [current and past issues]. Alexandria, VA: American Physical Therapy Association, Section on Education.

Kegan R. *In Over Our Heads: The Mental Demands of Modern Life.* Cambridge, MA: Harvard University Press; 1994: 274.

May WW et al. Model for ability-based assessment in physical therapy education. *J Phys Ther Educ*. 1995; 9(1): 3–6.

Millis B. *Helping Faculty Build Learning Communities Through Cooperative Groups.* College Park, MD: University of Maryland; 1988.

Newble DI. *Assessing Clinical Competence at the Undergraduate Level.* Dundee, Scotland: Association for the Study of Medicine; 1992.

Palloff RM, Pratt K. Building Learning Communities in Cyberspace: Effective Strategies for the Online Classroom. San Francisco: Jossey-Bass; 1999.

*The Blue MACS: Mastery and Assessment of Clinical Skills, 6th ed.* Austin, Texas: Texas Consortium for Physical Therapy Education; 1998.

## APPENDIX 2-1

# Evaluative Criteria for Accreditation of Education Programs for the Preparation of Physical Therapists*

## *With Interpretive Comments and Guidelines*

### INTRODUCTION

The Commission on Accreditation in Physical Therapy Education (CAPTE) is the only recognized agency in the United States for accrediting education programs for the preparation of physical therapists and physical therapist assistants. CAPTE is also involved in accreditation of established education programs in other countries at the request of the program and the sponsoring institution.

CAPTE attempts to assure that accredited programs prepare graduates who will be effective contemporary practitioners of physical therapy. The Commission acknowledges the critical role of the profession in defining the nature of contemporary practice and determining practice expectations and the demands that are placed on graduates. The Commission recognizes that institutional environments in which physical therapist education programs exist must ensure the opportunity for physical therapy to thrive as both an academic and professional discipline. An accredited program has the right to establish objectives, in addition to those in these *Evaluative Criteria,* that are in keeping with the mission and resources of the institution, as well as the mission of the program.

### A. THE PROFESSION AND THE PRACTICE ENVIRONMENT

Physical therapy, as a profession, dates from the beginning of the century, when the advances in health care made possible the survival of people affected by poliomyelitis and war injuries. Physical therapy has continued to evolve and to respond to the needs of society with physical therapists now practicing in a variety of clinical settings with unprecedented levels of professional responsibility. Physical therapists are integral members of the primary care team and are involved in prevention of disability and promotion of positive health, as well as acting as consultants in restorative care. Physical therapy practice today is based on a well-developed body of scientific and clinical knowledge. Physical therapists also apply knowledge from the basic, behavioral, and social sciences.

According to the *Model Definition of Physical Therapy for State Practice Acts,* a current definition of physical therapy is

> Physical therapy, which is the care and services provided by or under the direction and supervision of a physical therapist, includes: (1) examining and evaluating patients with health-related conditions, impairments, functional limitations, and disability in order to determine a diagnosis, prognosis, and intervention; (2) alleviating impairments and functional limitations by designing, implementing, and modifying therapeutic interventions; (3) preventing injury, impairments, functional limitations, and disability, including promoting and maintaining fitness, health, and quality of life in all age populations; and (4) engaging in consultation, education, and research. [Adopted by the American Physical Therapy Association (APTA) Board of Directors in March 1995 (BOD 03-95-24-64).]

In addition, two other documents which help to describe physical therapy as a profession were used in developing these *Evaluative Criteria*: *A Guide to Physical Therapist Practice, Volume 1: A Description of Practice* and *A Consensus Model of Physical Therapist Professional Education,* 3rd rev. Both of these documents were developed through lengthy, participatory processes. *A Guide to*

* Adopted October 30, 1996; effective January 1, 1988; revised August 2000.

*Physical Therapist Practice, Volume I: A Description of Practice*, including the patient management model, evolved through a project involving three outside reviews in 1993. A fourth and fifth review involved APTA chapter presidents and section presidents. Beginning in December 1994, a Board of Directors' subgroup met on five occasions to review the document before submitting a final version of the Guide to the March 1995 Board of Directors and the 1995 House of Delegates. The House of Delegates voted to endorse the patient management model and to disseminate the Guide to numerous stakeholder groups (RC 21–95, RC 35–95).

*A Consensus Model of Physical Therapist Professional Education* was developed through a consensus process that was approved by the APTA Board of Directors and implemented by the APTA Education Division in early 1994. The Third Revision of the Model was based on the results of two conferences (130 member consultants and observers) and written comments from forums held at the Combined Sections Meeting and Annual Conference, one thousand educators and clinicians who attended meetings in 38 cities across the country, an 800-member reader/reviewer group, and numerous program administrators, faculty members and clinicians in the course of program visits.

Professional education programs and the accreditation process must be responsive to the health care needs of citizens and communities as well as to the needs of the health care system. Practitioners must be prepared to participate in today's health care environment by providing direct services to individuals and groups and by contributing to improved health care delivery.

Provision of care is a collaborative process which requires recognition of the essential roles of the individual, families, insurers/payors, other consumers of physical therapy services, and other health care practitioners. Care givers must understand the continuing evolution of the health care system. Practitioners must be aware of the need to assure high quality care in the most efficient manner to realize societal goals for health care services and delivery.

Physical therapists provide health care to their patients/clients in a wide variety of settings, including, but not limited to, physical therapy office practices, hospitals, rehabilitation facilities, homes, long term care settings, schools, industrial settings and athletic/fitness centers.

## B. THE ACADEMIC ENVIRONMENT

The higher education environment is inherently conducive to physical therapy education for many reasons including the community of scholars, the balance of academic and community life, and the sharing of ideas within a dynamic collegial environment. Professional education programs for the preparation of physical therapists must be conducted in an environment that fosters the intellectual challenge and spirit of inquiry characteristic of the community of scholars and in an environment that supports excellence in professional practice. The institutional environment must be one that ensures the opportunity for physical therapy to thrive as both an academic and professional discipline. In the optimum environment, physical therapy upholds and draws upon a tradition of scientific inquiry while contributing to the profession's body of knowledge. The program faculty must demonstrate a pattern of activity that reflects a commitment to excel in meeting the expectations of the institution, the students, and the profession.

The academic environment must provide students with opportunities to learn from and be influenced by knowledge outside of, as well as within, physical therapy. In this environment, students become aware of multiple styles of thinking, diverse social concepts, values, and ethical behaviors that will help prepare them for identifying, redefining, and fulfilling their responsibilities to society and the profession. Of major importance is emphasis on critical thinking, ethical practice, and provision of service to meet the changing needs of society.

For this environment to be realized, the missions of the institution and the education program must be compatible and mutually supportive.

## C. HISTORY OF ACCREDITATION IN PHYSICAL THERAPY

Education programs for the preparation of physical therapists have been recognized in some manner since 1928, when the American Physical Therapy Association first published a list of approved programs in the June 1928 "Review." In 1936, at the request of the APTA, the American Medical Association (AMA) agreed to become involved in accreditation and recognition of programs in physical therapy. From 1936 to 1956 the AMA was solely responsible for accreditation activities. From 1957 to 1963, the AMA and the APTA shared an informal arrangement and, from 1964 to 1976, a formal collaborative arrangement existed for accreditation of physical therapy programs. In 1977, after APTA's withdrawal from the formal collaborative arrangement, the Commission on Accreditation in Education (CAE) was recognized as an independent accrediting body by the US Department of Education and the Council on Postsecondary Accreditation. Today, CAPTE, the current name for CAE, is recognized by the US Department of Education and the Council for Higher Education Accreditation as the sole agency in the United States for accrediting education programs for the preparation of physical therapists and physical therapist assistants.

The Commission on Accreditation in Physical Therapy Education makes autonomous decisions concerning the accreditation status of education programs for the preparation of physical therapists and physical therapist assistants. In 1989 the APTA House of Delegates voted to change the purpose and function of the Commission on Accreditation in Physical Therapy Education to include the formulation, adoption, and timely revision of the evaluative criteria for accreditation of all professional and paraprofessional education programs in physical therapy. Previously responsibility for those functions had been shared with the APTA House of Delegates and the APTA Board of Directors. The members of the Commission represent the communities of interest, including physical therapy educators, clinicians, consumers, employers, representatives of institutions of higher education, physicians, and the public.

Accreditation standards are periodically reviewed to assure their responsiveness to the changing and expanding nature of physical therapy. The development and promulgation of the *Evaluative Criteria* involve participation of the constituencies affected by the process. Major revisions were adopted in 1978 and in 1990. The revision that appears in this document pertains **only** to the evaluative criteria used in the accreditation of professional programs that prepare **physical therapists** for initial practice. Those evaluative criteria utilized in accreditation decisions for education programs that prepare **physical therapist assistants** may be found in the document entitled *Evaluative Criteria for Accreditation of Education Programs for the Preparation of Physical Therapist Assistants.*

## D. SPECIALIZED ACCREDITATION

Accreditation is essentially a voluntary process used to assess the quality of education programs. Ordinarily, institutions voluntarily seek accreditation to demonstrate to various constituencies that the specialized programs meet accepted standards and have a certain level of quality. Accreditation in physical therapy is linked to a required credentialing process, licensure. All states in the United States require licensure for practice, and graduation from an accredited program is a requirement for licensure. Institutions seeking to initiate or maintain a physical therapy education program, therefore, also seek accreditation because they wish to have their graduates become eligible for licensure.

The purposes of accreditation in physical therapy education, as defined by the scope of responsibility required of a recognized specialized accrediting agency, are to assure the quality of and to improve education programs for the preparation of physical therapists and physical therapist assistants. CAPTE, the recognized specialized accrediting agency in physical therapy education, is responsible for fulfilling these purposes that directly serve the interests of the students and the public. The institutions of higher education that house physical therapy programs benefit from self-evaluation and self-directed improvements which are stimulated by the accreditation process and by the counsel and advice from onsite visitors and the Commission. Through accreditation, professional education programs for the preparation of physical therapists and paraprofessional education programs for the preparation of physical therapist assistants are publicly recognized because they demonstrate levels of performance, integrity, and quality that entitle them to the confidence of the profession, the communities they serve, and the general public. The Commission attempts to assure that accreditation criteria for judging education programs reflect the preparation necessary for graduates to be effective as contemporary practitioners. An accredited program is acknowledged to have the right to establish objectives in addition to those in these *Evaluative Criteria* that are in keeping with the mission and resources of the institution, as well as the mission of the program. The accreditation process recognizes the role of innovation in identifying improved patterns of effectiveness in education and innovative approaches to patient care, as well as advancing the unique mission and goals of the institutions and programs.

In many institutions, the professional physical therapy program is the only physical-therapy–related endeavor. At other institutions, the professional program is part of a constellation of physical therapy activities, including other degree programs and clinical services. The accreditation process focuses on the quality of the professional program and concerns itself with other activities only as they affect the professional program.

Accreditation of education programs for the preparation of physical therapists is based on the mutual responsibility for the quality of professional education. Members of the profession, in collaboration with others in the community of interest served by the accrediting agency, have the responsibility for defining the profession and the roles and responsibilities for which the education programs prepare their graduates. The Commission recognizes that individual institutions have the responsibility for setting their own educational policies and the specific requirements leading to a post-baccalaureate degree and for providing an environment that promotes the high-quality professional education of physical therapists.

It is the intention of the Commission, with the adoption of these *Evaluative Criteria*, to limit its scope of accreditation activities related to professional education programs for the preparation of physical therapists to those programs culminating with a post-baccalaureate degree, effective January 1, 2002.

## E. DEFINITIONS

Documents, such as this one, are used by numerous constituencies, each of which may have its own interpretation of the terminology being utilized. This is often the result of the typical usage patterns at given institutions. It is important, therefore, that the authors of the document specify the definitions of terms as used so that misinterpretations can be minimized. While there are many other terms that could be defined, the terms included here are those that raised the most comment when these criteria were first circulated.

The Commission recognizes that individual institutions may have different definitions or faculty classifications than those identified below; however, for the purposes of this document and related accreditation activities, the following definitions are to be used:

- Core Faculty: those individuals appointed to and employed primarily in the program, including the program administrator and those who report to the program administrator. Members of the core faculty typically have full-time appointments, although some part-time faculty members may be included among the core faculty. The core faculty include physical therapists and may include others with expertise to meet specific curricular needs. As noted in Criterion 2.2.3., the core faculty have the qualifications and experience necessary to achieve the goals of the program through educational administration, curriculum development, instructional design and delivery, and evaluation of outcomes. The core faculty are generally the group with the responsibility and authority related to the curriculum. The core faculty may hold tenured, tenure track, or non-tenure track positions.
- Adjunct Faculty: those individuals who have classroom and/or laboratory teaching responsibilities in the program and who are not employed by the institution, though they may receive honoraria or other forms of compensation. The adjunct faculty may or may not be "appointed" to the faculty. The adjunct faculty may include, but are not limited to, guest lecturers, "contract" faculty, instructors of course modules, tutors, etc.

- Clinical Education Faculty: those individuals engaged in providing the clinical education components of the program, generally referred to as either Center Coordinators of Clinical Education (CCCEs) or Clinical Instructors (CIs). While these individuals are not usually employed by the educational institution, they do agree to certain standards of behavior through contractual arrangements for their services.
- Supporting Faculty: those individuals with faculty appointments in other units within the institution who teach courses which are part of the professional program, e.g., faculty from a biology department who teach physiology, or faculty from a School of Medicine who teach pathology, etc.
- Program Faculty: all faculty involved with the program, including 1) the Core Faculty, 2) the Adjunct Faculty; 3) the Supporting Faculty; and 4) the Clinical Education Faculty.
- Faculty [unmodified]: when the term faculty is used without a modifier (adjunct, core, supporting, clinical education or program) it can be interpreted generically. The Commission has modified the term in those cases when a specific faculty group is being addressed.
- Program Administrator: the individual employed full-time by the institution, as a member of the core faculty, to serve as the program's academic administrator: Dean, Chair, Director, Coordinator, etc.
- Library Systems: the mechanisms through which students and faculty gain access to current information. The access to information may be provided through electronic media, interlibrary loan as well as through the traditional books and journals.
- Diagnostic Process: the evaluation of information obtained from the patient or client examination, which is organized into clusters, syndromes or categories.
- Differential Diagnosis: the determination of which one of two or more different disorders or conditions is applicable to a patient or client.
- Foundational Sciences: the foundational sciences in physical therapy include: Anatomy, Histology, Physiology, Applied Physiology, Pathophysiology, Behavioral Sciences, Biomechanics and Kinesiology, Neuroscience, Pathology and Pharmacology.
- Clinical Sciences: the clinical sciences in physical therapy include content about the cardiovascular/pulmonary, endocrine, gastrointestinal, genitourinary, integumentary, musculoskeletal and neuromuscular systems and the medical and surgical conditions frequently seen by physical therapists. The clinical sciences also include content for individual systems related to the specific responsibilities of patient screening, examination, evaluation, diagnosis, prognosis, plan of care, intervention and outcome assessment, and evaluation.

## F. FORMAT AND UTILIZATION OF THE EVALUATIVE CRITERIA

The *Evaluative Criteria* which follow consist of several components: section preambles, evaluative criteria, and interpretive comments and guidelines.

The criteria are divided into four sections, each of which has a preamble. The purpose of the preamble is to provide an overview of the criteria included in the section and the rationale for their inclusion. In preparation of accreditation documents, programs are welcome to respond to the section preambles though the Commission does not expect that they do so.

Within each section, specific criteria elucidate the Commission's requirements in order for a program to be accredited. The Commission expects that programs will be in satisfactory compliance with the intent of each of the evaluative criteria. The Commission recognizes, however, that programs can be out of compliance with some criteria and still be accredited. In concert with US Department of Education requirements, the Commission expects that programs will come into satisfactory compliance with all criteria within two years of being determined to be out of compliance.

Each criterion has an interpretive comment and guideline (printed in italics) which serves to explain the intent of the criterion and may provide information about the types of evidence which the program can use to demonstrate compliance with the criterion. The interpretive comment and guideline does not substitute for the criterion per se but rather attempts to provide a demonstration of what factors may be in place if the program is in compliance with the criterion.

## SECTION 1: ORGANIZATION

### Preamble

**Physical therapists must work within the structures of their practice and of legal, social, and ethical environments; similarly, physical therapist education programs must function within the structure of the institutions in which they exist. Physical therapist education programs must be vital parts of the institutions in which they are located, and the existence of programs must be consistent with institutional missions and resources. Institutions that offer physical therapist education programs must do so because of their commitment to humanistic principles, scientific inquiry, and service to society. They must exhibit sensitivity to the role of health professions in society. Physical therapist education programs must be integral to institutional missions and be logical extensions of the institution's education and service programs.**

**Institutions must be committed to professional education and demonstrate awareness of the differences between professional education and traditional degree programs. Among the differences are the following: professional education requires the student to engage the entire body of knowledge related to the profession and to demonstrate accountability for the utilization of that knowledge; professional education is structured and focused on the knowledge and skills necessary for initial practice of the profession; emphasis is placed on socialization of the student into the profession, including the behavioral and ethical standards to be met; and, faculty are expected to serve as exemplary professional role models.**

**Through the structure and function of the institution, graduates must be made aware of their need to build on their liberal education, to incorporate the concepts of responsible citizenship into their professional lives, to interact with other professionals, to continue their education throughout their professional careers, and to be ethical and scientifically current in order to be responsible health care practitioners. Innovation and variations from traditional approaches to professional education are institutional prerogatives that are expected and encouraged when evidence is provided that they are effective and beneficial.**

**1.1. Institution**

**1.1.1. The sponsoring institution is authorized under applicable law or other acceptable authority to provide a program of postsecondary education. In addition, the institution has been approved by appropriate authorities to provide the professional physical therapy program.**

*The institution of higher education has been authorized to conduct business in the jurisdiction in which it is located. This authorization may be required by government or private sectors. In addition, the institution has been authorized to provide a physical therapy education program by meeting governing regulations required by the state, private sector, or the institutional accrediting agency. Programs in countries other than the United States that seek CAPTE accreditation must be established programs with authorization by the appropriate governing body to conduct business in the jurisdiction.*

**1.1.2. The education program for the physical therapist is provided by an institution accredited by an agency recognized by the U.S. Department of Education or by the Council for Higher Education Accreditation. [For programs in countries other than the U.S., the Commission will determine an alternative and equivalent external review process.]**

*The institution of higher education must have accreditation granted by the appropriate accrediting agency for the program to be eligible for CAPTE accreditation. In this way the program need not be evaluated for fundamental elements necessary in an institution of higher education, and the responsibility for such documentation and evaluation shifts from the program to the institutional level. Programs in countries other than the United States that seek CAPTE accreditation must be established programs in institutions of higher education that have a regular external review of the quality of its operation, the adequacy of its resources to conduct programs in professional education, and its ability to continue its level of operation.*

**1.1.3. Institutional and program policies and procedures are based on appropriate and equitable criteria and conform to applicable law.**

*The institution ensures that policies and procedures that affect all faculty and staff are clearly described, provided to the faculty and staff in a timely manner, and applied equitably.*

*The sponsoring institution must have nondiscriminatory policies and procedures that are applied equitably and conform to applicable law. The policies and procedures assure equal opportunity with respect to race, creed, color, gender, age, national or ethnic origin, sexual orientation, and disability or health status. This criterion, however, does not negate the program's right to act affirmatively for certain groups of people, identified by race, color, gender, national or ethnic origin, or disability or health status, nor does it prohibit institutions from activities associated with enhancing diversity among their faculty, students, or staff. Should the program elect to act affirmatively in any case, the Commission expects that the program describes its decision to do so in its publications available to the interested parties. The Commission also recognizes the right of programs and institutions to limit activities to certain groups if allowable by law, such as certain religious affiliated programs or those that serve only males or females.*

**1.1.4. Institutional and program policies protect the rights and safety of individuals in all activities associated with the education program.**

*The institution must have policies and procedures that are designed and implemented to protect the rights and safety of all individuals involved in any aspect of the physical therapy program. One such right is the opportunity to file grievances within the institution and program and to have such grievances processed in a timely manner.*

*Policies and procedures ensure due process in the handling of student and faculty concerns and/or complaints at all levels of the program and institution. The program has policies and procedures for handling complaints received from other sources such as clinical education sites, parents, etc.*

*The faculty and students are responsible for preserving the privacy, dignity, and safety of all people, including patients/clients, patients'/clients' families or care givers, students, faculty, and support staff who are involved in the classroom, laboratory, clinical, research, and administrative activities of the program.*

*The academic institution is responsible for ensuring that students are informed of potential health risks they may encounter throughout the education program, and in clinical practice. Safety regulations and emergency procedures, including access to emergency services, regulations outlining universal body precautions and governing the use of equipment, and the storage and use of any hazardous materials, are posted, reviewed periodically, and distributed to all appropriate parties, such as faculty and students.*

*The institution, the program, and each clinical education site have policies describing confidentiality of records and other personal information, as well as policies and procedures on the use of subjects in research if applicable. The program and each clinical education site have guidelines on the use of human subjects in demonstrations and practice for educational purposes. Procedures exist for obtaining the informed consent of people to participate in demonstrations and studies and the authorized use of any material portraying information about or images of individuals.*

**1.1.5. Institutional and program policies and procedures provide for compliance with accreditation policies and procedures, including**

*The institution and program have policies and procedures which are designed to facilitate the program's continued accreditation status.*

**1.1.5.1. timely submission of required fees and documentation, including reports of graduation rates, performance on state licensing examinations, and employment rates,**

*The institution and program are responsible for submitting requested documentation, and fees, by the established deadlines. Requested documentation includes but is not limited to, progress reports, Biennial Accreditation Reports, and reports of graduation rates, performance on state licensing examinations, and employment rates.*

**1.1.5.2. timely notification of expected or unexpected substantive change(s) within the program, and of any change in institutional accreditation status or legal authority to provide postsecondary education,**

*The institution and program are responsible for notifying CAPTE of all substantive changes in the program prior to implementation. Unexpected substantive changes are to be reported immediately after they occur. Substantive changes to be reported include, but are not limited to, change in program leadership, change in the administrative structure in which the program is housed, significant decreases in resources available to the program (faculty, staff, space, equipment, funding, etc.), increases (greater than 25%) in the size of classes to be admitted, major curricular changes, and establishment of an expansion program. Additionally, the institution and program are responsible for notifying CAPTE of any threatened or actual change in institutional accreditation status or legal authority to provide postsecondary education immediately upon notification of this change in status. CAPTE's response to such notification will be to investigate further the implications of such changes on the program.*

**1.1.5.3. mechanisms for handling complaints about the program and maintaining records of complaints about the program, and**

*The institution and program have identified procedures for handling complaints about the program. Records of complaints about the program, including the nature of the complaint and the disposition of the complaint, are maintained by the program.*

**1.1.5.4. coming into compliance with accreditation criteria within two years of being determined to be out of compliance.**

*The institution and program are responsible for bringing the program into compliance with the* Evaluative Criteria *within two years after the determination that the program is out of compliance.*

**1.1.6. Written agreements between the institution and the clinical education sites describe the rights and responsibilities of both, including those of their respective agents.**

*The program is responsible for arranging and maintaining clinical education agreements. A written agreement, in a format acceptable to both parties, exists between the institution and each clinical education site accepting students for clinical education. Minimally, the written agreement states the following: the purpose(s) of the agreement; the objectives of the institution and the clinical education site in establishing the agreement; the rights and responsibilities of the institution, the clinical education site, and the student; and the procedures to be followed in reviewing, revising, and terminating the agreement.*

**1.2. Program Authority, Goals, and Objectives**

**1.2.1. The program's mission reflects and adds to the mission of the institution.**

*The professional physical therapy program is recognized by the institution for its contribution to the achievement of the institution's mission.*

**1.2.2. The goals and objectives of the physical therapy program are an integral part of the mission of the institution.**

*The program mission, goals, and objectives are compatible with the mission of the institution in which the program is offered and address the physical therapy needs of the community that the institution serves. The program has a written statement of philosophy which relates to the program's mission. The philosophy describes the program's basic beliefs about education and learning, the role of the profession, and the interrelationship of these beliefs. The program's mission is the basis for the development of the curricular philosophy, goals, and purpose around which the curriculum is designed. The program may be unique in its design and mission; however, this does not relieve the program of its responsibility to provide a program that is consistent with the mission of the profession of physical therapy and these* Evaluative Criteria.

**1.2.3. The core faculty have responsibility for the governance of the program and the authority to ensure that its policies are implemented.**

*The institution provides opportunity for the program to be responsible for governance of the physical therapy education program. The core faculty's responsibility and authority in the program also require them to operate within the institution's established governance processes.*

**1.2.4. The program faculty, using institutional guidelines, establish, assess, and uphold academic regulations including those that are specific to the program. These regulations include, but are not limited to, admission criteria, grading policies, minimum performance criteria, and student progression through the academic, clinical, and other components of the curriculum.**

*Using institutional guidelines and procedures, core faculty initiate, adopt, evaluate, and uphold academic regulations that are specific to the program. All program faculty uphold the established regulations. The regulations are compatible with institutional rules and practices and include, but are not limited to, grading policy, minimum performance levels including those relating to professional and ethical behaviors, and student progression through the program. The institution supports the program faculty's professional judgment in upholding these academic regulations.*

*Policies exist to guide the dissemination and implementation of all established regulations which affect the program faculty and/or students.*

**1.2.5. There is evidence of ongoing communication among all program faculty and other people directly involved with the program. There is evidence that effective communication is used to coordinate the efforts of all people and departments directly involved with the program.**

*There are mechanisms that facilitate and maintain coordination and communication among all program faculty and departments, including clinical education sites, directly involved with the program. The program has procedures with specified lines of communication and with clearly delineated responsibilities to enable effective interactions among all individuals and groups involved with the program. Procedures are established for effective communication between students and the program faculty.*

**1.3. Program Faculty Policies and Procedures**

**1.3.1. Policies and procedures that directly affect program faculty are described, applied equitably, and provided to prospective and current program faculty in a timely manner.**

*Institutional and programmatic policies and procedures that affect program faculty are available, as appropriate, to all program faculty. Policies and procedures related to appointment, tenure, and promotion are clearly described and available, as appropriate, to program faculty. Information about academic regulations, due process for program faculty and students, and other policies and procedures, including those related to accreditation activities, is provided, as applicable, to all program faculty.*

**1.3.1.1. Core faculty have the same rights and privileges as other faculty with similar rank and responsibilities within the institution.**

*The institution ensures that rights and privileges that affect all other faculty within the institution are extended and applied equitably to the core faculty. The institution provides the core faculty with opportunities to participate in the governance of the institution, as well as that of their own program, following guidelines that are applicable to all faculty in that institution. People with ongoing academic and administrative responsibilities hold academic appointments in the institution in which the program is located in accordance with institutional policies.*

**1.3.1.2. The rights and privileges of adjunct faculty are delineated and communicated to the program faculty as appropriate, and evidence is provided that these rights and privileges are based on their level of participation in the program.**

*The rights and privileges of adjunct faculty are appropriate for their participation in the program and similar to the rights and privileges afforded to the adjunct faculty in other programs throughout the institution. The rights and privileges of the adjunct faculty are communicated to them and to other members of the program faculty as appropriate. Adjunct faculty participation in program governance and curriculum review is consistent with institutional policy and with their level of participation in the program.*

**1.3.1.3. The rights and privileges of clinical education faculty and policies and procedures related to clinical education are delineated and communicated to all program faculty.**

*The rights and privileges of clinical education faculty are appropriate for their participation in the program and are similar to the rights and privileges afforded those people with similar responsibilities in other programs throughout the institution. Policies and procedures related to clinical education are provided to clinical education faculty. Clinical education faculty participation in program activities and curriculum review is consistent with institutional policy.*

**1.3.2. Faculty policies and procedures ensure that regular evaluation of the core faculty occurs and that these include assessments of teaching, scholarly activity, and service.**

*Students, faculty, and administrators contribute to the assessment of the effectiveness of each core faculty member. The regular and ongoing faculty evaluation program is designed to assess and improve the effectiveness of teaching, scholarly activity and service of each core faculty member, including the program administrator, in order to maximize the faculty member's viability in the academic setting particularly in regard to tenure and promotion. The assessment of core faculty is based on defined goals that are measurable and attainable.*

**1.3.3. The program faculty meet their responsibilities by:**

**1.3.3.1. maintaining their competence and knowledge levels by remaining current in their areas of responsibility, and**

*Individual faculty members are responsible for remaining current in all areas where they are expected to contribute expertise to the program. This may be in areas of teaching, clinical practice, research participation and/or supervision, other scholarly activities, administration, or curriculum management (development and review). Competence may be maintained through use of primary literature, participation in symposia, professional or scientific forums, research, clinical practice, or participation in other scholarly activities. In academic environments, particularly those associated with professional education, levels of competence are determined by peer determinations. Although a variety of means may be available to demonstrate current competencies, including the use of any of the mechanisms described here a primary means of showing competence is through the traditional academic indicator of peer reviewed publications (research, clinical, or otherwise).*

**1.3.3.2. engaging in ongoing faculty development that is based on program needs identified in the evaluative process and evaluations of individual faculty members,**

*The program supports, and the program faculty participate in, continuing development activities directed toward improving faculty effectiveness. The development activities are linked to the results of the assessments of faculty effectiveness and the identified needs of the program. Development also is based on the expectation that faculty remain current in their content areas and takes into consideration the faculty member's level of contribution to the program. Effective development of program faculty is enhanced by setting measurable and attainable goals. Methods for achieving the goals and a timetable for accomplishing the goals are stated, and both are reviewed regularly. The development activities reflect an overall plan for improvement in program faculty effectiveness and the growth of and changes in the program. Resources for development need not be limited to money, but may include time for activities such as faculty mentoring, extramural collaboration, and sharing of clinical and teaching expertise.*

**1.3.3.3. participating in the governance of the institution and/or program to the degree allowed by institutional guidelines.**

*Institutions may fulfill their responsibilities for faculty governance by making opportunities available to faculty to participate in governance, but the faculty must in turn avail themselves of these opportunities. In institutions where faculty governance is encouraged and expected, program faculty must fulfill this obligation to the institution by demonstrating, collectively and individually, patterns of involvement similar to those of faculty members with equal ranks and responsibilities.*

**1.4. Student Policies and Procedures**

**1.4.1. Student recruitment, admission, and retention procedures are based on appropriate and equitable criteria and applicable law, and the policies and procedures assure nondiscrimination and equal opportunity to all students. This does not preclude a program's right to act affirmatively for certain groups of people.**

*Policies and procedures applied in student selection, evaluation, and retention do not discriminate on the basis of race, creed, color, gender, age, national or ethnic origin, sexual orientation, and disability or health status. The establishment and consistent application or use of academic regulations, student-oriented objectives, and documentation of student achievement of the objectives insure nondiscrimination.*

*This criterion, however, does not negate the program's ability to act affirmatively for certain groups of people, including those identified by race, color, gender, national or ethnic origin, or disability or health status, nor does it prohibit institutions from activities associated with enhancing diversity among their student populations; however, it is expected that all published materials related to admissions policy and practice includes information about the program's decision to act affirmatively for the selected groups. The Commission also recognizes the right of programs and institutions to limit activities to certain groups if allowable by law, such as certain religious affiliated programs or those that serve only males or females.*

**1.4.2. Students are provided with the current policies, procedures, and information about the institution and program that may affect them, including, but not limited to catalogs, academic calendars, and grading policies.**

*The institution ensures that policies and procedures that directly affect prospective and enrolled students, including accreditation status and activities, are clearly described, are applied equitably, and are provided so that materials (such as those with specific deadlines) are received in a timely manner.*

*The program provides prospective and enrolled students with access to or copies of rules and regulations related to admissions, matriculation, progression through the program, withdrawal and dismissal procedures, due process, clinical education, and other academic policies and procedures. Materials related to institution and program policies are accurate, comprehensive, current, and provided to students in a timely manner. The program provides students with information about career opportunities, costs of the program (including tuition, fees and refund policies), academic and clinical education sites, accreditation status of the institution and the program, and health and professional liability insurance requirements.*

*Students are informed about policies and procedures for obtaining and financing their health care during their participation in the program, including during clinical education.*

## SECTION 2: RESOURCES AND SERVICES

### Preamble

**The professional physical therapy education program is an integral part of the institution of higher education. Students enrolled in the program have completed prerequisite courses and experiences designed to lead to their successful completion of the program. The program faculty present a broad spectrum of teaching, research, and clinical expertise. Resources necessary to support all facets of the professional physical therapy education program, including human resources, fiscal support, facilities and equipment, and support services, are planned for, secured, and well managed.**

**The Commission recognizes that the professional program may be administratively located in a unit that engages in activities in addition to the professional program (e.g., post-professional education, clinical services and/or primary research). The intent of CAPTE accreditation activities, however, is to focus on those resources and services available to the professional education program.**

**2.1. Students**

**The program admits and graduates students consistent with its mission and the needs of society.**

*The program considers its mission and the mission of the institution when decisions are made related to admission. Activities designed to retain and graduate students also reflect the mission of the institution and program. In addition, the program considers the needs of society in relation to its decisions concerning admission, retention and graduation of students.*

**2.2. Program Faculty**

**2.2.1. The core faculty:**

**2.2.1.1. Is sufficient in number and possesses the expertise to assure instructional design, content delivery and curricular evaluation;**

*The core faculty consists of physical therapists, and may include others, with expertise to meet specific curricular needs. The core faculty are employed primarily to work in the program and report to the program administrator. The core faculty have the qualifications and experience necessary to achieve the goals of the program through educational administration, curriculum development, instructional design and delivery, and evaluation of outcomes.*

*A sufficient number of core faculty exist so that teaching loads are consistent with others throughout the institution and are reflective of similar professional programs nationally. Contact hours should be considered along with credit hours when determining faculty teaching loads. The complexity of the material being taught, the teaching methodology being used, the number of students per class, and the experience of the core faculty members must be considered when planning for a sufficient number of core faculty. In addition, physical therapy education programs have unique needs, similar to those of other professional education programs, where core faculty must counsel students, develop and maintain relationships with all program faculty, develop clinical sites, and supervise students in clinical practice.*

*Therefore, an adequate number of core faculty is required so that these roles may be carried out. Determinations of adequate core faculty size can only be made with these responsibilities in mind and comparisons across faculty units within an institution are only relevant when these factors are taken into account.*

**2.2.1.2. is sufficient in number and time commitment to engage in research, other scholarly activities, governance, administration, and other activities (e.g., clinical practice and service to professional organizations);**

*There is an adequate number of core faculty to allow for adequate time to engage in research or other scholarly activity, involvement in program and institution committee responsibilities, admissions, administration, and activities, such as clinical practice and participation in professional organizations, that contribute to individual professional growth and development.*

**2.2.1.3. is sufficient in number to provide collegial interaction and professional growth of faculty and students.**

*In higher education faculty members are expected to be content experts and to contribute to the growth of knowledge in their areas of expertise. In addition, all faculty are expected to develop professionally. The development and maintenance of faculty competence and capability requires colleagues who represent a diversity of ideas and who can serve as mentors, peer counselors, and as colleagues for teaching, research or other scholarly activities, and clinical projects. The number of core faculty is sufficient to allow this to occur.*

**2.2.2. The program administrator (e.g., dean, chair, director, coordinator, etc.) is a physical therapist who has qualifications comparable to other administrators who manage similar units within the institution; senior faculty status; and relevant experience in higher education requisite for providing effective leadership for the program, its faculty, and its students.**

*The program administrator is a physical therapist who gives evidence of and demonstrates the following: proven educational leadership, including, but not limited to, (a) a vision for physical therapist professional education, (b) understanding of and experience with curriculum content, design and evaluation, (c) employing strategies to promote and support professional development, (d) proven effective interpersonal and conflict management skills, (e) abilities to facilitate change, (f) negotiation skills (relative to planning, budgeting, funding, faculty and program status, employment and termination, space, and appropriate academic and professional benefits), and (g) experience in strategic planning; teaching and research qualifications comparable to those of senior full-time faculty members in the institution; senior faculty status; a post-professional academic doctoral degree; active service on behalf of physical therapist professional education, higher education, the larger community, and organizations related to their academic interest; effective management of human and fiscal resources; commitment to lifelong learning; active role in institutional governance.*

**2.2.3. The program faculty as a unit, including the program administrator and the academic coordinator of clinical education, have the qualifications and experience necessary to achieve the program goals through effective processes of curriculum development, instructional design, and evaluation of outcomes. The program faculty, in the aggregate, give evidence of and demonstrate the following:**

*Faculty function both as individuals and collectively within a program. To achieve program goals, specific activities must be accomplished. The program faculty must, therefore, as a group, demonstrate ability to develop curriculum, design and implement instructional activities, and evaluate outcomes.*

**2.2.3.1. expertise in teaching and content to design, implement, and evaluate the curriculum and to ensure that educational outcomes corresponding to entry-level practice expectations are being achieved;**

*Faculty expertise in the aggregate must cover all areas of content in the curriculum. The program faculty as a group must have skills and knowledge necessary to design and implement a curriculum and to evaluate its outcomes in terms of entry-level practice expectations.*

**2.2.3.2. ability to identify performance deficits and unsafe practices of students and to determine the student's readiness to engage in clinical education;**

*The faculty's collective responsibility is to determine whether students are prepared for practice, both during various phases of the education program and when students are assigned to clinical education experiences. Mechanisms must be in place where faculty can communicate concerns in these areas to one another so that the faculty can act collectively to determine safety and readiness.*

**2.2.3.3. ability to coordinate and conduct the clinical education portion of the curriculum;**

*Individual faculty may have assigned roles in a program's clinical education program, but the faculty as a whole must assume responsibility for the coordination and conduct of clinical education activities. Toward that end the faculty in the aggregate must have adequate number of personnel with adequate levels of expertise to develop, maintain, and evaluate clinical education.*

**2.2.3.4. ongoing communication among all faculty, including clinical instructors, to ensure continuity and consistency between program goals and clinical education outcomes;**

*Communication with clinical education faculty may be primarily a task of specific faculty, but the program faculty as a whole must be staffed with people adequate in number and expertise to achieve effective ongoing communication regarding program goals and clinical education expectations. Responsibility for ongoing communication with clinical education faculty is a responsibility of the faculty in the aggregate although not all faculty may be involved in this activity.*

**2.2.3.5. ability to monitor and facilitate ethical and professional behaviors.**

*The faculty have a collective responsibility to identify whether students exhibit behaviors which suggest that they may not be capable of meeting ethical and professional standards for membership in the profession. Mechanisms must be in place where faculty can communicate concerns in these areas to one another so that the faculty can act collectively on concerns regarding ethical and professional behaviors.*

**2.2.4. Individual faculty members are qualified to fulfill their assigned responsibilities.**

*The physical therapist professional education faculty include a blend of expert clinicians and doctorally prepared faculty who give evidence of and demonstrate the following:*

- *post-professional academic and/or clinical credentials consistent with roles and responsibilities, with a doctorate and/or clinical specialization expected;*
- *research, other scholarly activity, or clinical practice or both, that contribute to teaching, the institutional mission, and the physical therapist professional education program;*
- *activity related to current and theoretically based approaches to teaching, the evaluation of teaching effectiveness, and student learning;*
- *oral and written communication skills, including the ability to address difficult issues and diverse populations;*
- *effective interpersonal skills,*
- *professional and ethical behavior;*
- *currency in content expertise.*

*In their professional activities and communication, the academic faculty serve as professional role models for students.*

**2.2.4.1. Each faculty member has documented expertise in all areas of assigned teaching, and demonstrated effective teaching and student evaluation skills.**

*Judgment about faculty competence in an area of the curriculum for which a faculty member (either academic or clinical) is responsible is based on past and current involvement in: advanced degree courses; clinical experience; research or other scholarly activity; and teaching (i.e., classroom, clinical, in-service and/or continuing education, and presentations) and attendance at in-service or continuing education courses. Competence in the area of the curriculum for which the program administrator and the academic coordinator of clinical education are responsible is judged in accordance with guidelines for determining competency of the rest of the faculty. When determining teaching effectiveness, multiple sources of data are used, including evaluations by students.*

**2.2.4.2. Each faculty member has a record of ongoing scholarly and professional accomplishments and community service consistent with the philosophy of the program and institution.**

*Each faculty member is involved, to a degree compatible with the institutional and program mission and philosophy, in research and/or other scholarly activity and in service to the community.*

**2.2.5. The clinical education faculty demonstrate clinical expertise in their area of practice and the capacity to perform as effective clinical teachers.**

*The clinical education faculty are those clinicians who have the responsibility for education and supervision of students in the clinical education sites. Members of the clinical education faculty serve as role models for students in scholarly and professional activities. Judgment about clinical education faculty competence is based on appropriate past and current involvement in: in-service or continuing education courses; advanced degree courses; clinical experience; research experience; and teaching experience (e.g., classroom, clinical, in-service and/or continuing education). Clinical education faculty must have a minimum of one year of professional experience (two years of clinical experience are preferred). Their continued ability to perform as clinical education faculty is assessed based on the individual's prior performance as a clinical educator, as well as other criteria established by the program.*

**2.3. Student Services**

**2.3.1. Information about the types of, qualifications for, and procedures to apply for financial aid through the institution and program is available to all students. Information about the existence of financial assistance from sources external to the institution and program is made available to the students as the institution or program become aware of these opportunities.**

*Information is made available in an accurate and timely manner to facilitate the students' ability to apply successfully for financial aid. Students are advised to seek appropriate counsel before entering into any legal obligation for financial assistance.*

**2.3.2. Students have access to counseling and testing services.**

*Professional counseling and testing services are available to students enrolled in the program and assistance is provided in obtaining those services. Academic advising and career counseling, as well as enrollment, matriculation, withdrawal and dismissal policies and procedures are provided.*

**2.3.3. The program provides students with regular reports of their academic and clinical performance and progress.**

*Students have scheduled opportunities to discuss academic performance and progress with faculty. The students have regularly scheduled opportunities to review and discuss clinical performance and progress with the clinical instructors or center coordinators of clinical education. Documentation of performance and progress are used in reviews and discussions.*

**2.4. Fiscal Planning and Management**

**2.4.1. There are adequate financial resources to achieve the program's stated objectives and to assure the continuing operation of the program.**

*An adequate budget is essential to meet programmatic goals and needs, including faculty and staff salaries, materials and equipment, faculty development, curricular development, program facilities, and the facilitation of scholarly activities of the faculty (e.g., research). Financial resources available to the program support the continuing operation of the program at an acceptable level. The program's budget reflects adequate support of essential program and faculty needs and ensures that obligations to potential and enrolled students are met. The program's projected budget reflects adequate support of the program's goals and objectives which are based on long-range planning and anticipated changes in program needs, faculty needs, and obligations to students. Institution and program budgets include, but are not limited to, faculty and staff salaries; funds for professional activities and development; supplies; equipment acquisition, repair, and replacement costs; and clinical visitation costs and other related clinical education costs.*

**2.4.2. Using institutional budget guidelines and faculty input, the program administrator has the responsibility and authority for planning and allocating the program's financial resources.**

*The program administrator, applying institutional policies and procedures and with input from the program faculty, establishes the priorities on which budget planning and allocation of program resources are based. The education program may be located in any one of various settings within or affiliated with the institution, but the resources to support the program's activities must be available from the institution directly or through an affiliated setting or from additional sources.*

**2.4.3. The program employs a fiscal plan that supports attainment of the program's short-and long-term goals and objectives.**

*The program conducts its planning for fiscal support with a knowledge of the institution's overall system for planning and budgeting. The budget plan is designed to protect the longevity and academic integrity of the program. The program administrator works with administrative officials of the institution in long range planning to assure that there is financial support for current and anticipated program needs, including support for the unique demands of clinical education, the admissions process, faculty development, and support for scholarly activities.*

**2.5. Administrative and Support Services**

**The program has, or has access to, administrative, secretarial, and technical support staff to meet its professional education, research, and service goals and objectives, including the specialized needs of physical therapy programs in the areas of admissions and clinical education.**

*The number and skills of administrative, secretarial and technical personnel assigned to provide supportive services for the program will vary in relation to the operational requirements of the program. The number of supportive personnel required will be determined by the size and activities of the faculty and student body and may include information management, printing/duplication, and assistance with instructional media.*

*The institution assures that support services facilitate the ability of students and faculty to meet their obligations.*

**2.6. Learning Resources and Library Systems**

**The resources of the institutional library system and related learning resource centers are adequate to support the educational and research goals of the program.**

*The library system provides access to current information in the fields of physical therapy, biomedical sciences, and related areas. This may be through holdings of books, journals, or electronic media within the facility or through alternative mechanisms to access information from other sources. Through the library system or learning resource centers, faculty and students have access to non-print materials, such as audiovisual aids and computer-based materials. The students and faculty are aware of the methods available to them to access information and have adequate access to these resources during non-class time.*

**2.7. Facilities**

**2.7.1. The program has offices and space for faculty and staff and access to classrooms and laboratories of sufficient quality and quantity to carry out program goals.**

*Classrooms of adequate size are available for scheduled use by the program. The number and size of the classrooms accommodate the number of students in courses and the scheduling requirements of the courses. Other factors that affect the amount and type of space necessary for the program are the number of concurrently scheduled courses, class sizes in those courses, format of various courses (e.g., seminar, lecture, and demonstration), student research requirements and accessibility for faculty, students and/or patients with disabling conditions. One or more classroom laboratories are available for laboratory practice by students. Students have opportunities for learning with access to equipment and supplies at times other than during regularly scheduled classes.*

*Adequate space for storage of equipment and teaching aids is provided in proximity to the classroom(s) and laboratory(ies). Dressing areas, lockers, lavatories, and toilets are readily accessible to the laboratory area. Offices for the program administrator, faculty, and supportive personnel are adequate in size, design, and location to enable these people to function effectively and efficiently. Office and meeting space is adequate to accommodate regular faculty and administrative activities and admissions, and administration of clinical education. Faculty and staff offices provide adequate space, privacy, and security for preparing instructional materials, advising students, and storing records and materials. Work areas are provided for supportive activities, including the preparation of instructional media. The institution maintains all spaces in a good state of repair and cleanliness and conducive to learning (e.g., with adequate lighting and electrical power, suitable furnishings, necessary water and waste lines, suitable floor coverings, and adequate heating, ventilation, and air conditioning.)*

**2.7.2. There is a sufficient quality and quantity of clinical education experiences to prepare students for practice.**

*The clinical education experiences are adequate in number and appropriate in scope to meet the objectives of clinical education, to reflect the stated mission of the program, and to reflect current physical therapy practice arenas. In addition to well-planned patient care and teaching experiences, the clinical education program includes opportunities for students to participate in diverse practice settings.*

**2.7.3. The program has, or has access to, space for core faculty to fulfill their role as scholars.**

*Core faculty are expected to contribute to the scholarship of the profession and to be viable academicians. They therefore must have access to adequate space that is appropriate for their research or other scholarly needs. Space in which to conduct research activities approved by the program and institution is available to meet the needs of the core faculty.*

**2.8. Equipment and Materials**

**2.8.1. The program has, or has use of, equipment and materials necessary to meet the goals and objectives of the program.**

*Supplies and equipment are available and in good repair and safe operating condition for: laboratory experiences; teaching; research; and supportive activities, such as preparation of instructional materials, correspondence, administrative materials, and special projects. The program is responsible for assuring that these supplies and equipment are reflective of contemporary practice in physical therapy, are sufficient in amount, and are available when needed.*

**2.8.2. The program has, or has use of, equipment and materials for core faculty to fulfill their role as scholars.**

*Core faculty are expected to contribute to the scholarship of the profession and to the mission of the institution. They therefore must have adequate equipment and materials that are appropriate for their scholarly needs. In addition, technological support and equipment are adequate to meet the needs of the core faculty to conduct research and other scholarly activities approved by the program and institution.*

## SECTION 3: CURRICULUM DEVELOPMENT AND CONTENT

### Preamble

**A curriculum is a plan for learning, designed by the program faculty in consultation with practitioners and members of communities of interest, to achieve explicit educational goals and objectives for preparation of a physical therapist. In addition to preparing practitioners, one goal of physical therapy education is to build on the liberal education of the student by incorporating the concepts of responsible citizenship into the professional curriculum. The curriculum sets forth the knowledge, skills, attitudes, and values needed to achieve these goals.**

**The professional program is built on a foundation of liberal arts, and social and basic sciences. Course work within the professional curriculum includes a balance of foundational and clinical sciences; critical inquiry; clinical practice; and studies of society, health care delivery, and physical therapy practice. The educational philosophy and values of the institution, the program, and the individuals who teach in it and the knowledge of and beliefs about learning are central aspects of the curriculum.**

**The educational outcomes are entry level and are based on practice expectations that are congruent with and reflect current physical therapy practice, emerging trends in health care delivery, and advances in physical therapy theory and technology.**

**3.1. Core faculty assume primary responsibility for curriculum development with input from all program faculty as well as from students enrolled in the program.**

*Curriculum development is the responsibility of the core faculty. The core faculty develop the curriculum using information about the contemporary practice of physical therapy; standards of practice; and, current literature, documents, publications and other resources related to the profession, physical therapy professional education, and educational theory. Input from program faculty, the clinical community, and students is utilized in this development process.*

**3.2. There is a formal curriculum plan.**

*The curricular plan developed by the faculty is documented and includes the components listed below.*

**3.2.1. The curriculum plan states the philosophy and the principles and values of the program and reflects the nature of professional education in physical therapy.**

*There is a formal statement of the philosophy, principles, and values on which the curriculum plan is based.*

**3.2.2. The curriculum plan includes the conceptual bases of the curriculum, the educational principles on which the curriculum is built, and statements of the expected student outcomes.**

*The conceptual bases of the curriculum are apparent in the description of the curriculum plan. The curriculum plan and expected student outcomes are formally presented and understood by all communities of interest including students.*

**3.2.3. The curriculum plan includes a series of organized, sequential, and integrated learning experiences.**

*The curriculum design is a well-planned and organized approach to the accomplishment of the program's mission utilizing sound principles of education. The comprehensive curriculum plan is designed in such a manner that the performance of the expected student outcomes is facilitated. Throughout the curriculum, opportunities are provided for students to explore areas of interest or to pursue in greater depth topics in which they wish to become more proficient or knowledgeable.*

*The comprehensive curriculum plan includes the development of instructional courses or units (both required and elective; both academic and clinical) which will be used in the implementation of the curriculum design. The didactic content of the instructional courses or units and the learning experiences should be those which will facilitate the attainment of the expected student outcomes.*

**3.2.4. The curriculum plan includes instructional units with objectives stated in behavioral terms that are reflective of the depth and breadth of the content and of the level of student performance expected.**

*The objectives of the instructional courses, units, and learning experiences should be stated in terms of what the student will be able to do or demonstrate upon successful completion of each course, unit, or experience. There should be a variety of effective methods, reflecting specific course didactic and/or skill content, by which the students achievement of the objectives and competencies can be measured.*

**3.3. The curriculum encompasses a variety of instructional methods selected to maximize learning.**

*There is evidence of consideration of a variety of instructional methods. Methods employed are chosen based on the philosophy of the curriculum plan, the content, the needs of the learners, and the defined outcomes expected of the students.*

**3.4. Faculty use evaluation processes to determine whether students are competent and safe to progress through the curriculum, including the clinical education component.**

*The program faculty utilize a variety of effective methods to assess student competence, safety, and readiness to progress through the curriculum. Evaluation of student performance occurs regularly. At a minimum, performance evaluation must occur at the end of each term of the curriculum and include assessment of performance in both academic and clinical course work. Student progression is based on demonstrated competencies. Students receive regular formal feedback about their performance.*

**3.5. Clinical experiences selected by the program reflect a variety of practice settings and provide the students with professional role modeling, and access to patients representative of those commonly seen in practice.**

*Clinical experiences required of students are planned based on student progression in the curriculum and are based on the type of supervision required, the variety of experiences needed, and the complexity of clinical problem solving to be accomplished. In planning clinical education programs, the collective experiences provided allow opportunities in patient care and teaching, as well as opportunities for students to learn through observation of and participation in administrative activities, quality assurance activities, clinical research, and supervision of physical therapist assistants and other supportive personnel.*

**3.6. The clinical experiences selected by the program ensure that the type and amount of clinical supervision are appropriate for the student's experience, ability and point of progression in the program, and that appropriate guidance and feedback are provided to the student.**

*The program provides a formally designed program of clinical education coordinated with all course work in the program. This is communicated to the clinical education faculty to facilitate their planning of appropriate clinical experiences for students and to ensure that the clinical education faculty appreciate the level of supervision needed by individual students at various phases throughout the curriculum. The program establishes policies and procedures with the clinical education faculty which assure that students receive planned guidance and formal and regular assessment of their clinical performance.*

**3.7. Physical therapy education is built on a balance of course work in social sciences, humanities, and natural sciences, that is appropriate in depth and breadth, to develop**

**the ability in students to think independently, to weigh values, to understand fundamental theory, and to develop skills for clinical practice, including critical thinking and communication.**

*Prerequisite course work for the professional program assures that the student has acquired a comprehensive background in the liberal arts and sciences. This includes study in social sciences, humanities and natural sciences which results in a broadly educated student. Students enter the professional program with skills which include being able to think independently, demonstrate problem solving techniques for solving complex and simple problems, weigh values and set priorities, understand fundamental theory, exhibit responsible social behavior, demonstrate professional collegiality and good citizenship, and effectively communicate both orally and in writing as expected of all students. These attributes are typically exemplified by students who have a baccalaureate degree.*

**3.8. The curriculum incorporates a combination of didactic, clinical, and research learning experiences that are reflective of contemporary physical therapy practice, and includes:**

**3.8.1. instruction in the foundational sciences, including laboratory or other practical experiences involving quantitative and qualitative observations;**

*Learning experiences are designed to (1) provide basic knowledge in the sciences related to normal and abnormal human structure, function, and response to injury and disease; (2) enhance the students' ability to make quantitative and qualitative observations; and, (3) facilitate understanding of the clinical sciences.*

**3.8.2. instruction in the clinical sciences, including laboratory or other practical experiences;**

*Theory and practical learning experiences are designed to (1) build on the foundational sciences; (2) develop the knowledge necessary to generate a diagnosis, prognosis and plan of care; and (3) develop the knowledge necessary for understanding, presenting rationale for, and applying intervention strategies.*

**3.8.3. learning experiences designed to achieve educational outcomes required for initial practice of the profession of physical therapy. Graduates of the program are prepared, in the following area, to:**

**Communication**

**3.8.3.1. Expressively and receptively communicate with all individuals when engaged in physical therapy practice, research, and education, including patients, clients, families, care givers, practitioners, consumers, payers, and policy makers.**

**Individual and Cultural Differences**

**3.8.3.2. Incorporate an understanding of the implications of individual and cultural differences when engaged in physical therapy practice, research, and education.**

**Professional Behavior**

**3.8.3.3. Demonstrate professional behaviors in all interactions with patients, clients, families, care givers, other health care providers, students, other consumers, and payers.**

**3.8.3.4. Adhere to legal practice standards, including all federal, state, jurisdiction, and institutional regulations related to patient or client care, and to fiscal management.**

**3.8.3.5. Practice ethical decision making that is consistent with applicable professional codes of ethics, including the APTA's Code of Ethics.**

**3.8.3.6. Participate in peer assessment activities.**

**3.8.3.7. Participate in clinical education activities.**

**Critical Inquiry and Clinical Decision-making**

**3.8.3.8. Participate in the design and implementation of decision-making guidelines.**

**3.8.3.9. Demonstrate clinical decision-making skills, including clinical reasoning, clinical judgment, and reflective practice.**

**3.8.3.10. Evaluate published studies related to physical therapy practice, research, and education.**

3.8.3.11. Secure and critically evaluate information related to new and established techniques and technology, legislation, policy, and environments related to patient or client care.

3.8.3.12. Participate in scholarly activities to contribute to the body of physical therapy knowledge (e.g., case reports, collaborative research).

Education

3.8.3.13. Educate others using a variety of teaching methods that are commensurate with the needs and unique characteristics of the learner.

Professional Development

3.8.3.14. Formulate and implement a plan for personal and professional career development based on self-assessment and feedback from others.

Screening

3.8.3.15. Determine the need for further examination or consultation by a physical therapist or for referral to another health care professional.

Examination

3.8.3.16. Independently examine and re-examine a patient or client by obtaining a pertinent history from the patient or client and from other relevant sources, by performing relevant systems review, and by selecting appropriate age-related tests and measures. Tests and measures (listed alphabetically) include, but are not limited to, the following:

a. aerobic capacity and endurance
b. anthropometric characteristics
c. arousal, mentation, and cognition
d. assistive and adaptive devices
e. community and work (job, school or play) reintegration
f. cranial nerve integrity
g. environmental, home, and work barriers
h. ergonomic and body mechanics
i. gait, assisted locomotion, and balance
j. integumentary integrity
k. joint integrity and mobility
l. motor function
m. muscle performance (including strength, power, and endurance)
n. neuromotor development and sensory integration
o. orthotic, protective, and supportive devices
p. pain
q. posture
r. prosthetic requirements
s. range of motion (including muscle length)
t. reflex integrity
u. self care and home management (including activities of daily living and instrumental activities of daily living)
v. sensory integrity (including proprioception and kinesthesia)
w. ventilation, respiration, and circulation

Evaluation

3.8.3.17. Synthesize examination data to complete the physical therapy evaluation.

Diagnosis

3.8.3.18. Engage in the diagnostic process in an efficient manner consistent with the policies and procedures of the practice setting.

3.8.3.19. Engage in the diagnostic process to establish differential diagnoses for patients across the lifespan based on evaluation of results of examinations and medical and psychosocial information.

3.8.3.20. Take responsibility for communication or discussion of diagnoses or clinical impressions with other practitioners.

Prognosis

3.8.3.21. Determine patient or client prognoses based on evaluation of results of examinations and medical and psychosocial information.

Plan of Care

3.8.3.22 Collaborate with patients, clients, family members, payers, other professionals, and individuals to determine a realistic and acceptable plan of care.

3.8.3.23. Establish goals and functional outcomes that specify expected time duration.

3.8.3.24. Define achievable patient or client outcomes within available resources.

3.8.3.25. Deliver and manage a plan of care that complies with administrative policies and procedures of the practice environment.

3.8.3.26. Monitor and adjust the plan of care in response to patient or client status.

Intervention

3.8.3.27. Practice in a safe setting and manner to minimize risk to the patient, client, physical therapist, and others.

3.8.3.28. Provide direct physical therapy intervention, including delegation to support personnel when appropriate, to achieve patient or client outcomes based on the examination and on the impairment, functional limitations, and disability. Interventions (listed alphabetically) include, but are not limited to:

a. airway clearance techniques
b. debridement and wound care
c. electrotherapeutic modalities
d. functional training in community and work (job, school or play) reintegration (including instrumental activities of daily living, work hardening, and work conditioning)
e. functional training in self care and home management (including activities of daily living and instrumental activities of daily living)
f. manual therapy techniques
g. patient-related instruction
h. physical agents and mechanical modalities
i. prescription, application, and as appropriate fabrication of adaptive, assistive, orthotic, protective and supportive devices and equipment
j. therapeutic exercise (including aerobic conditioning)

3.8.3.29. Provide patient-related instruction to achieve patient outcomes based on impairment, functional limitations, disability and patient satisfaction.

3.8.3.30. Complete thorough, accurate, analytically sound, concise, timely, and legible documentation that follows guidelines and specific documentation formats required by the practice setting.

3.8.3.31. Take appropriate action in an emergency in any practice setting.

Outcomes Measurement and Evaluation

3.8.3.32. Implement an evaluation of individual or collective outcomes of patients or clients.

Prevention and Wellness

3.8.3.33. Identify and assess the health needs of individuals, groups, and communities, including screening, prevention, and wellness programs that are appropriate to physical therapy.

3.8.3.34. Promote optimal health by providing information on wellness, disease, impairment, functional limitations, disability, and health risks related to age, gender, culture, and lifestyle.

Management in Various Care Delivery Systems

3.8.3.35. Provide primary care to patients with neuromusculoskeletal disorders within the scope of physical therapy practice through collaboration with

**other members of primary care teams based on patient or client goals and expected functional outcomes and on knowledge of one's own and other's capabilities.**

**3.8.3.36. Provide care to patients referred by other practitioners, independently or in collaboration with other team members, based on patient or client goals and expected functional outcomes and on knowledge of one's own and other's capabilities.**

**3.8.3.37. Provide care to patients, in collaboration with other practitioners, in settings supportive of comprehensive and complex services based on patient or client goals and expected functional outcomes and on knowledge of one's own and other's capabilities.**

**3.8.3.38. Assume responsibility for the management of care based on the patient's or client's goals and expected functional outcomes and on knowledge of one's own and other's capabilities.**

**3.8.3.39. Manage human and material resources and services to provide high-quality, efficient physical therapy services based on the plan of care.**

**3.8.3.40. Interact with patients, clients, family members, other health care providers, and community-based organizations for the purpose of coordinating activities to facilitate efficient and effective patient or client care.**

Administration

**3.8.3.41. Delegate physical-therapy-related services to appropriate human resources.**

**3.8.3.42. Supervise and manage support personnel to whom tasks have been delegated.**

**3.8.3.43. Participate in management planning as required by the practice setting.**

**3.8.3.44. Participate in budgeting, billing, and reimbursement activities as required by the practice setting.**

**3.8.3.45. Participate in the implementation of an established marketing plan and related public relations activities as required by the practice setting.**

Consultation

**3.8.3.46. Provide consultation to individuals, businesses, schools, government agencies, or other organizations.**

Social Responsibility

**3.8.3.47. Become involved in professional organizations and activities through membership and service.**

**3.8.3.48. Display professional behaviors as evidenced by the use of time and effort to meet patient or client needs or by providing *pro bono* services.**

**3.8.3.49. Demonstrate social responsibility, citizenship, and advocacy, including participation in community and human service organizations and activities.**

*The curriculum includes content and learning experiences designed to prepare students to exhibit the above practice expectations upon graduation from the program. The expected student outcomes include those sets of knowledge and skills which the graduates are prepared to demonstrate upon successful completion of the required academic and clinical portions of the education program. The practice expectations are drawn from the* Normative Model of Physical Therapist Professional Education *(1996) and the* Guide to Physical Therapist Practice, Volume I *(1995, and early drafts of the 1997 revision).*

*In determining the specific content to be included, the program faculty utilize information about the contemporary practice of physical therapy; standards of practice; and current literature, documents, publications and other resources related to the profession, health care delivery, physical therapy professional education, and educational theory. The Commission recognizes that the documents referenced above are subject to periodic review and revision. In view of the changing nature of health care delivery and of the profession, the Commission expects that the program faculty will keep abreast of any and all changes in professional physical therapy practice as reflected in future revisions of these documents and will make appropriate adjustments in curricular content and expectations, whether or not these criteria have been formally revised.*

*The program faculty evaluate students in a variety of ways during the academic and clinical education aspects of the program to ascertain each student's preparation for physical therapy practice.*

**3.9. The first professional degree for physical therapists is awarded at the postbaccalaureate level at the completion of the physical therapy program.**

*The institution is responsible for naming the degree at the post baccalaureate level that is awarded after the completion of the education program. A program located in an institution which is not a degree granting institution must demonstrate that it has an agreement with one or more accredited institutions which will grant the first degree, at the postbaccalaureate level, to the student upon completion of the physical therapy program.*

## SECTION 4: PROGRAM ASSESSMENT

### Preamble

**Physical therapy education programs are accountable for an ongoing process of assessment of educational outcomes and for continuous improvement in all aspects of the program.**

**In judging compliance with the following evaluative criteria, the Commission on Accreditation in Physical Therapy Education and the on-site review team will seek evidence that the program is involved in an on-going effort to determine the effectiveness of the program. The information collected about the performance of program graduates related to the practice expectations of the curriculum as well as evidence that supports the relevance of the program philosophy and the attainment of the program's mission, goals and objectives is obtained through ongoing outcome assessment efforts and used to support future changes in all aspects of the program. The ongoing process of assessment includes collection of information on a regular basis with input from multiple sources and using a variety of methods to gather data.**

**Although the curriculum must include learning experiences that lead to the attainment of the educational outcomes in Section 3.8.3., the Commission recognizes that the complexity and variety of physical therapy practice is such that program graduates may engage in those activities to varying degrees. The Commission expects that the program will determine the extent to which this variety in graduate practice warrants changes in the program, particularly in light of the need to prepare graduates for practice in any setting or location.**

**4.1. Assessment is part of a systematic and formal approach to continuous improvement. There is an ongoing process of assessment to determine the effectiveness of the program that includes, but is not limited to, the following (listed alphabetically):**

*The program is engaged in collecting information on a regular and ongoing basis. The collection of information uses multiple approaches to assessment and includes data from a variety of sources. Such sources should include but not be limited to: program graduates, their coworkers and/or employers, the students enrolled in the program, and clinical education faculty who supervise the students during all aspects of their clinical education experiences. Program faculty, administrators, support staff, graduates and students are involved in the regular assessment about whether institution and program policies, procedures and resources facilitate or hinder the attainment of the program mission and goals.*

**4.1.1. adjunct and supportive faculty**

*The performance of adjunct and supportive faculty is assessed at the completion of their teaching assignments. The assessment includes review of teaching effectiveness and may include review of other aspects of performance related to other responsibilities as appropriate. This evaluation is expected to be used to determine appropriate faculty development activities, and to be considered when determining whether to continue using these faculty members.*

**4.1.2. admissions criteria and prerequisites**

*The faculty regularly assess the appropriateness of both the admissions criteria and the admissions process to determine the adequacy of each for selecting students who are able to successfully complete the program and whose performance as graduates reflect the mission of the program as well as the practice expectations. The program faculty regularly review the prerequisites for the program to determine if the required background is appropriate in depth and breadth to prepare students for physical therapy professional education.*

**4.1.3. clinical education faculty**

*Clinical education faculty are evaluated in those years during which they have clinical education responsibilities in the program. This evaluation is expected to be used by the program to determine the clinical faculty development activities.*

**4.1.4. clinical education program**

*There is an assessment of the clinical education program as a whole to determine the adequacy of the program in meeting the needs of the students and mission and objectives of the program. As an important aspect of the entire curriculum review special emphasis is placed on the adequacy of the clinical education aspect of the curriculum. This assessment is linked to the evaluation of the variety of sites, the quality of student supervision, the availability of learning experiences in all practice expectations and the communication among and between all involved individuals associated with the program.*

**4.1.5. core faculty**

*Core faculty are evaluated at a minimum of once per year. The review includes assessments of teaching, research and other scholarly activity, and service as well as evaluations of any specific functions of their responsibilities within the program, such as administration of the program and clinical education, committee functions, student advisement, or as a member of a faculty practice. The program's analysis of the strengths and weaknesses of the core faculty is used in planning both individual and collective faculty development activities as well as in the faculty recruitment process.*

**4.1.6. curriculum**

*The curriculum is assessed by all individuals who are involved with the program and the process includes input from program faculty, graduates from the program, employers of graduates and students. Individual courses within the curriculum, and well as the curriculum as a whole, are assessed. The focus of curriculum assessment is determination of strengths and weaknesses of the program and whether the practice expectations and specific mission, goals and objectives of the program are met. The individual courses and the full curriculum are also assessed in light of the changing roles and responsibilities of the physical therapist practitioner; the dynamic nature of the profession and the health care delivery system; and, the analysis of current literature, documents, publications and other resources related to the profession, physical therapy professional education, and educational theory.*

**4.1.7. institutional policies and procedures**

*The program faculty regularly review the institutional policies and procedures to determine their effectiveness in facilitating the achievement of the program's mission, goals and objectives.*

**4.1.8. mission, philosophy, goals and objectives**

*Utilizing the analyses of outcome assessments in the context of contemporary physical therapy practice, the program faculty regularly determine the extent to which the mission, philosophy, goals and objectives are met. During this analysis process the program determines if the program's philosophy, mission, goals and objectives, continue to be appropriate for the program and are in concert with the mission of the institution.*

**4.1.9. performance of recent graduates**

*The program faculty regularly assess the performance of recent graduates related to the practice expectations of the curriculum as well as the specific expectations linked to the program's unique mission, goals and objectives. Analysis of the results of outcome measures are used by the faculty to make judgements about the strengths or weaknesses of the program and/or to support assessment of other aspects of the program.*

**4.1.10. program policies and procedures**

*The program faculty regularly review the program policies and procedures to determine their effectiveness in facilitating the achievement of the program's mission, goals and objectives.*

**4.1.11. resources**

*The program faculty regularly review the program resources such as budget, space, equipment and supplies to determine whether the resources available to the program are used effectively to facilitate the achievement of the program's mission, goals and objectives. The process includes an assessment of whether the human resources available to the program are sufficient in number and are used effectively.*

## Focus on a Leader

**MARY JANE HARRIS, MS, PT**
**DIRECTOR, COMMISSION ON ACCREDITATION IN PHYSICAL THERAPY EDUCATION**
**AMERICAN PHYSICAL THERAPY ASSOCIATION**
**ALEXANDRIA, VIRGINIA**

*1. Mary Jane, please briefly capsulize for readers your credentials, professional chronology, and current and recent professional activities.*

I graduated from Ithaca College with a Bachelor of Science in Physical Therapy in 1969. My first position was one that provided multidimensional experiences, which I believe to be critically important for new physical therapist clinicians. I began my clinical career at Saint Francis Hospital, Pittsburgh, PA, where I stayed for approximately 10 years. I started clinical work as a staff physical therapist, where I rotated through a variety of clinical experience settings, including rehabilitation, which was my area of interest. After several years, I became the Center Coordinator for Clinical Education (CCCE), and was responsible for the clinical education of student physical therapists from five colleges and universities. Approximately 15 professional, entry-level physical therapy students per year rotated through our facility, most of whom did rehabilitation rotations with me.

During that time, I went back to school and obtained my Master of Science degree in physical therapy education at the University of Pittsburgh, where I did some part-time teaching in proprioceptive neuromuscular facilitation, my primary area, and the management of spinal cord injury patients. I aspired at that time to become an Academic Coordinator of Clinical Education (ACCE), thanks in part to modeling and mentoring by the late Professor Vicki Greene, Physical Therapy Department, University of Pittsburgh.

For my last 2 years at Saint Francis, I moved out of clinical practice in the rehabilitation department and became the administrative assistant to the medical director of the rehabilitation unit.

Dr Rosemary Scully, EdD, PT, of the Physical Therapy Department of the University of Pittsburgh, was on my master's degree thesis committee and recommended me as a potential faculty member to Judy Anderson, who was starting a new physical therapy education program at Northern Illinois University. In 1979, I accepted her invitation and left Saint Francis Hospital to become the ACCE at Northern Illinois University. I was excited to be there at the advent of a new program, to develop the clinical education program with my own original ideas. I had a year before we enrolled professional students in the program, so that I had sufficient time to develop the clinical education program.

I remained at Northern Illinois University for exactly 15 years (to the day). During that time, I moved from being the ACCE to being program director.

Regarding mentors, I consider Rosemary Scully to be one of my most important mentors. She was mentor to so many physical therapists. She was highly influential in helping guide my career path, as was Dr Anne Pascasio, Dean, School of Health-Related Professions, University of Pittsburgh. Anne helped me with my master's degree plan and career planning. She guided me into specific course work to help me fulfill my aspiration to become an ACCE. It is amazing how Rosemary and Anne were able to simultaneously mentor multiple protégées so well.

Clinically, my physical therapy mentor was Tom Winner, Director of the Physical Therapy Department at Saint Francis Hospital. I and others were always reluctant to allow Tom to take over our patient load while we were away, not because he did not manage their care well, but because he managed them too well. His superlative techniques and rapport with patients made him so well liked that patients were "spoiled" by the time we got them back! He is a wonderful person and physical therapist. I had the pleasure of attending his retirement party, honoring his 44 years of service to the profession in the same position at the same institution. He never aged over the decades.

Another important mentor to me was Mary Elizabeth Kolb, whom I also met while at Saint Francis. She was a past president of the American Physical Therapy Association (APTA). She also had been director of the D.T. Watson School in Pittsburgh. She was in the process of earning an advanced degree in information sciences at the University of Pittsburgh. While at Saint Francis, she worked on the clinical trials for dantrolene sodium, an antispasticity drug. She was wonderful to work for and with. Dr Kolb went on to be director of clinical studies for Norwich Pharmaceuticals. She was a clinical physical therapist, not a basic scientist, but found her niche in clinical research and profoundly influenced those of us whom she touched.

All in all, I was fortunate to have educational, clinical, and research mentors early in my professional development. I view mentorship in physical therapy as more informal than formal in nature. I have found that multiple mentors, helping me with different aspects of my career ladder, have made my progression much smoother. Now I have the privilege of mentoring others who are working their way through the profession.

All during my early professional career, I was involved in the professional association. As center coordinator for clinical education at Saint Francis, I became responsible for an instructional course for physical therapy aides. Saint Francis had a nationally renowned physical therapy aide education program. Physical therapy aides from all over the northeast region attended the course, which consisted of 4 weeks of classroom instruction and 4 weeks of on-the-job training. In that capacity, I became the de facto chair of the physical therapy aide committee in the Southwestern District, Pennsylvania Physical Therapy Association. I went on to be secretary and held other leadership positions in the Southwestern District.

When I moved to Illinois, I continued my involvement in the Illinois Chapter and the APTA. I was Illinois chapter president for 2 years, from 1991–1992. During this time, I was selected and trained as an on-site evaluator for the Commission on Accreditation in Physical Therapy Education. I became involved in on-site evaluations, and, at one point, was appointed to the Commission. I served on the Commission for 2 years, then resigned that post to take a staff position on the Commission in August 1994. I am currently Director, Department of Accreditation, APTA.

My broad clinical, academic (as student and faculty), and administrative experience gave me a complete perspective of the profession, which has been very helpful to me in all the roles I have had the privilege to serve in.

*2. What are the salient education and accreditation problems, issues, and dilemmas facing the physical therapy profession?*

Physical therapy education is in crisis today. A primary reason for this state of affairs is the growing number of developing education programs. The Commission's role in this process is *not* to limit the number of new programs, but to ensure that high-quality community standards are being met by all. If these standards are met, programs will be accredited; if not, they will not be accredited. I get a bit defensive when professionals attempt to assign blame to CAPTE for the large and increasing numbers of education programs.

Since the APTA House of Delegates resolution of 1998 disfavoring new and expanded education programs, the number of new programs has lessened, but I do not think that there is necessarily a cause-and-effect phenomenon between these two events. Two years ago, the Commission received 72 new Declarations of Intent to start new education programs; this year, we expect to receive only four for physical therapist and physical therapist assistant programs.

Existing programs, too, are scaling back, even ceasing to exist. In some cases, these decisions are facilitated by CAPTE decisions; in others, institutional considerations drive the closures. It is happening more in the physical therapist assistant education community than in the physical therapist education community.

The new *Evaluative Criteria*, adopted in 1996 and effective 1998, have substantially changed accreditation standards for new and existing education programs. The new standards set a significantly higher quality bar for program accreditation. One difference from previous accreditation standards is the requirement that physical therapist education programs award a postbaccalaureate degree. As a result, all baccalaureate programs are in the process of converting to graduate-level programs and must complete that process no later than January 1, 2002. Additionally, under curricular content, there is enhanced overt emphasis on prevention and wellness and management at all levels and in all settings. Lastly, there is a greater expectation that all faculty engage in scholarly activity. Graduate education requires graduate-level-educated faculty, who compete with colleagues for tenure and promotion on the basis of peer-recognized scholarly activity. These faculty must, in turn, have the time to carry out such scholarly activity. They cannot spend all their time in the classroom; they need time to do many diverse things related to their development. On average, physical therapy faculty spend less than 10 hours weekly in the classroom. In programs where they must devote greater time to classroom work, program accreditation may suffer.

Regarding Criteria 3.7, physical therapists need to be educated broadly, not just in the natural sciences. CAPTE firmly believes that physical therapy education program graduates need to be educated citizens of the world, not just narrowly educated as physical therapist–scientists. However, the Commission is also cognizant of the fact that developing the didactic physical therapy–specific knowledge base takes substantial time. We try to help set the appropriate required balance of educational experiences for development of the Renaissance person.

CAPTE does not specifically require that professional physical therapy students have a baccalaureate degree prior to commencing professional-phase study. However, if such students do not possess baccalaureate degrees, then they must have the requisite skills typically achieved through the earning of a baccalaureate degree. These skills include, but are not limited to, citizenship and the ability to weigh values and make judgments. To deal effectively with a rapidly changing global health care market, physical therapists need these broad skills and educational background, in addition to their physical therapy-specific education, to be optimally effective.

Another educationally related problem is a relative dearth of qualified, doctoral level physical therapy faculty. As a result, many educators and policy experts state, and I agree, that the quality of physical therapy education generally may be declining. Under the new *Evaluative Criteria*, education programs are evaluated every 8 years. Six years remain until all programs have been evaluated under the new standards, and we can determine whether this is fact or not. The Vector Study aftermath may actually increase the number of qualified physical therapy faculty, as clinicians leave that aspect of practice in favor of education opportunities. CAPTE is currently collecting data in this area.

Regarding clinical education, constituting approximately one third of aggregate professional education, factors such as managed care and its push for greater productivity on the part of clinicians have adversely affected the quality and quantity of clinical experiences available to professional students. Again, this problem is exacerbated by the growing number of developing programs and by program expansion.

The power of clinical education in role-modeling for novice physical therapists and assistants is critically important. When I was a professional student, I had three short clinical experiences with relatively little supervision. They were not good experiences. I did not want the same for my students. However, once a clinical instructor, I had to make a conscious effort to change from that deleterious model, which had been almost ingrained in me from my past experiences. If we do not put students in excellent clinical environments with high-quality teaching, learning, and care standards, then they may model what they get and function at a lower level in their early clinical experiences postgraduation.

There is discussion in the APTA to adopt the medical model for clinical education, so that professional students are matched centrally with clinical sites. Another model, similar to what exists in nursing, is for academic faculty to carry out clinical education. The latter proposal would require larger core faculty in academic institutions. Approximately one fifth of physical therapist education programs report having in place faculty practices. All faculty in any discipline need to have some time to consult or practice as "free time." Such free time is critical to their professional and personal development.

In the United States, our professional education programs are creating a different physical therapist than is educated and prepared around the world. I had the opportunity 7 years ago to consult with physiotherapists in Africa, and found their models, like many in Europe and throughout the rest of the world, to be more technical and less independent.

Distance education is another salient education issue. Distance education, in my opinion, is just another education delivery method. As such, it must be evaluated just like any other education delivery method, by the same exacting standards. Are there objectives? Do students achieve objectives, i.e., is there an appropriate evaluative component? Do the students express in course and program evaluations that they have had good learning experiences?

When the Commission examines distance learning models, it will utilize the same criteria that are used to evaluate traditional teaching–learning models. To date, physical therapy distance education programs have met these high standards.

*3. Where do you believe physical therapy education will be in the year 2050? What needs to be accomplished to get the profession where you envision it being in 2050?*

By 2050, doctoral-level professional physical therapist education will predominate. This doctoral education will be professional in nature, similar to the Juris Doctor and Medical Doctor, not purely academic like the PhD or EdD degrees. Approximately one fifth of professional programs are currently in transition toward doctoral entry-level professional education. The Commission takes the official position that the criteria it has promulgated are appropriate for either master's or doctoral levels of preparation, and that is the decision of individual education institutions to decide which is appropriate for them. The same criteria are used to evaluate baccalaureate (those still in existence), master's, and doctoral-level programs.

Anecdotally, there are differences between master's and doctoral entry-level programs. The DPT programs tend to be a little longer; have more clinical education; and a slightly greater emphasis on basic sciences.

Clinical education may by then include sophisticated virtual reality experiences, as technology permits. This is not so unimaginable, considering that much of airline pilot psychomotor skills education takes place in simulators.

In a similar vein, accreditation activities, such as site visits, may be carried out via computer. For such to be effective, programs must remain honest, open, and desirous of complying with known standards.

Finally, concerning the status and numbers of physical therapy and related professionals and professional and support disciplines, I cannot predict what the future may hold. It wouldn't surprise me, however, if physical therapy, occupational therapy, and athletic training were all one profession.

## Focus on a Leader

**Mary Ann Wharton, MS, PT**
**Associate Professor and Curriculum Coordinator**
**Department of Physical Therapy,**
**Saint Francis University**
**Loretto, Pennsylvania**

1. *Mary Ann, please briefly capsulize for readers your credentials, professional chronology, and current and recent professional activities.*

I am currently associate professor and curriculum coordinator, Department of Physical Therapy, Saint Francis University, Loretto, PA. I was invited to Saint Francis in 1991 to serve as a consultant to assist the University in assessing the feasibility of developing a Master of Physical Therapy program, and have been associated with the program since that time. Early duties included directing the activities of an Advisory Committee, assisting in implementing CAPTE guidelines, and serving on search committees for the Program Chairman and ACCE. When the first class of students began the professional phase of the curriculum, I joined the faculty as a part-time professor and curriculum coordinator. I served as the initial course coordinator for a physical therapy procedures course. In 1997, I increased my time to one-half time to continue as curriculum coordinator, assist the accreditation self-study, and teach the first health care systems course, consisting of professional issues and clinical documentation. In 1998, I increased my status to full time to continue responsibilities of coordinating the curriculum, and to assume teaching responsibilities for the entire health care systems track, which consists of four three-credit courses that address ethics and legalities and a seminar that studies current issues in health care delivery. I also teach geriatric curriculum content and coordinate several other courses.

In the capacity of curriculum coordinator I am responsible for facilitating the integration of the curriculum. I work with the entire full-time faculty and many of the adjunct faculty, including guest lecturers and those teaching elective courses on special topics. This role is essential to assure that the goals of our integrated curriculum model are achieved.

To fulfill service to the University, I currently serve as secretary of an interdisciplinary Problem-Based Learning Task Force, whose purpose is to develop and deliver an interdisciplinary course for students enrolled in physical therapy, occupational therapy, physician assistant, and nursing majors. A case-based course was developed and offered for the first time during the Spring 2001 semester. This course successfully achieved the goal of facilitating interdisciplinary case-based problem solving by both students and faculty.

Concurrently with my faculty responsibilities, I am actively involved in the American Physical Therapy Association (APTA) and its components. I chair the Ethics Committee for the Pennsylvania Chapter of the APTA, a position that I have held since 1994. In this capacity, I educate members and the public about ethical issues in physical therapy; field and answer ethical questions from members and the public; mentor new committee members on how to understand the complex APTA Procedural Document and the implications of the Code of Ethics and Standards of Practice; adjudicate legitimate ethical complaints and cases brought to the state-level committee; and refer, where appropriate, persons with related questions to other regulatory and related entities, such as the State Physical Therapy Licensure Board and State Insurance Commission, as well as to other committees of the Pennsylvania Chapter and the APTA. Since 1993, I have served as a charter member of the Editorial Advisory Group for *PT: The Magazine of Physical Therapy*. I am also an active member of the Geriatric, Education, and Neurology Sections of APTA.

In addition to faculty responsibilities at Saint Francis University, I am an adjunct associate professor in physical therapy, Community College of Allegheny County, Boyce Campus. I teach geriatrics, ethics, and legalities to physical therapist assistant students. I also provide consultation for geriatric clinical practice. My areas of interest in geriatric physical therapy include balance and falls, osteoporosis, cerebrovascular accidents, and Parkinson's disease.

My educational background includes a professional degree from Ithaca College in 1970 with a Bachelor of Science degree in Physical Therapy, and a Master of Science degree from the University of Pittsburgh's School of Health Related Professions in Leadership, Education, Administration and Development, with an emphasis in geriatric physical therapy. During the course of my graduate studies at the University of Pittsburgh, I completed a research thesis that identified advance-level competencies in geriatric physical therapy and the accompanying knowledge, skills, and attitudes. That thesis was used by the University of Pittsburgh to assist in developing an advanced master's degree program in geriatric physical therapy and by the Geriatric Section, APTA, as part of the proposal for geriatric clinical specialization and board certification in 1985.

2. *What are the salient education problems, issues, and dilemmas facing the physical therapy profession?*

I believe that it is critically important for physical therapist and physical therapist assistant students to have general, broad-based clinical experiences during affiliations, and, as graduates, to have similar first-job experiences. This type of exposure acclimates them not only to the profession and the range of physical therapy clinical activities, but also exposes them early on to the dynamics of the interdisciplinary patient care team.

I believe that there are great problems with mentoring in physical therapy. Everyone is potentially adversely affected by a relative dearth of mentors; professionals, students, academic and clinical educators, educational and clinical institutions, and patients/clients. I have always been fortunate enough to have a mentor or multiple mentors. I started my career as a physical therapy volunteer in high school. The physical therapists at local hospitals first introduced me to the physical therapy profession. Within legal limits, I engaged in both observation of, and participation in, clinical patient care activities. During physical therapy school, my professors, especially Professor Bob Grant, encouraged me to persevere if I became discouraged or if the going got rough. When I began clinical practice, the most important mentors that I had were Emil Furlong, a staff physical therapist at a rehabilitation center, who encouraged me to attend professional meetings and planted the seed in me for later professional service, and Archibald Simons, now a retired physical therapist, who got me involved in leadership positions in the professional association. Archie was an APTA Lucy Blair Service awardee and was involved in the Pennsylvania Physical Therapy Association's leadership circle for many decades. I later was privileged to be named a Lucy Blair Service awardee in 1994.

Two very significant professional mentors were Dr. Rosemary Scully and Dr. Anne Pascasio. I first met Dr. Rosemary Scully, Chair of the Physical Therapy program at the University of Pittsburgh in 1979 at the APTA annual conference in Atlanta. She encouraged me to pursue advanced formal education to augment my credentials so that I could exert greater influence within the profession. She also gave me the opportunity to be a full-time faculty instructor in the physical therapy program at the University of Pittsburgh while I pursued graduate education. At this time, I also met Dr. Anne Pascasio, Dean of the School of Health Related Professions. Together Anne and Rosemary facilitated the vision and created the opportunity for me to explore geriatric physical therapy practice and education. There were no comparable postprofessional geriatric physical therapy programs anywhere at that time. Clinical physical therapists, however, had begun to move into this field, due to the increasing geriatric population, and, in part, to a favorable Medicare reimbursement climate. Simultaneously, leaders like Joan Mills, Bette Horstman, Dr. Carole Lewis, Osa Jackson, and numerous others began developing the Geriatric Section of the APTA. Their models, encouragement, and facilitation helped me to explore, grow, and pursue my interests in and contributions to geriatric physical therapy.

As I became more involved in the professional association, I developed so many mentors that they became too numerous to count. And I began to mentor others, especially physical therapist and physical therapist assistant students. I am an active member of APTA Members Mentoring Members Task Program. I have retained Rosemary Scully and Anne Pascasio as personal mentors to this day. They continue to advise me personally and professionally, and exert strong influence on my professional work in higher education. Rosemary was my consultant in the Saint Francis Master of Physical Therapy program. She helped lay the foundation for the professional education curriculum.

Why is this rendition of my mentoring history important? It is important because mentoring is crucial to individual professional development and evolution of the profession itself. I sincerely believe that there is a lack of mentors today, especially in the clinic. Today many senior clinicians are moving into academia, leaving a dearth of potential mentors for junior clinicians. Clinical specialization was devised in part as a way to keep master clinicians in place to mentor subordinates, as well as to model the most efficacious treatment for patients. The special recognition of board certification in part serves as a reward for their recognized expertise.

Without effective mentoring, I fear that we cannot move to a higher level of autonomous clinical practice. Clinical physical therapists are struggling at the advent of their careers with inexperience, a more precarious job market, and fewer role models to mold them into master clinicians.

Another salient issue in physical therapy involves coming to grips with the Doctor of Physical Therapy (DPT) issue and related terminal PT degree/credentials issues. For me, the question is: What are we educating the physical therapist to be? We need to bridge the gap between academia's perception of the need for the DPT and the clinical reality. It is a good thing to augment credentials and skills, but we need to approach it thoughtfully and cautiously. The end result should be that the clinical and academic environments should be in sync with their definitions of appropriate degrees for both entry-level and master clinicians. The goal of an entry-level DPT to create a clinician who is capable of making independent decisions while still working as a team player is a good one.

Another issue facing the physical therapy profession is meeting the ongoing need to produce quality, committed graduates from our educational programs. I firmly believe that we need to return to a time when we developed altruism, empathy, and compassion as primary professional character traits in graduates rather than having (or letting) them focus on how much money they will earn after graduation. It is what they can do for others that really counts.

We also need to define what we are as clinical health professionals, e.g., identify ourselves as experts in the human movement system, as Dr. Shirley Sahrmann espouses, and then defend our defined scope of practice based on our expertise. We cannot just provide the public with a laundry list of modalities and procedures as the definition of our professional practice. Today, most physical therapists and physical therapist assistants cannot articulate a good concise working definition of our profession. We need to better educate professional students to be able to do so, and ground that definition in expertise in the human movement system.

3. *Where do you believe physical therapy education will be in the year 2050? What needs to be accomplished to get the profession where you envision it being in 2050?*
In 2050, physical therapy education will include a stronger link between and among basic sciences, clinical science, and clinical physical therapy practice. There will be greater emphasis on the clinician's ability to make independent judgments, so as to make him or her a logical point of entry into the health care system for patients with neuromusculoskeletal dysfunction. We will teach physical therapist and physical therapist assistant students to work more effectively within the context of an interdisciplinary health care delivery team. We will be more autonomous in reaching focused physical therapy diagnoses and in designing specific interventions for patients and clients of all ages and status. We will focus on prevention and wellness to a greater degree than we do now, although this and the aforementioned trends have already begun to develop into the curricula of professional and clinical education. I cannot predict whether professional physical therapist education will be carried out exclusively at the doctoral level, although I suspect that it will be so done. The academic environment is driving it that way, in part because of competition for students and the need to offer higher-level credentials upon graduation to meet the defined entry level for autonomous clinical practice.

To get to these ends, we must create (just as Dr. Helen Hislop said in 1975) a pool of specialists in the foundational sciences, and continue to draw on information from the foundational sciences in developing our educational curricula. We need to develop master clinicians who utilize this vision of point-of-entry patient management so that it becomes the norm. We need to improve the inputs and outcomes of professional education so that we are perceived by the public and complementary professionals as independently respected for our expertise in the movement system. Our internal association and accreditation processes should continue to drive our development rather than external factors and forces, e.g., the political health care system, reimbursement environments, and the opinions of a few influential physical therapists to the exclusion of majority opinion.

CHAPTER 3

# Clinical Practice: Practice Settings

RON SCOTT

## Key Words and Phrases

American Board of Physical Therapy Specialties (ABPTS)
Cardiopulmonary Practice Patterns
Clinical Examination Data Set
Clinical Specialist
Diagnosis
Direct Access Practice
Disability
Documentation
Evaluation
Examination
Evidence-Based Practice
Functional Limitation
Impairment
Integumentary Practice Patterns
Intervention
*Guide to Physical Therapist Practice*
Mentoring
Military Practice Model
Musculoskeletal Practice Patterns
Neuromuscular Practice Patterns
Preferred Practice Patterns
Prognosis
Protégé, Protégée
Outcomes

*This chapter describes physical therapy clinical practice, the mainstay of physical therapy professional practice. The newly implemented* Guide to Physical Therapist Practice, *2nd ed., has changed the physical therapy clinical practice paradigm by modifying the parameters of practice. They are, under the* Guide: *patient/client examination, evaluation, diagnosis, prognosis, and intervention. Goals have been replaced with care outcomes and impairment-based cardiopulmonary, integumentary, musculoskeletal, and neuromuscular diagnoses. Novice clinicians progress into master clinicians through effective mentoring and facility/system support for continuing education and professional development. The military model of advanced direct access practice (which includes first-contact patient care, credentialing and privileging, follow-on referral, and limited radiograph and prescription writing) is an excellent prototype for doctoral level (DPT) and direct-access-based physical therapist clinical practice.*

## DOMAINS AND SCOPE OF PRACTICE

The clinical practice of physical therapy is as multifaceted as is the practice of physical therapy globally. Globally, physical therapy practice entails clinical practice, clinical and basic science research, education-based practice, health care administration and policy practice, among other possible parameters of practice. The clinical practice of physical therapy may be categorized in several ways: by patient/client populations within a given practice (e.g., geriatric, neurologic, orthopedic, pediatric); by practice-related theories or approaches (e.g., Bobath, McKenzie); by emphasis along a health and wellness continuum (e.g., prevention, post-injury care, pathology-based); and by other possible categorizations.

Clinical physical therapists clearly are primary health care providers, i.e., health professionals who provide first-line clinical health services within an autonomous scope of professional practice. The American Physical Therapy Association (APTA) defines and describes primary care and the expected role for clinical physical therapists therein in the *Guide to Physical Therapist Practice* as:

> the provision of integrated, accessible health care services by clinicians who are accountable for addressing a large majority of personal health care needs, developing a sustained partnership with patients, and practicing within the context of family and community. . . . As clinicians involved in examination and in the evaluation, diagnosis, prognosis, intervention and prevention of acute musculoskeletal and neuromuscular disorders, physical therapists are well-positioned to provide these services as part of the primary health care team. . . . For acute musculoskeletal and neuromuscular conditions, triage and initial examination are appropriate physical therapy responsibilities. The primary care team may function more efficiently when it includes physical therapists who can recognize musculoskeletal and neuromuscular disorders, perform examinations and evaluations, and intervene without delay.

As of the writing of this text, direct access by patients and clients to clinical physical therapist primary care providers exists in 33 states. By direct access, the meaning intended is that patients and clients may seek the professional services of a clinical licensed physical therapist without a referral from any referring entity. Depending on state law, referring entities may include other primary health care professionals such as physicians and surgeons, dentists, chiropractors, podiatrists, nurse practitioners, and physician assistants.

In 19 jurisdictions that allow physical therapy direct access practice, there are legislative restrictions on the direct access practice, including, but not limited to, the privilege to examine, but not to intervene, on behalf of patients; the requirement for a medical examination and diagnosis prior to direct access care; special qualifications for direct access practitioners; and so forth. The three branches of the military—Air Force, Army, and Navy—allow the most extensive express direct access authority for military physical therapists, pursuant to their federal constitutional "Supremacy Clause" authority. Military physical therapy direct access practice is described in greater detail at the end of this chapter.

Table 3-1 gives the direct access status for the 50 states and the District of Columbia. It is reprinted from the *2000 State Licensure Reference Guide*, and is used with permission from the American Physical Therapy Association.

TABLE 3-1

**A Summary of Direct Access Language in State Physical Therapy Practice Acts Direct Access to Physical Therapy Laws April 2000**

| State & Year Obtained | Omission/ Provisions | Practice Act Language Summary |
|---|---|---|
| AL | | No Direct Access |
| AK–1986 | Omission | ■ License revocation or suspension when failure to refer a patient to another qualified professional when the patient's condition is beyond PT training. |
| AZ–1983 | Omission | ■ Lawful practice—A physical therapist shall refer a client to appropriate health care practitioners if the PT has reasonable cause to believe symptoms or conditions are present that require services beyond the scope of practice and if physical therapy is contraindicated. |
| AR–1997 | Omission | No Restrictions |
| CA–1968 | Omission | ■ Prohibits diagnosis of disease. Attorney General ruled that an initial diagnosis by a physician or other licensed diagnostician is required before physical therapy can commence. |
| CO–1988 | Omission | ■ Disciplinary action when failure to refer a patient to another qualified professional when the patient's condition is beyond PT training.<br>■ Prohibits diagnosis of disease. |
| CT | | Evaluation Only |
| DC | | Evaluation Only |
| DE–1993 | Provisions | ■ Permits treatment with or without referral by a licensed medical or osteopathic physician.<br>■ Must refer patient if symptoms are present for which treatment is outside scope of PT.<br>■ May treat a patient for up to 30 days, after which a physician must be "consulted."<br>■ Prohibits substantial modification of prescriptions accompanying a patient. |

*continued*

TABLE 3-1

**A Summary of Direct Access Language in State Physical Therapy Practice Acts Direct Access to Physical Therapy Laws April 2000** (Continued)

| State & Year Obtained | Omission/ Provisions | Practice Act Language Summary |
|---|---|---|
| FL–1992 | Provisions | ■ Must refer patient or consult with health care practitioner if the patient's condition is outside scope of PT.<br>■ If physical therapy treatment is required beyond 21 days for a condition not previously assessed by a practitioner of record, the PT shall obtain a practitioner of record who will review and sign the plan.<br>■ Prohibits PTs from implementing plan of treatment for patients in acute care settings including hospitals, ambulatory surgical centers, and mobile surgical facilities. |
| GA | | Evaluation Only |
| HI | | No Direct Access |
| ID–1987 | Omission | ■ Prohibits the use of radiology, surgery, or medical diagnosis of disease.<br>■ Must refer when patient condition is outside PT scope of practice. |
| IL–1988 | Provisions | ■ Must refer to a physician, dentist, or podiatrist when patient condition is beyond scope of practice.<br>■ Must have documented referral or documented current and relevant diagnosis from a physician, dentist, or podiatrist to treat.<br>■ Must notify physician, dentist, or podiatrist that established the diagnosis that the patient is receiving physical therapy pursuant to that diagnosis. |
| IN | | No Direct Access |
| IA–1988 | Provisions | ■ Permits evaluation and treatment with or without a referral from a physician, podiatric physician, dentist, or chiropractor, except that a hospital may require that PT evaluation and treatment provided in the hospital be done only upon prior review by and authorization of a member of the hospital's medical staff.<br>■ Prohibits PTs from practicing operative surgery or osteopathic or chiropractic manipulation or administering or prescribing drugs or medicine. |
| KS | | Evaluation Only |
| KY–1987 | Provisions | ■ Definition of "physical therapy" includes PT treatment performed upon referral by a licensed doctor of medicine, osteopathy, dentistry, chiropractic, or podiatry. Law permits direct access to treatment. |

TABLE 3-1 CONTINUED

| State & Year Obtained | Omission/ Provisions | Practice Act Language Summary |
|---|---|---|
| | | ■ Must refer to a physician or dentist when patient condition is beyond scope of practice.<br>■ When basis for treatment is referral, the PT may confer with the referring physician, podiatrist, dentist, or chiropractor. |
| LA | | Evaluation Only |
| ME–1991 | Provisions | ■ When treating a patient without referral from a doctor of medicine, osteopathy, podiatry, dentistry, or chiropractic, the PT: (1) cannot make a medical diagnosis; (2) must refer the patient to a licensed doctor of medicine, osteopathy, podiatry, dentistry, or chiropractic if no improvement in the patient is documented within 30 days of initiation of treatment; (3) must consult or refer the patient to a licensed doctor of medicine, surgery, osteopathy, podiatry, dentistry, or chiropractic if treatment is required beyond 120 days.<br>■ Without a referral, PT may not apply manipulative thrust to the vertebrae of the spine or administer drugs.<br>■ Employers are not liable for charges under workers' compensation for services unless the employee has been referred to the PT.<br>■ Must make referral when beyond the scope of PT practice. |
| MD–1979 | Omission | ■ Grounds for license revocation if PT is practiced inconsistently with any written or oral order of a physician, dentist, or podiatrist. |
| MA–1984 | Omission | ■ Regulation sets PT Code of Ethics as standard for referral relationships. PT will refer to a licensed practitioner of medicine, dentistry, or podiatry if symptoms are present of which physical therapy is contraindicated or which symptoms are indicative of conditions for which treatment is outside scope of PT practice. PT will also provide ongoing communication with the licensed referring practitioner.<br>■ PT must disclose to patient any financial interest if the referring source derives income from the PT services. |
| MI | | Evaluation Only |
| MN–1988 | Provisions | ■ Medical diagnosis prohibited.<br>■ Must have order or referral by a physician, chiropractor, podiatrist, or dentist to continue treatment after 30 days.<br>■ Must practice for 1 year under a physician's orders before treating without referral.<br>■ Must consult with patient's health care provider before altering provider's original written order. |

*continued*

TABLE 3-1

**A Summary of Direct Access Language in State Physical Therapy Practice Acts Direct Access to Physical Therapy Laws April 2000** (Continued)

| State & Year Obtained | Omission/ Provisions | Practice Act Language Summary |
|---|---|---|
| | | ■ Must refer to a licensed health care professional when condition is beyond scope of practice.<br>■ Must report other PTs who fail to comply with practice act.<br>■ Must submit reports to a licensed health care provider for periodic review at least every 2 years.<br>■ PT with more than 1 year of clinical experience may initiate treatment of a patient for a condition not previously diagnosed for up to 30 calendar days once within a 4-month period without referring to a licensed health care provider. Does not apply to patients initially referred by provider.<br>■ PT with more than one year of clinical experience may initiate treatment of a patient for a lifelong and ongoing previously diagnosed condition warranting physical therapy treatment. Verification of diagnosis must be obtained by licensed health care provider within 30 days of initial admission<br>Evaluation Only |
| MS | | Evaluation Only |
| MO | Provisions | ■ Law states that PT evaluation and treatment procedures may be performed by a licensed PT without referral.<br>■ License revocation if PT practices beyond the scope and limitation of training and education. |
| MT–1987 | | |
| NE–1957 | Omission | Performing procedures outside of the scope of PT practice constitutes unprofessional conduct. |
| NV–1985 | Omission | Prohibits diagnosis of physical disabilities, massage of superficial soft tissue, and chiropractic adjustment. |
| NH–1988 | Provisions | Physical Therapist I<br>May not practice without a written prescription or referral from a person licensed to practice medicine, dentistry, podiatry, chiropractic, or naturopathy, or from a person licensed as a physician assistant or advanced registered nurse practitioner.<br>Physical Therapist II<br>Permitted to evaluate and develop a working diagnosis for treatment without referral with the following considerations:<br>■ Must obtain consultation with a person licensed in medicine, and qualified to refer to a PT, in order to continue treatment beyond 75 consecutive days. |

TABLE 3-1 CONTINUED

| State & Year Obtained | Omission/ Provisions | Practice Act Language Summary |
|---|---|---|
| | | ■ Must refer patient when condition is outside the scope of physical therapy or if a patient requires further medical evaluation or diagnostic testing, or if there is no documented improvement within 30 days of the initiation of treatment.<br>■ Must have at least 2 years' experience as a licensed PT.<br>■ Must be engaged in continuing education.<br>■ Must have submitted references from two physicians. |
| NJ | | Evaluation Only |
| NM–1989 | Provisions | ■ A PT shall not accept a patient for treatment without an existing medical diagnosis for the specific medical or physical problem made by a licensed primary care provider except for children in special education programs and for acute care within the scope of PT practice.<br>■ Must communicate to the patient's primary health care provider PT diagnosis and plan of treatment every 60 days unless otherwise indicated by the primary care provider. |
| NY | | Evaluation Only |
| NC–1985 | Provisions | ■ Manipulation of the spine must be prescribed by a physician.<br>■ Medical diagnosis of disease prohibited.<br>■ Unlawful practice when failure to refer to a licensed medical doctor or dentist when patient's condition is beyond scope of PT practice. |
| ND–1989 | Omission | ■ License revocation when failure to refer to a licensed health care professional any patient whose medical condition is beyond the scope of PT practice. |
| OH | | No Direct Access |
| OK | | Evaluation Only |
| OR–1993 | Provisions | To practice without referral a licensed PT must:<br>■ Hold a Level C CPR certificate.<br>■ Complete a course, of at least 18 hours, designed to enable the PT to identify signs and symptoms of systemic disease, particularly those that can mimic neurological or musculoskeletal disorders, and to recognize conditions that require timely referral to a medical doctor, osteopathic physician, chiropractic physician, podiatrist, dentist, licensed physician assistant, or licensed nurse practitioner.<br>■ Within 3 years of compliance with the previous requirements, a PT practicing without referral must complete at least 32 hours of continuing education. Thereafter the PT must complete at least 50 hours of continuing education every 3 years. |

continued

TABLE 3-1

**A Summary of Direct Access Language in State Physical Therapy Practice Acts Direct Access to Physical Therapy Laws April 2000** (Continued)

| State & Year Obtained | Omission/ Provisions | Practice Act Language Summary |
|---|---|---|
| | | ■ PTs qualified to practice without prior diagnosis or referral must refer a patient when signs and symptoms are present that would require treatment beyond the scope of PT practice, or if physical therapy is contraindicated, or if 30 days have passed since the initial physical therapy treatment; unless:<br>■ The patient is a child or student eligible for special education.<br>■ The patient is a student athlete seeking treatment in the role as athlete.<br>■ The patient is a resident of a long-term care facility, a residential facility, an adult foster home or an intermediate care facility for mental retardation.<br>Personal injury protection benefits are not required to be paid for physical therapy treatment of a person covered by the applicable insurance policy unless the person is referred to a PT. |
| PA | | Evaluation Only |
| RI–1992 | Provisions | ■ Must disclose to the patient in writing the scope and limitations of the practice of physical therapy and shall obtain their consent in writing.<br>■ Must refer the patient to a doctor of medicine, osteopathy, dentistry, podiatry, or chiropractic within 90 days after the treatment commenced (unless the treatment has concluded).<br>■ Must have 1 year of clinical experience to practice without referral. |
| SC–1998 | Provisions | ■ In the absence of a referral, must refer the patient to a licensed medical doctor or dentist if providing PT services beyond 30 days after the initial evaluation.<br>■ Must refer patient to a licensed medical doctor or dentist if patient's condition is beyond scope of physical therapy. |
| SD–1986 | Omission | No Restrictions |
| TN–1999 | Provisions | ■ Evaluation permitted without referral.<br>■ PT may treat a patient for an injury or condition that was subject of a prior referral if all the following conditions are met: (1) within 4 days of the commencement of therapy the PT consults with the referring practitioner; (2) the PT must confer with the referring practitioner in order to continue treatment after 10 treatment sessions or 15 consecutive calendar days, whichever comes |

TABLE 3-1 CONTINUED

| State & Year Obtained | Omission/ Provisions | Practice Act Language Summary |
|---|---|---|
| | | first; and (3) the PT commences any episode of treatment within 1 year of the referral by the referring practitioner.<br>■ PTs must be licensed for 1 year prior before utilizing the direct access provisions of the practice act.<br>■ A licensed PT may provide physical assessments or instructions including recommendation of exercise to an asymptomatic person without referral.<br>■ PTs may provide services without referral in emergency circumstances. |
| TX–1991 | Provisions | Prohibits the diagnosis of disease.<br>After holding a license for 1 year, physical therapists may treat a patient for an injury or condition that was the subject of a prior referral if the following conditions are met:<br>■ The PT notifies the referring licensed practitioner within 5 business days of the commencement of therapy.<br>■ Must confer with the referring practitioner after 20 treatment sessions or 30 consecutive calendar days, whichever comes first.<br>■ Treatment is commenced within 1 year of the referral.<br>May provide physical assessments or instructions to an asymptomatic person without referral. |
| UT–1985 | Omission | Prohibits diagnosis of disease, surgery, acupuncture, or x-ray for diagnostic or therapeutic uses. |
| VT–1988 | Omission | No Restrictions |
| VA | | No Direct Access |
| WA–1988 | Provisions | ■ A physical therapist may only provide treatment utilizing orthoses that support, align, prevent, or correct any structural problems intrinsic to the foot or ankle by referral or consultation from an authorized health care practitioner.<br>■ No restriction on the ability of any insurance entity or any state agency or program from limiting or controlling the utilization of physical therapy services by the use of any type of gatekeeper function.<br>■ Must refer patients when symptoms or conditions are beyond scope of PT practice. |
| WV–1984 | Provisions | ■ Prohibits electromyography examination and electrodiagnostic studies other than the determination of chronaxia and strength duration curves except under the supervision of a physician electromyographer and electrodiagnostician. |

*continued*

TABLE 3-1

**A Summary of Direct Access Language in State Physical Therapy Practice Acts Direct Access to Physical Therapy Laws April 2000** (Continued)

| State & Year Obtained | Omission/ Provisions | Practice Act Language Summary |
|---|---|---|
| | | ■ Referral requirement removed from practice act in 1984 session. However, due to an oversight, language remains that considers practice without referral grounds for license revocation. Despite this oversight, the State Board of Physical Therapy operates under the assumption that the legislative intent of the bill was to permit direct access. |
| WI–1989 | Provisions | Written referral of a physician, chiropractor, dentist, or podiatrist required except if a PT provides services:<br>■ In schools to children with exceptional education needs.<br>■ As part of a home health care agency.<br>■ To a patient in a nursing home pursuant to the patient's plan of care.<br>■ Related to athletic activities, conditioning, or injury prevention.<br>■ To an individual for a previously diagnosed medical condition after informing the individual's physician, chiropractor, dentist, or podiatrist who made the diagnosis. |
| WY | | Evaluation Only |

## GUIDE TO PHYSICAL THERAPIST PRACTICE

In November 1997, the APTA published Parts I (basic physical therapy patient/client management and examination parameters) and II (preferred practice patterns) of its *Guide to Physical Therapist Practice* (hereinafter *Guide*), which was intended to minimize unwarranted variation in physical therapy care delivery, to improve the overall quality of care rendered and patient/client satisfaction with services, and to promote reimbursement for physical therapy services. The second edition of the *Guide* was published in January 2001. The new edition clarifies terminology and consolidates several practice patterns. The *Guide* categorizes professional clinical practice by licensed physical therapists into five distinct practice parameters, applicable to all patients and clients in all clinical settings:

- Examination
- Evaluation
- Diagnosis

- Prognosis
- Intervention

Each of these clinical practice parameters is briefly described below.

Patient/client *examination* includes all of the traditional components of examination from the classic medical model, including patient/client intake, observation, communication, history, and physical examination. Patient/client examination is a prerequisite to diagnosis and intervention in physical therapy. (Fig. 3-1). A physical examination includes not only a pertinent, succinct, detailed history, but also a global systems review and focused tests and measurements designed to lead to accurate and reliable evaluative findings, impairment-based diagnosis, and optimal intervention(s).

*Evaluation* in clinical physical therapy practice entails the skilled analysis of patient/client history and examination findings and the formulation of clinical judgments about patient/client (systemic) impairments, functional limitations particular to individuals, and disabilities and their consequences for major life activities.

*Diagnosis* is the scientific labeling of patient/client conditions for the purposes of ascertaining optimal interventional strategies and succinctly communicating vital patient/client information to relevant others. *Prognosis*

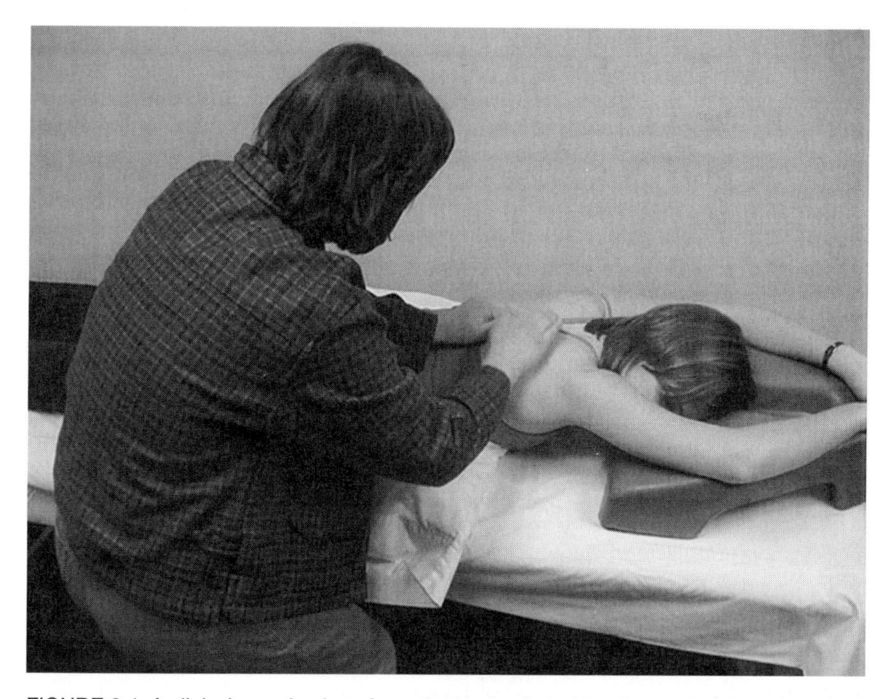

FIGURE 3-1 A clinical examination of a patient is the first of the five parameters of physical therapy practice.

entails predicting patient/client improvement over a specified time, based on an established physical therapy plan of care that contains specific short- and long-term interventional expected outcomes (goals) of remediation and/or prevention.

*Intervention* involves directed professional interaction by physical therapists toward their patients and clients to effect beneficial changes in their health status, based on predetermined impairment-based diagnoses and in support of established prognoses.

Preferred practice patterns provide comprehensive, evidence-based physical therapy management strategies for ameliorating specific musculoskeletal, neuromuscular, cardiopulmonary, and integumentary conditions. Preventive strategies to ameliorate injury or disease are included for each practice area.

*Musculoskeletal diagnostic groups include*:

- Skeletal demineralization
- Impaired posture
- Generalized impaired muscle performance
- Impaired joint mobility, motor function, muscle performance, and/or range of motion associated with:
  —local inflammation
  —connective tissue dysfunction
  —fracture, arthroplasty, or other surgical procedures
  —spinal dysfunction
  —amputation.

*Neuromuscular practice patterns address*:

- Impaired motor function and/or sensory integrity associated with:
  —congenital or acquired disorders of the central nervous system in infancy, childhood, or adolescence
  —acquired progressive and nonprogressive disorders of the central nervous system in adulthood
  —peripheral nervous system injury
  —acute, subacute, or chronic polyneuropathy or
  —nonprogressive disorders of the spinal cord
- Impaired arousal, range of motion, sensory integrity associated with coma, near-coma, or a persistent vegetative state.

*The cardiopulmonary practice patterns include*:

- Impaired aerobic capacity and endurance:
  —secondary to deconditioning associated with systemic disorders
  —associated with cardiovascular pump dysfunction or failure
- Impaired ventilation, respiration and aerobic capacity associated with:
  —airway clearance dysfunction

—ventilatory pump dysfunction or failure
—respiratory failure in the neonate

- Impaired ventilation with mechanical ventilation secondary to ventilatory pump dysfunction or failure
- Impaired ventilation and respiration with:
  —potential for respiratory failure
  —mechanical ventilation secondary to respiratory failure.

*The integumentary preferred practice patterns include* (in addition to primary prevention and risk factor reduction inherent in all area practice patterns):

- Impaired integumentary integrity secondary to:
  —superficial skin involvement
  —partial- or full-thickness skin involvement and cicatrix (scar) formation
  —involvement extending into fascia, muscle, and/or bone, and scar formation (Fig. 3-2)
- impaired circulation and anthropometric (physical) dimensions secondary to lymphatic system disorders.

Parts III and IV of the *Guide* are currently in development and in the field for comments, and are expected to address comprehensive clinical exami-

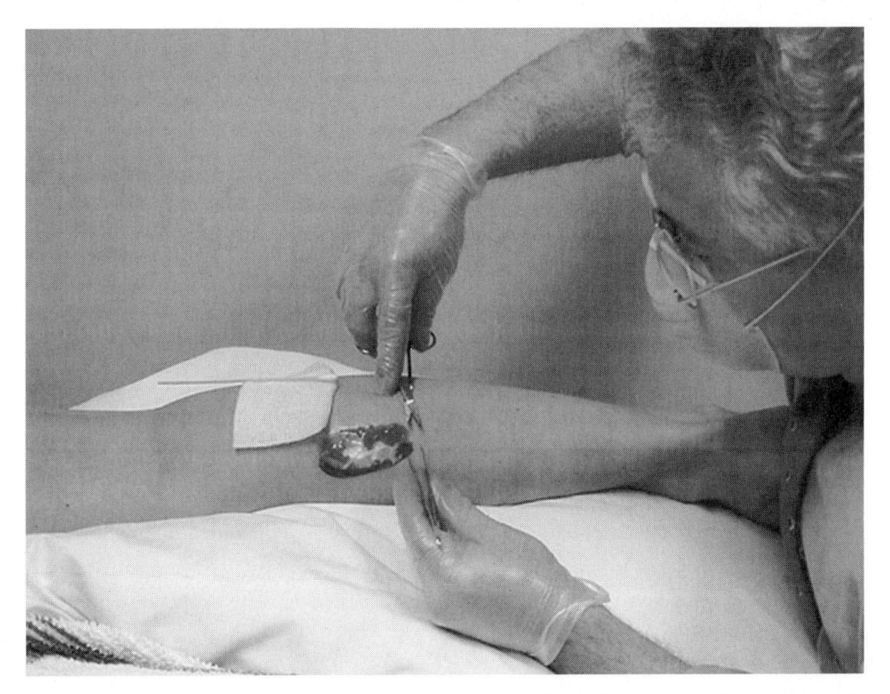

FIGURE 3-2 A simulation of sharp wound debridement of right lower leg under sterile conditions is shown (from the *Guide to Physical Therapist Practice*, 1997, with permission of the American Physical Therapy Association).

## PATIENT/CLIENT MANAGEMENT FORM

DATE:______________

NAME:______________________________ LOCAL ADDRESS:______________

LOCAL PHONE:______________________ E-MAIL:______________________

PERMANENT ADDRESS AND PHONE:______________________________

REASON FOR VISIT:______________________________________

______________________________________________________

REFERRING MD/DO:__________________ MED DX:__________________

MEDICATIONS:__________________________________________

SYSTEM REVIEWS:

EXAMINATION (INCLUDING TESTS & MEASUREMENTS):

EVALUATION/PT (IMPAIRMENT) DX:

PROGNOSIS:

INTERVENTION:

MISC. HEALTH INFORMATION:

DISCLAIMER/INFORMED CONSENT:____________________, PT, communicated the following to me: PT evaluate findings & diagnosis, recommended intervention & goals, material risks of harm/complication, & reasonable alternatives, and solicited & satisfactorily answered my questions, if any. I agree to actively cooperate with the agreed intervention.

Pt/Client Signature__________________________

FIGURE 3-3 Generic physical therapy documentation forms based on examples from the *Guide to Physical Therapist Practice*. (*continued*)

**PROGRESS NOTE** **DATE**__________ **PT NAME**__________________

**PROBLEM:**

**STATUS:**

**PLAN**

---

**DISCHARGE NOTE** **DATE**__________ **PT NAME**__________________

**STATUS:**

**PLAN:**

---

FIGURE 3-3 *Continued*

nation data sets for specific impairments and standardized tests, measurements, and instrumentalities to measure defined outcomes for particular impairments.

The following is a shell exemplar of physical therapy documentation forms for initial and periodic/discharge examinations, which may be expanded or modified for specific systemic impairment diagnoses and clinical practice settings (Fig. 3-3).

## MENTORING

Through formal and informal professional and continuing education, hands-on experience and mentoring, the novice physical therapist clinician develops into a master clinician who is capable of more expeditiously moving through the patient/client examination to a precise, accurate diagnoses. The same evolution applies to physical therapist assistants within their domain of professional clinical practice. This evolutionary process requires all three developmental components: education, experience, and mentoring to be optimally effective.

## A PERSPECTIVE ON MENTORING

Mentoring is a well-established and validated process in interpersonal business relations within which a teacher, or mentor, serves as a catalyst to facilitate the professional (and often personal) growth of a protégé. In Maslow's and Aldefer's hierarchy of human needs, the mentor assists the protégé in achieving self-esteem and self-actualization.

A given mentor and protégé may or may not derive from a strict organizational superior-subordinate relationship. Whether a mentor is a master clinician, a current or former educator, a consultant or friend, or any other person, every physical therapist and physical therapist assistant (especially including those in clinical practice) needs a mentor or multiple mentors in order to maximize self-potential.

The roles of a mentor range from technical education, training, and development to coaching and feedback to role-modeling, motivation, and counseling. A protégé's attributes should include: being an andragogical (self-directed) learner; having the ability to trust the mentor and to confide in and communicate openly with, him or her; and possessing the willingness to learn and to have an innate drive to succeed.

The mentor-protégé relationship is a "win-win" symbiotic one, within which both mentor and protégé gain and grow. The mentor achieves satisfaction in part from fulfilling the generativity need of imparting acquired skills and insight to someone else who will integrate them into his or her own professional persona. No mentor is infallible, and occasional failings, except perhaps for breaches of trust, are readily remediable within the relationship.

Female protégées may experience relative difficulty in establishing relationships with male mentors, in part because of male socialization of sex stereotyping of male and female roles. Many prospective male mentors lack relevant interpersonal experiences with women outside of traditional roles of spouse, child, other relative, or lover. Yet mentoring is as, or more, critical to female protégées as to men, so that women should actively and assertively seek out mentors—male or female—to facilitate their growth and development. Prospective male mentors should be (or become more) sensitive to the needs of female protégées, and foster their development just as they do or would for male protégés. Similar considerations apply to mentors and protégés from different racial or ethnic backgrounds.

Organizations without formal mentoring programs should expeditiously initiate them in consultation with human resource management specialists. From sponsorship programs for new employees to community outreach efforts that target disadvantaged persons (and positively affect a business' goodwill and revenue), mentoring is a social responsibility as well as a requisite for business success.

## PHYSICAL THERAPY CLINICAL MANAGEMENT

Physical therapy clinical management is a multidimensional specialized area of advanced practice, within which well-educated and highly trained clinical managers oversee clinic operations (including procuring and maintaining equipment, supplies, quality, information, and risk management); lead human resources (professionals, support, administrative, and clerical personnel) responsible for providing patient care; budget and allocate fiscal resources; and interact with internal and external entities affecting clinic operations on an ongoing basis.

Of the myriad administrative duties incumbent upon physical therapy clinic managers, unarguably the most important is human resource management. In a managed care era characterized by down-sizing, diminution of employee benefits, outsourcing, and deflated employee morale in the face of patient care reimbursement cut-backs, physical therapy clinical managers face the herculean task of continuing to recruit; assign and promote; train, educate, and develop; discipline (where required); and foster the self-determination and self-actualization of professional human resources who make the discipline the highly respected profession that it is.

Fiscal clinical management is another important area of physical therapy clinical management. From forecasting to budgeting to appropriating to allocating monies for vital clinical endeavors, managers bear front-line responsibility for the ongoing financial viability of the clinic.

Quality, information, and liability risk management are additional dimensions of physical therapy clinical management that bear mentioning. Quality management and oversight has risen to prominence over the past several decades as a means to attempt to optimize internal (patient/client) and internal and external satisfaction (by staff, peers, accreditation and review entities, and others) of patient care activities carried out within the clinic and facility. Information management is a complex responsibility, involving the management of patient care documentation; dissemination of policies and procedures, compliance with governmental and accreditation entity standards and mandates, and respect for patient/client privacy and dignity. New federal HIPPA standards require that even greater attention be paid to patient-informed consent and privacy of health-related patient data. Liability risk management entails tactics and strategies undertaken to prevent and mitigate iatrogenic patient injuries, and to meet the duty owed by the clinic manager to the employer to dampen malpractice and general liability exposure. Proactive and ad hoc consultation with facility attorneys is routine for clinic managers, who may lack formal legal education and training.

Physical management is the final area of physical therapy clinical management to be addressed. Physical, or facilities management, encompasses activities as disparate as equipment procurement, calibration, and maintenance to janitorial services to community relations—all part of this complex, critical, detail-focused aspect of management.

Anyone can be taught to manage, but not all managers are leaders. Leadership, the process of acting as a catalyst to effect positive change through others within a business organization, is crucial to business success. Leadership by clinical managers may range from highly directive (e.g., in times of cataclysmic change) to decentralized, supportive management in times of stability and in the face of maturity of the professional workforce. Physical therapy clinical management is as important a calling as is any other aspect of practice. Many or most physical therapy managers undertake specialized graduate education and post-professional training in business administration or in human resources or general management. Professional organizations, such as the American Management Association and the Society for Human Resource Management, offer excellent support to physical therapy clinical managers, through publications, courses, conferences and consultation.

## GENERAL PRACTICE AND PRACTICE SPECIALTIES

The clinical practice of physical therapy parallels that of medicine, with congruous general practice and practice specialty categories. The American

Physical Therapy Association describes clinical physical therapy in the *Guide* as:

> Care management for patients and clients with impairments, functional limitations, disabilities, and adverse changes in physical function and health status associated with injury, disease, or other etiology. Physical therapists also are involved in prevention and wellness activities, screening, and the promotion of positive health and wellness behaviors and activities.

Physical therapy clinical practice may be visualized along multidimensional intersecting planes. It may be delineated according to patient age groupings (i.e., pediatric, adolescent, young adult, middle-aged, geriatric), patient gender (e.g., women's health practice), or by a systems approach (cardiopulmonary, integumentary, neurologic, orthopedic). On another plane, practitioner specialization within a classification (e.g., limited scope practice according to an approach, such as McKenzie-based practice) may be used to define a physical therapy clinical practice. The experience level of a clinician or clinicians within a practice may rightly describe the practice (e.g., novice to master clinicians; presence and numbers of board-certified clinical specialists within the practice). Finally, geographic practice setting (hospital-based, home health, private clinic, etc) may be used to describe a given practice. Figure 3-4 illustrates this concept.

The clinical practice of physical therapy was not always as broad and autonomous as it is now, and is ever-evolving. In 1927 in *Hygeia* (precursor to the *Journal of the American Medical Association*), the profession was described in an article titled "Uses and Abuses of Physical Therapy" as the "employment of physical forces in the treatment of diseases and injuries." The scope of physical therapy practice was described as entailing primarily electrotherapy, and also including heliotherapy, hydrotherapy, the employment of artificial sunlight and radiant light and heat, massage, and medical gymnastics. Close physician oversight was recommended to optimize quality and patient safety.

## AMERICAN BOARD OF PHYSICAL THERAPY SPECIALTIES

The American Board of Physical Therapy Specialties (ABPTS) is a component of the American Physical Therapy Association, and is responsible for developing and overseeing administration of certification examinations to physical therapists seeking formal recognition for advanced clinical practice competencies. The ABPTS certifies physical therapists in the following practice specialty areas:

- Cardiovascular and pulmonary physical therapy
- Clinical electrophysiology

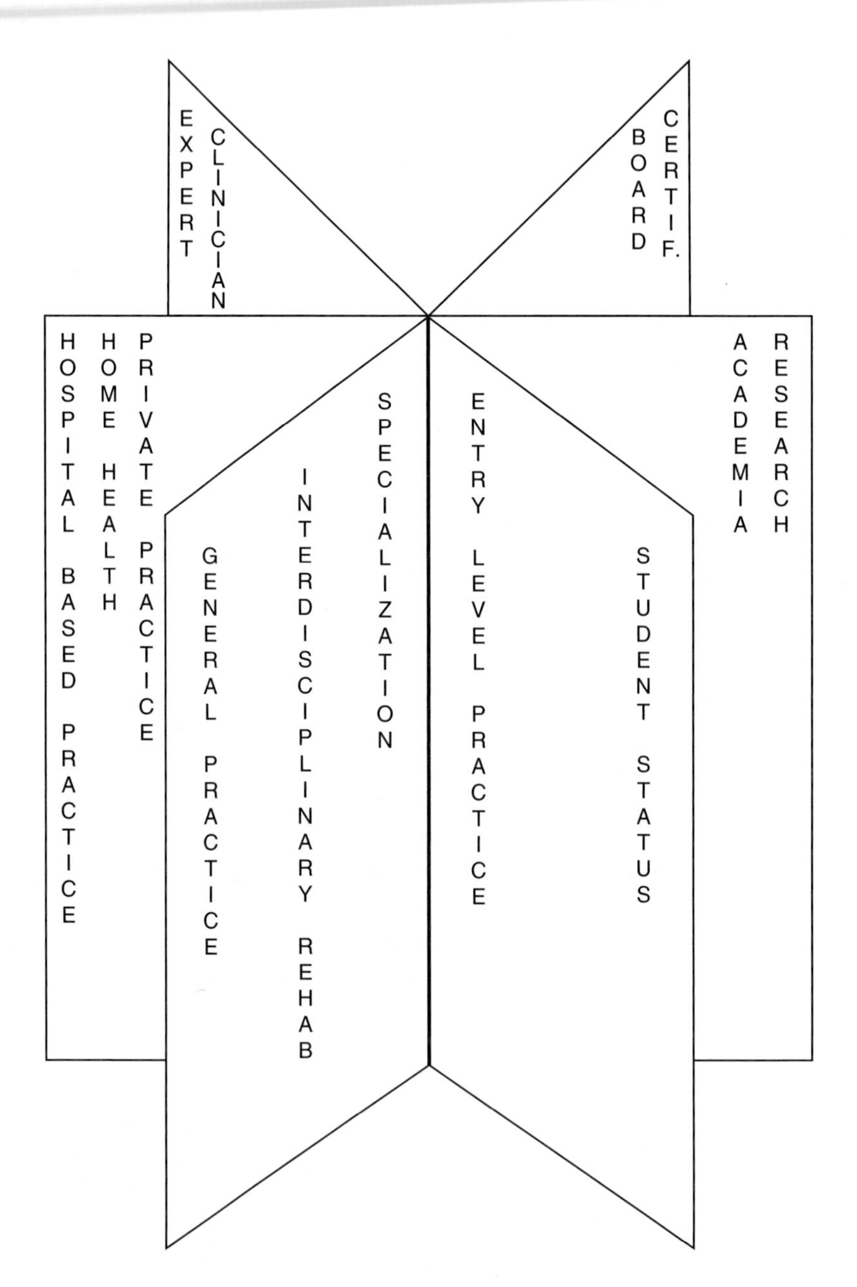


FIGURE 3-4 Multidimensional attributes of physical therapy clinical practice (drawn by Paul S. Scott).

- Geriatric physical therapy
- Neurologic physical therapy
- Orthopedic physical therapy
- Pediatric physical therapy
- Sports physical therapy

Specific requirements for precertification years of clinical practice experience and for supporting evidence of advanced competency, such as clinical research and teaching, vary from specialty to specialty, as do conditions for recertification. As of October 2000, there were a total of 3,205 ABPTS board-certified physical therapist clinical specialists, 1,653 of whom are orthopedic-certified clinical specialists. Only ABPTS-certified physical therapists are entitled to use the designator "_CS" after their professional credentials (e.g., John Doe, PT, OCS, for an ABPTS-certified orthopedic physical therapist).

## EVIDENCE-BASED PRACTICE

The precipitating event that accelerated the current strong emphasis on evidence-based practice in physical therapy was investigative reporter Lisa Miller's 1994 news article describing five different approaches by New York physical therapists to the care of mechanical knee dysfunction. That report was disconcerting, not so much because any approach or advice was incorrect, but because the discipline had so much variation in practice. As a result, the implementation of the *Guide* was accelerated, as were educational efforts to promote evidence-based practice.

Evidence-based practice involves supporting or justifying the parameters of clinical practice (examination procedures, tests and measurements, and interventions) with scientific evidence. Justification of the parameters of health professional clinical practice is not done to promote conformity among practitioners, but to optimize the quality of individualized patient care and to minimize health care costs at the macro- and micro-levels.

Evidence supporting valid clinical health clinical practice may derive from the peer-reviewed literature, from clinical practice guidelines and protocols, from textual references, and from other objective sources. The use of such scientific evidence in legal proceedings has been in effect for decades, from expert witnesses testifying in health care malpractice trials routinely justify their expert opinions with such evidence.

## MILITARY PRACTICE MODEL

The military physical therapy clinical practice model differs from civilian practice in several key respects. Military physical therapists are not constrained in their federal practice on federal enclaves by state practice acts. They are governed in their physical therapy practice by federal statutes and regulations.

In the early 1970s, the military suffered an acute shortage of primary care active-duty physicians. A policy was enacted that created nonphysician extenders to fill the need for primary care, first-line providers. Physical therapists, along with occupational therapists, physician assistants and nurse practitioners, were recruited for these positions.

The requirements for serving in the military as a primary care physician surrogate vary from service to service (Army, Navy, Air Force). For the Army, the governing regulations are Army Regulation 40–48 and 40–68.

Licensed military physical therapist–physician extenders present their credentials, and are granted formal practice privileges in a particular military medical facility, similar to the process employed for physicians and dentists. Such physical therapists are credentialed to examine, evaluate, and intervene on behalf of patients without referral who present with acute, subacute, or chronic minor neuromusculoskeletal conditions. They may order radiographic studies and initiate follow-on referrals to other primary or consulting providers. In some cases, they may also be privileged (based on education and experience) to write patient prescriptions for nonsteroidal antiinflammatory medications. Practice privileges are subject to periodic review and renewal.

## Activities, Cases, and Questions

1. **Activity**: Interview five physical therapists in clinical practice. Discover their opinions on direct access practice and the military practice model.
2. **Case**: X. is newly licensed physical therapist. She is employed by ABC Medical Center, and is assigned to be a wound care therapist, a position that includes 24-7-365 on-call duties on a rotating basis. X. does not feel personally competent to independently carry out sharp debridement of wounds. What steps, if any, should she take to apprise her supervisors of this situation? What steps should X.'s supervisors take to assess her competency to carry out wound care and to develop her cognitive and psychomotor skills in this area of practice?
3. **Questions**: What is your personal opinion about the propriety of a DPT-educated clinical physical therapist being called "doctor"? What steps can and should be taken to minimize patient/staff misunderstandings about such a physical therapist's status and credentials?

**Acknowledgments** Special thanks to photo models Heather Richardson, Jill Seibert, and Kris Zwemer.

## ADDITIONAL READINGS

Bernhart-Barbridge D. What's New: *Guide to Physical Therapist Practice*, 2nd ed. *PT: Magazine of Physical Therapy*. 2001;9(3):34–37.

Dininny P. More than a uniform: the military model of physical therapy. *PT: Magazine of Physical Therapy*. 1995;3(3):40–48.

Duncan PW. Evidence-based practice: a new model for physical therapy. *PT: Magazine of Physical Therapy*. 1996;4(12):44–48.

Greathouse DG, Schreck RC, Benson CJ. The United States Army physical therapy experience: evaluation and treatment of patients with neuromusculoskeletal disorders. *J Ortho Sports Phys Ther*. 1994;19:261–266.

*Guide to Physical Therapist Practice*. Alexandria, VA: American Physical Therapy Association; 1997.

Hartwick AMR. *The Army Medical Specialist Corps: The 45th Anniversary*. Washington, DC: Center of Military History (US Army); 1993.

Johns G. *Organizational Behavior: Understanding and Managing Life at Work*, 4th ed. New York: HarperCollins College Publishers; 1996: 617–620.

Kovacs R. Uses and abuses of physical therapy. *Hygeia*. 1927 (Dec):614–616.

Lewis CB, Bottomley JM. *Geriatric Physical Therapy: A Clinical Approach*. East Norwalk, CT: Appleton & Lange; 1994.

Magee DJ. *Orthopedic Physical Assessment*, 3rd ed. Philadelphia, PA: WB Saunders; 1997.

McFarland B. Mentor programs benefit students, professionals. *HR News*. 2000; 9(10):27.

Miller L. One bum knee meets five physical therapists. *Wall Street Journal*. September 24, 1994: B1, B6.

Putting it into practice: A Guide Q&A. *PT: Magazine of Physical Therapy*. 2000; 8(12):40–43, 86.

Smith C. Strength in numbers: the clinical research agenda and physical therapy's future in science. *PT: Magazine of Physical Therapy*. 2000;8(9):52–54.

Tecklin JS. *Pediatric Physical Therapy*, 3rd ed. Philadelphia: Lippincott Williams & Wilkins; 1999.

Wong R, Barr J, Farina N, Lusardi M. Evidence-based practice: A resource for physical therapists. *Issues on Aging*. 2000;23(3):34–44.

Wynn KE. A guide to the 'guide.' *PT: Magazine of Physical Therapy*. 1997;5(11):58–63.

## Focus on a Leader

**RICK RITTER, MA, PT, OCS**
**PRIVATE PRACTICE, SAN FRANCISCO, CALIFORNIA**

1. *Rick, please briefly capsulize for the readers your credentials, professional chronology, and current and recent professional activities.*
I received my BS degree in PT at Marquette University in 1967 and my MA in Human Resources Management from Pepperdine University in 1981. I entered the Army in 1967, and began a 20-year career. The focus of my postprofessional education has been orthopaedics and sports physical therapy. I have held various staff and leadership positions throughout my Army career, including co-development of the first course to teach Army physical therapists neuromusculoskeletal screening in 1989. I concluded my Army career with a 6-year assignment as Chief, Physical Therapy, United States Military Academy, West Point, NY. I entered private practice as an associate in 1987 and later entered a partnership that developed a large orthopaedic/sports-oriented private practice. I am currently associated with a small private practice with a large HMO population. I am also an Assistant Clinical Professor in the UCSF/SFSU graduate program in physical therapy. I have served the Orthopaedic Section on the Nominating Committee 1983–1986, and the Orthopaedic Specialty Council 1988–1994 (Chair, 1991–1993); as co-editor of *Orthopaedic Physical Therapy*; I developed the Description of Advanced Clinical Practice in 1994; and I received the Section's Paris Distinguished Service Award in 1997. I have served as delegate to the APTA House of Delegates from various states where I have lived, and for the last 7 years as a delegate from California. I was elected to the Chapter Board, CCAPTA, in 1996, and reelected to a 2-year term as Director in 1998, then elected as Secretary in 2000. I am also Chair, Government Affairs Committee and a member of the Diagnosis Task Force. I am simultaneously a member of the Board of California PT Fund, a research grant, professional scholarship, and student loan organization.

2. *What are the salient problems, issues, and dilemmas affecting clinical physical therapists and assistants as we enter the 21st century?*
For me the central challenge is that of true independent practice for physical therapists, meaning that an individual consumer can access the expertise of the physical therapist directly without any conditions or restrictions. As long as the "usual way" that a consumer accesses our services is by

referral, we will find that our viability as a professional will continue to be challenged. *Consumers* is a term that is used on purpose to indicate that not all those who come to see us will be seeking to address impairments, dysfunction, or disabilities. Some may seek advice on wellness and prevention, performance enhancement, second opinions, or other areas of our expertise. Although we have the knowledge and skill to serve the general population, we seem to be the only ones that know it. As good as the few public relations steps we have taken as a profession have been, we cannot be satisfied with our current "recognizability." We must focus our message and continue our efforts to inform the public as well as our colleagues who we are and what we do. One of the positive impacts that the HMO/managed care model of care has had is that patients have had to learn and learn fast about insurance benefits. Many have discovered that limited access or controlled access to physical therapy has had a negative impact on their rehabilitation outcome. I am seeing a realization and recognition from the consumer that we offer a valuable service, and they would like to be able to have more direct access. At least in my present situation, consumers express a solid satisfaction with the service we provide that is at least equal to, if not greater than in, past years. I often wonder if we value our professional selves and the service we provide as much as those who receive the service value what we do. Our unique set of knowledge and skills is unmatched in health care professions, yet we find ways to refer to ourselves as "just a PT." That makes me crazy! We are experts in addressing impairments, functional limitations, and disabilities or changes in physical function as a result of injury, disease, or changes in health status from other causes. Our greatest challenge is to "self-actualize" the profession of physical therapy so that consumers/patients/clients can readily access our expertise.

3. *Where do you believe physical therapy will be in the year 2050? What needs to be accomplished to get the profession where you envision it being in 2050?*
Predicting the future is best undertaken by those who are smart enough to look far enough ahead to a time when accountability will not be an issue. That being said, I think of myself as a realistic optimist. I expect we will be in a much better position then than we are now. One fact stands out to me when looking at the difference between where we are and where I expect us to be. We have too good a "product" or professional knowledge and skill set to not do well. Our underpinnings, A Normative Model of Physical Therapist Professional Education, A Normative Model for Physical Therapist Assistant Education, Standards for Clinical Education, Standards for Residency Programs, and the *Guide to Physical Therapist Practice*, first and second editions, are sound and yet flexible enough to allow further refinement and growth. In the legislative/regulatory arena, we have the Model Practice Act. There is an increasing body of literature that indicates what we do is effective

and worthwhile. There does need to be more evidence, and we seem more focused on that challenge and blessed with more dedicated individuals as well as more funds available for research than ever before. Most important is the easing of tension between the clinical practitioner, researcher, and academician; that tension must continue to melt into nonexistence.

We in 2050 will be practicing in a collegial medical model including clinical and nonclinic-based practice, and our services will be accessed directly by consumers, although referral relationships will certainly continue to exist. One of the differences in the referral relationships will be that it will be a "two-way" relationship. The physical therapist will become an important referral source for those who in the past have only referred patients to us; they will now receive patients from us. Consumers will value the component of their health care that we provide equally with other providers. I expect long before 2050 we will be preparing physical therapists at the professional doctorate level, and physical therapist assistants at the baccalaureate level.

One of the prices for this newfound professional freedom will be an even greater level of professional responsibility. The academic preparation for this level of practice is much farther along than the "system" of preparing individuals for the professional social environment of independent practice. What was once built into practice settings has become a victim of the changes in health care delivery. It was most common for a physical therapist, upon completion of their professional preparation, to spend a year or two with a more senior staff. Typically, there would be an individual that would mentor the new PT in those first several months and beyond. Now it is not unusual for a new PT to become a "senior" staff in a matter of months. It is not that we do not recognize the need and value of the mentoring relationship; we began a program in the Orthopaedic Section several years ago. What must happen now is that we find a way to refashion the formation of mentoring relationships that were so easily facilitated by organizational structure. I believe that these relationships will be critical for our future independent practice. Certainly academic programs will continue to integrate professional behaviors into professional preparation, but living the behaviors, having the behaviors shaped and focused by personal relationships, is ultimately how the individual will capture the art of physical therapy practice.

The only thing I can say for sure about 2050 is that things will be different from what they are today. Technology in so many fields will impact what we do, how we do it, how we record and transmit the information, and how we provide follow-up. I am sure that there will be things that will happen that only a few among us can dream about at this time. I expect us to thrive as a profession in the future, and feel comfortable saying that there are individuals, some not yet discovered, that have the professional and political will to lead us on this journey.

CHAPTER 4

# Clinical Practice: Neurologic Physical Therapy

KRISTIN ZWEMER

*Neurologic physical therapy* is a general term used to describe the complex physical therapy management of persons who demonstrate some type of neurologic dysfunction. Most people think of stroke or closed head injury when thinking of an ailment involving the nervous system; however, there are many other forms of neurologic dysfunction, including, but not limited to, amyotrophic lateral sclerosis (Lou Gehrig's disease), multiple sclerosis, spinal cord injury, and Parkinson's disease. This chapter serves as an introduction to the principles of the physical therapy management of adults demonstrating neurologic impairments, and will review general physical therapy management strategies as they relate to specific neurologic rehabilitation practices. It is assumed that the reader will appreciate the importance of integrating various practice strategies into all specialty areas.

## MOTOR DEVELOPMENT

To develop a treatment approach for individuals with neurologic dysfunction, a therapist must have a working knowledge of motor development and motor control (broadly defined as the control of movement and posture). Generally, three main models of motor development exist: the hierarchical, reflex, and systems models. All three models offer insight into the processes of human movement, and we have gained an in-depth understanding of the nervous system and its relation to motor function from them.

One of the pioneers who studied the maturation of the nervous system and its relation to behavior was G. E. Coghill. Coghill's studies were the first to offer insights into the anatomy of the nervous system, specifically his conclusion of 1:1 mapping of the nervous system to movement,[1] which paved the way for later developmental theorists like Myrtle McGraw and Arnold Gesell.

Following in Coghill's footsteps, McGraw applied Coghill's idea of a 1:1 relationship between the nervous system and movement to humans. Her classic experiment involved the study of identical twins. She trained one of the twins for certain activities and did not train the other to determine whether training influenced the development of certain behavior patterns.[2] The foundation of McGraw's neural-maturationist view was based on her theory that as the cortex developed primitive behavior patterns disappeared and were replaced with more functional mature behaviors.[2] Because the cerebral cortex developed later than other divisions of the brain, the behaviors displayed as development progressed became more varied and functional. When after injury primitive behavior patterns returned, McGraw explained that the injury had affected cortical functioning. As a result, the cerebral cortex was no longer able to control or suppress the subcortical nuclei, and, therefore, the primitive behavior patterns emerged.[3]

Gesell took the neuromaturational view formulated by Coghill and McGraw a step further in investigating other behaviors in addition to motor functioning. His main advance to motor development theory was his belief that as the neuromotor system grew and matured there was a continual readjustment in the relationship between flexor-extensor and symmetric-asymmetric control. According to Gesell, the environment and experience played minor roles in motor development.[4]

Yet another contribution to motor development was the reflex-based description of development. According to this view, infants exhibited primarily simple reflexes. As the cerebral cortex developed and began to inhibit primitive behavior patterns, the simple reflexes diminished or became integrated into more mature motor behaviors. This theory correlated with McGraw's findings that when the central nervous system was damaged these infantile simple reflexes returned.

All of the advances in motor development discussed thus far offer insight into the organization of the nervous system, and thus motor control. The work of McGraw and Gesell gives therapists an understanding of the milestones of motor development, which is valuable in the physical therapy management of pediatric patients and those adults exhibiting primitive behavior patterns as a result of an injury. In addition, reflex testing is a significant component of the physical therapy examination of a client with neurological dysfunction. Overall, the work of these developmental theorists offers physical therapists a set of norms that are an integral component in the physical therapy management of individuals with neurologic dysfunction. The theories mentioned thus far, however, fail to capture the richness of development. The linking thread in the work of Coghill, Gesell, and McGraw is an assumption that the nervous system is the sole controller of motor development. Why do infants, as well as individuals recovering from injury, often adapt so well to their specific environmental circumstances? If physical therapists relied only on these theories as a framework for therapeutic interventions, they could be seriously limiting the treatment options available to their clients due to the strict acceptance of the manner in which the brain affects development. According to these theories, the patient is the passive recipient of therapy.[5]

The more recent Dynamical Systems approach to motor development addresses the importance of other factors (subsystems) to the developmental process. This approach brings with it a whole different set of assumptions than the theories discussed previously. The Dynamical Systems theory contends that motor development proceeds through the interaction of many subsystems within and outside of the body.[6] Because of the interdependence of subsystems on each other to produce a movement, it is not surprising that when one subsystem undergoes changes, the entire movement will change and readjust to the interaction that results.[6] By integrating Dynamical Systems theory into the framework of physical therapy management strategies, a therapist must evaluate all of the subsystems involved in a movement as they relate to each other and to the task in question. Although many questions regarding motor development continue to be debated, the Dynamical Systems theory offers several intervention options unrelated to direct manipulation of the nervous system. Thelen states, "A dynamical systems perspective would agree that CNS damage places constraints on the system but also recognizes that other subsystems influence the behavior as well."[6]

All of the developmental theories discussed offer specific elements to the development of physical therapy management strategies, whether it is reflex testing, developmental norms, or developmental milestones. Because of the unique context of every individual's circumstances, the clinical presentation of the patient population as a whole is highly variable, and this variability must be accounted for. The theories described above assist in explaining this variability; however, the picture of movement control is not yet complete and remains an ongoing process, explored generally in this chapter.

## PHYSICAL THERAPY MANAGEMENT: EVALUATION COMPONENTS

Physical therapists are one member of a team of health care professionals involved in the rehabilitation of individuals with neurologic dysfunction.

This team most often includes occupational therapists, speech pathologists, neuropsychologists, counseling psychologists, nurses, physicians, case managers, and respiratory therapists. It is crucial for all members of the team to engage in active discussion with one another, as each team member has individual expertise and insight into patient and family issues.

## Cognition/Attention

The initial interaction with a patient is an excellent opportunity to assess the patient's cognitive status, as well as to gain insight into the patient's perspective of his or her impairment. Often times this interaction is centered on discussing the individual's past medical history. Although an individual who has sustained a spinal cord injury generally does not present with cognitive impairment, a physical therapist can gain a psychosocial perspective into how the individual is coping with his injury during the initial meeting. On the other hand, someone who has sustained a stroke or closed head injury may be inaccurate or completely unable to provide information related to her past medical history. From the review of the particular disease, a therapist learns, generally, what to expect from specific neurologic diseases or injuries, realizing that every individual's situation is unique.

When considering the cognitive status of an individual who demonstrates a neurologic deficit, involve the speech pathologist, neuropsychologist, and occupational therapist to assist with developing a dynamic picture of the patient's perceptual and cognitive functioning level. Typical questions asked to assess cognition revolve around current events or orientation to person, place, and time. Not only are the answers themselves important, but how the answers are given is also important. Does the individual take a long time to answer a question? Is the language intelligible? Is the individual able to attend to the questions or easily distracted? It is essential for the physical therapist to discuss his or her impressions with the other members of the health care team who have expertise in these areas to confirm their thoughts and gain information on the most appropriate means of interacting with the patient.

## Sensation/Proprioception

It is important to assess the patient's sensation during the examination process, as this is often impaired in individuals with neurologic dysfunction. Light touch, deep pressure, pinprick, and temperature sensations should all be assessed as well as proprioception and kinesthesia. The quality of the individual's sensation is also important. The results of the sensory evaluation are critical to the physical therapy management techniques a therapist will be able to employ, and offer insight into what deficits to expect as therapy progresses.

## Tone

Tone, defined as the resting tension exhibited in a muscle, is critically important in neurologic rehabilitation because, by and large, every person presenting with a neurologic impairment will exhibit some variation of abnormal tone. The ability to skillfully assess muscle tone and spasticity is crucial for physical therapists working with individuals with neurologic dysfunction. There are several characteristics to consider when evaluating muscle tone. A therapist moves the individual's limbs passively through the range of motion and feels for any resistance or heaviness at various joints, as well as noting where in the range of motion the resistance is felt. The next step is for the therapist to consider if there is a pattern to the tone felt, and then the therapist attempts to detect at which joints and in which specific muscle groups the tone is present.

## Movement Strategies

The quantity and quality of volitional movement is also an essential aspect of the physical therapy evaluative process. Is the patient able to move through the entire available range of motion? Is the limb being moved in a position where gravity is assisting the movement, is the limb being moved against gravity, or in a position where the effects of gravity are essentially eliminated? Is the individual able to isolate movement at each joint, or is the movement part of a synergistic pattern that incorporates movement at several joints at one time? Is the movement coordinated? The physical therapist must also assess the speed and accuracy of the path the limb or body part is taking. If an individual demonstrates the ability to selectively isolate motor activity, an assessment of strength should then be performed. It is important to ask the patient to move his extremities, head, and trunk in different positions and then document clearly what was observed. For example, a patient may not experience difficulty moving her lower extremity while seated in a supportive chair, but may demonstrate significant difficulty when asked to move her lower extremity while lying supine on a mat table.

## Postural Control/Balance/Righting Reactions

Another important aspect of a neurologic examination is whether an individual is capable of achieving and maintaining certain postures. If a patient is unable to maintain upright sitting, attempting to assess limb movement in this position may be futile. Static and dynamic balance must be assessed in various positions to determine when and where balance is impaired. Is the individual capable of attaining upright sitting and maintaining this position throughout various challenges? Is the individual capable of shifting weight from one body part to another while sitting or standing? Many tests for assessing balance have been designed over the past several years in an attempt to objectify the physical therapy evaluation of balance and to serve as a means of predicting falls.

### Reflexes

At some point in the evaluation process a physical therapist must check for the presence of primitive reflexes and for the quality of deep tendon reflexes. The results of the reflex testing portion of the physical therapy examination offer insight into the extent of central nervous system damage.

These evaluative components do not stand alone as a complete physical therapy examination and evaluation. These components are integrated with basic evaluative techniques to create a physical therapy management framework for individuals with neurologic impairments. Keep in mind that these physical therapy management strategies require significant elaboration or minimization depending on individual patient presentation. The most important thing to remember in treating neurologically involved patients is that the evaluative process does not end after the initial session. The evaluative process continues throughout the duration of treatment in an effort to continually reassess the physical therapy management strategies employed.

## TREATMENT COMPONENTS

Physical therapy management techniques for the treatment of individuals with neurologic impairments must focus on functional activities if the eventual goal is functional independent living. In addition to focusing on functional activities, the issue of tone must be addressed throughout treatment as well. The abnormal tone demonstrated must be normalized in conjunction with, or prior to, working on functional activities. Several basic techniques follow for facilitating or inhibiting muscle tone. Performing a quick stretch of a particular muscle or muscle group will, for physiologic reasons beyond the scope of this chapter, facilitate increased muscle tone. Alternatively, a slow prolonged stretch is one of the most effective techniques used to inhibit muscle tone and is the premise behind inhibitory or serial casting. The type of manual contacts applied to an individual will also affect muscle tone. Quick short contacts, such as brushing or vibration, facilitate muscle tone, whereas slow deep pressure, such as slow stroking or compression, serves to inhibit muscle tone. Traction (the act of separating two points), when used over a joint, tends to increase muscle tone, whereas joint approximation is an ideal technique for relaxing muscles surrounding a joint. In looking at how other body systems affect the neuromuscular system, the vestibular system has a dramatic effect on muscle tone. Rapid movements or changing direction and frequency quickly tend to facilitate an increased motor response, whereas slow repetitive movements are calming and tend to inhibit motor responses. Ask yourself, do you tend to relax more when you are rapidly shaken or gently rocked?

If the tonal management techniques discussed above are unsuccessful or if an individual's tone is particularly high, medications and other medical interventions are often used in conjunction with physical therapy management techniques to effectively reduce spasticity. Again, the communication between the health care team members is essential in determining if further medical interventions are necessary.

## NEUROLOGIC DISORDERS/INJURIES

### Stroke

Stroke or cerebrovascular accident (CVA) is a disturbance in brain function lasting more than 24 hours, caused by an impairment of blood flow to the nervous system.[7] This nervous system damage can be caused by cerebral ischemia (inadequate blood flow and thus inadequate oxygen) or cerebral hemorrhage (heavy blood flow). Stroke is the third most common cause of death in developed countries, and of those who survive, 50% are permanently disabled.[7] The physical therapy management strategies for individuals who have suffered a stroke focus initially on positioning and passive range of motion. As recovery progresses the focus shifts to include functional training, tone management techniques (to facilitate or inhibit muscle tone), endurance training, and patient and family education.

### Traumatic Brain Injury

In the United States one person will die and another will be permanently disabled as a result of a traumatic brain injury (TBI) every 5 minutes.[8] Head injury is the leading cause of death among young adults.[8] The most common cause of TBI is automobile accidents. Often an individual who sustains brain injury due to trauma has other injuries as well that complicate the rehabilitation process. The initial focus is preserving life and preventing further damage or injury. Physical therapists are concerned with multiple issues when treating individuals with TBI, including, but not limited to, the patient's arousal level, cognitive status, medical complications, fractures, muscle tone impairments, activity tolerance, and sensory impairments. The clinical presentation is varied and complex in individuals with TBI, and thus necessitates a dynamic individualized treatment plan integrating multiple physical therapy management strategies. The importance of a multidisciplinary team in brain injury rehabilitation cannot be stressed enough.

## Amyotrophic Lateral Sclerosis

Amyotrophic lateral sclerosis (ALS), also known as Lou Gehrig's disease after the baseball player who developed the disease, is a rapidly progressive neurologic disease that invariably leads to death from respiratory failure.[8] ALS is characterized by degeneration of motor neurons, and is one of the most common motor neuron diseases, with an incidence of 1 to 2 per 100,000.[8] Individuals with ALS develop motor weakness, muscle cramping and twitching combined with spasticity and hyperreflexia. The goals of physical therapy intervention are adjusted to meet the needs of the individual as the disease progresses. Initially, physical therapy focuses on energy conservation training; this focus shifts to introducing adaptive equipment, stretching, and low-level strength training for unaffected muscle groups as the disease progresses. With continued disease progression, the goals continue to shift and include appropriate wheelchair seating and positioning to maximize independence, stretching, passive range of motion, and breathing exercises. Patient and family education is crucial at every stage in the disease process to maximize independent functioning.

## Multiple Sclerosis

Multiple sclerosis (MS) is a progressive disease characterized by demyelination in the central nervous system.[8] The demyelination is a random process and, therefore, the disease symptoms are variable. In advanced cases of MS, weakness, spasticity, sensory loss, fatigue, urinary incontinence, and visual disturbances are often present.[8] The clinical course is divided into distinct patterns and overall prognosis is difficult to predict. As a result, the clinical manifestations of the disease differ greatly between individuals. Physical therapy intervention is important at all stages of the disease, initially to educate individuals on exercise tolerance. Often, individuals with MS require bracing and tone management interventions as well as functional training and proper wheelchair positioning as the disease progresses.

## Spinal Cord Injury

An individual who sustains a traumatic spinal cord injury often sustains other serious associated injuries, such as fractures, closed head injuries, or internal organ damage.[8] Initially, the primary medical goal is preserving life. Other methods of spinal cord damage are nontraumatic in origin and include circulatory compromise, compression of the spinal cord, tumors, abscesses, and congenital malformations of the vertebral canal.[8] The physical therapy intervention strategies differ depending on the degree and location of damage to the spinal cord; however, certain aspects of care are fundamental regardless of the extent of injury. It is crucial for early passive range of motion and stretching to be performed to maintain muscular elasticity and prevent contractures. Functional training takes on increased importance as the rehabilitation process progresses. Generally, physical therapy intervention strategies include gait training, wheelchair training, strengthening the unaffected muscles, transfer training, endurance activities, and positioning. Again, patient and family education is crucial to the overall physical and psychological recovery process.

### Parkinson's Disease

Parkinson's disease is one of the most common involuntary movement disorders, affecting approximately 1% of people over 50 years. It results from a loss of dopaminergic neurons in the substantia nigra. The clinical manifestations of Parkinson's disease include tremor, shuffling (often festinating) gait, rigidity, dysarthria, and forward trunk flexion. Physical therapy interventions include balance training, passive and active range of motion, muscle stretching to improve or maintain flexibility, and functional training (gait, transfer training). The goal is to keep individuals with Parkinson's disease as mobile as possible for as long as possible to prevent associated medical complications.

## SUMMARY

It is imperative for physical therapists engaged in managing individuals with neurologic dysfunction to integrate all aspects of their knowledge into developing a dynamic examination and treatment framework. Because no two individuals with the same medical diagnosis demonstrate the same clinical manifestations, the therapist's ability to alter physical therapy management techniques to meet individual needs is crucial. This chapter introduced the reader to several basic concepts involved in the physical therapy management of individuals with neurologic impairments, beginning with an introduction to motor development and how it serves as a basis for the physical therapy management of individuals with neurologic dysfunction and continuing with a discussion of neurologic physical therapy evaluative and treatment components. Several neurologic impairments and general physical therapy management strategies were reviewed to give the reader insight into how different injuries or disease processes are managed. Physical therapists working with individuals with neurologic dysfunction find it very challenging and rewarding. It is an area of physical therapy that is continually changing as scientists gain a better understanding of the nervous system.

## REFERENCES

1. Coghill GE. *Anatomy and the Problem of Behaviour*. New York: Cambridge University Press; 1929.
2. McGraw M. *Growth: A Study of Johnny and Jimmy*. New York: D. Appleton Century Company; 1935.
3. McGraw M. *The Neuromuscular Maturation of the Human Infant*. New York: Columbia University Press; 1943.
4. Gesell A. Reciprocal interweaving in neuromotor development. *J Comp Neurol*. 1939; 70(5):161–180.
5. Barnes MR et al. *Reflex and Vestibular Aspects of Motor Control, Motor Development and Motor Learning*. Atlanta: Stokesville Publishing; 1990.
6. Jenson J et al. A dynamical systems approach to motor development. *Phys Ther*. 1990; 70(12)763/17–774/28.
7. Swash M, Schwartz, M. *Neurology: A Concise Clinical Text*. London: WB Saunders; 1989.
8. Umphred DA. *Neurological Rehabilitation*. Baltimore: Mosby; 1995.

CHAPTER 5

# Clinical Practice: Orthopaedic Physical Therapy

PENNY SAMUELSON

Orthopaedic physical therapy is one of the seven identified areas of physical therapy specialty recognized by the Board of Specialties of the American Physical Therapy Association. It also is the focus area of the Orthopaedic Section of the American Physical Therapy Association. In seeking to define it, the Section identifies it as "the evaluation and treatment of musculoskeletal disorders, prevention of disability related to the dysfunction of the musculoskeletal system, and enhancement of the performance of the musculoskeletal system."

This definition, however, only tells part of what the study of orthopaedic physical therapy was, is, and seeks to be. This is not a static field entrenched in muscle insertions and kinesiology (as the beginning student may see it) but a dynamic field ever challenged to better its understanding of human neuromusculoskeletal workings within our internal and external environments. It is a quintessential example of applied science utilizing physics, chemistry, anatomy, physiology, pathology, and biomechanics, tempering this mix with psychology, sociology, and education. These working sciences are applied to situations that demand attention. The motivating factors may be pain, limited function, or the potential of injury. As such, it is a branch of physical therapy that encompasses many of the basic principles of the profession as a whole.

Orthopaedic physical therapy is an evolving science, one that owes much to the pioneers on whose efforts the field has been built and continues to grow. The American Physical Therapy Association (APTA) recognized the Orthopaedic Section as a special interest area in 1974 along with Pediatrics and Clinical Electrophysiology.[1] There was some initial reluctance to add additional sections because there was some concern that this would cause division in the organization. Fortunately, this has not been the case. By facilitating communication among therapists with similar interests, there has been a sharing of ideas and enthusiasm, which has enhanced the field.

One of the prime movers for the establishment of the Orthopaedic Section was Stanley Paris. He was interested in promoting manual and manipulative therapy to be a viable part of the field of physical therapy in the United States. Other countries had already embraced manipulation as part of physical therapy, but in the United States these techniques were primarily utilized by chiropractors and osteopaths. In 1968 Paris facilitated the formation of the North American Academy on Manipulation Therapy. This group provided educational seminars and interested many physical therapists in their manual approach. Paris continued his efforts to promote mobilization and manipulation techniques in becoming the first president of the Orthopaedic Section in 1974. In 1975 the APTA acknowledged mobilization as an appropriate treatment procedure for physical therapy.[2] In 1992, mobilization was noted as one of the skills that graduate physical therapists should possess as part of the *Evaluative Criteria for Accreditation of Educational Programs for the Preparation of Physical Therapists*.[3] That year also marked the establishment of the American Academy of Orthopaedic Manual Therapists.[4]

Mobilization, however, is not the only focus within today's Orthopaedic Section. There are special interest groups, which include Foot and Ankle, Performing Arts, Pain Management, Occupational Health, and Animal Physical Therapist (the last of these represents a developing area of the field that is generally not acknowledged as within the scope of present physical therapy practice). The section has grown to include over 11,000 members and deals with all areas that address orthopaedic physical needs. In doing so, there is overlap in areas specifically addressed by other sections: pediatrics, geriatrics, sports and hand rehabilitation, among others. Rather than compartmentalizing and limiting interaction, these overlaps are welcomed and the bodies of knowledge amassed by the efforts of those in other sections work to enhance rather than detract from an understanding of human function in different stages of their life and environment. The Sports and Orthopaedic Sections share a common research journal.

## MANUAL THERAPY

The manual therapy component of orthopaedic physical therapy was initially built on the work of physicians and clinicians that identified methods of evaluation and treatment for musculoskeletal disorders. Some of the more notable contributors to this body of knowledge include Dr James Cyriax, author of *Textbook of Orthopaedic Medicine*, and Dr James Mennell, author of *The Science and Art of Joint Manipulation* published in the 1950s. Mennell's son, John authored *Joint Pain*, which built on his father's work. Robert Maigne proposed that interventions should not be painful in his work *Les Manipulations Verebrales*.[5] Janet Travel (personal physician to three American presidents and acknowledged as the proponent of JFK utilizing a rocking chair) initially opposed physical therapists using the diagnostic skills inherent in evaluation for mobilization and manipulation, but she later embraced and taught the profession these skills. She is particularly known for her work on trigger point treatment. Geoffrey Maitland, a South Australian physiotherapist authored *Vertebral Manipulation* and *Peripheral Manipulation* and suggested carefully graded movements. Freddy Kaltenborn, a Norwegian practitioner, strongly emphasized the importance of joint surface interaction in the understanding of the joint movements.[3,5] Robin McKenzie, a New Zealand physiotherapist, devised an approach to back pain that emphasized the active role that patients needed to take in treatment of their back pain and specific movement and positioning techniques. Stanley Paris developed a curriculum of mobilization and manipulation for the spine and extremities. As the science of manipulation and mobilization became more accepted, many other names became more familiar as they provided continuing education courses for physical therapists in an effort to expand therapists' understanding and skills. Brian Mulligan, a New Zealand therapist, introduced a system of apophyseal gliding that emphasized self-mobilization techniques. Diane Lee, a Canadian therapist, wrote extensively on the lumbar spine and pelvic girdle. Olga Grimsby and Dos Winkle (a founder of the International Academy of Orthopaedic Medicine) provided additional insights to the growing body of knowledge of joint movement and soft tissue interaction.[6] Others that helped found the Orthopaedic Section and those who received training in the early years provided courses for the growing demand. Sandy Burkhart, the second president of the Orthopaedic Section, has taught extensively. Duane Saunders facilitated the concepts of "Back School." The American Academy of Orthopaedic Manual Therapists provided other opportunities for therapists looking to refine their skills in manual therapy by sponsoring continuing education courses and a research journal.[7]

Despite the notable contributions that many physicians, clinicians, and researchers have provided, there is no consensus on appropriate approaches to evaluation and treatment. This lack has led to the development of followings within manual therapy related to the theoretical constructs proposed by different authors. Some therapists develop an eclectic approach, choosing the elements of each approach that seem to work for their particular situation or patient. In spite of this lack of agreement, all the approaches have encouraged clinicians to thoroughly know their neuromusculoskeletal anatomy and consider the implications of structural interactions. This increased demand for this intricate knowledge level has provided the incentive for many to move beyond their initial training to develop additional expertise.

## PERIOPERATIVE CARE

Another major area of orthopaedic physical therapy is perioperative care. The association between orthopaedic surgeons and physical therapists is a natural and expected part of the field. This requires a knowledge and understanding of the surgical techniques used and of healing tissue response to allow development of the appropriate rehabilitation plan. As in all fields of medicine, this presents a challenge to the clinician to stay abreast of changing techniques. Physicians such as Frank Noyes and Neer have provided research and development of protocols for postoperative rehabilitation.

New technology can drastically change the role of the physical therapist. For example, the advent of arthroscopic knee surgery significantly shortened the rehabilitation timeline. More recently, techniques that use controlled heat to shrink loose tissues suggests that there is less need for extensive rehabilitation, but the exact reactions of this shortened tissue have not been fully determined over time. Artificial discs may represent another leap forward in the treatment of back pain and change the field again. Gene therapy is being investigated as a possible future of articular cartilage repair—an area that currently creates a need for numerous knee surgeries.

When dealing with the postoperative patient, like those who present in many other situations, surgery is not the only aspect of care to be considered. Additional diagnoses may confound what may be the preferred approach. A wrist fracture complicates the care of a patient who requires the use of a walker or crutches to walk. Cardiac or circulatory concerns may limit intensities of exercises that may be used. Nerve injuries can make a marked difference in the ability to rehabilitate a replaced joint. As most clinicians can readily attest, patients rarely have only one concern. Other factors to consider may be economic in nature, environmental, or societal. A worker who is to return to a difficult work situation may have little motivation to progress. An elderly person living alone may have difficulty managing independently but may not feel that he or she is able to afford or need intermediate care. A student athlete may feel that chances for scholarships are at risk if he or she do not participate in a particular game.

Therapists need to keep abreast of medications and their effects and be alert to adverse drug reactions in order to aid the physician in the coordination of the patient's care. The therapist may be the first one to identify signs of infection or other complications because she sees the patients on a regular basis. The therapist works as a part of the rehabilitation team, coordinating services with other professionals, family members, and the patient.

Reasonable goals have to be articulated based on the ongoing evaluation of the patient. Reestablishing a patient's maximum strength, range of motion, and function are major areas of focus. Delayed healing, adhesions, neural entrapment, excessive scarring, additional injuries, or a host of other problems may complicate attainment of these goals. All of these concerns speak to the need for the therapist to have a broad-based in-depth understanding of medical developments.

## GENERAL ORTHOPAEDICS

The third focus of orthopaedic physical therapy includes a plethora of neuromusculoskeletal concerns. Fracture care, ergonomics, shoe and extremity orthotics, gait deviations, treatment of localized inflammation, or overuse syndromes are some of the areas of expertise that the orthopaedic therapist needs to possess. Significant contributors to general orthopaedics have included Jennie McConnell, an Australian physiotherapist, who pioneered taping techniques to aid in treating muscular imbalances, Joanne Posner-Meyer and Caroline Creager, who highlighted the use of the Swiss ball in stabilization programs, and David Butler, whose work *Mobilization of the Nervous System* increased awareness of neural flexibility issues. The list of approaches and techniques seems ever-growing and includes positional release, craniosacral therapy and strain-counterstrain. Robert Donatelli and Michael Wooden's various editions of *Orthopaedic Physical Therapy* acknowledge the wide variety of skills and theory that form the basis for this field.

Some of the problems may have straightforward answers, others may require more investigative work. The apparently insidious onset of hamstring origin sensitivity might be attributable to a recent trip to a mountainous area and excessive uphill climbing. The headaches that only present themselves in the fall for an otherwise healthy teenager could be related to TMJ (jaw) pathomechanics that are aggravated by playing saxophone in marching band. The hip discomfort on one side of the body may be due to compensatory motion to make up for excessive pronation of the opposite foot. A change in job status requiring heavier lifting, compounded with excessive weight gain and poor posture, could be the precipitating factors for back discomfort. A poorly designed workstation and increased computer utilization combined with a new prescription for bifocals can be the cause of neck pain. To adequately treat these problems that may be expressed to the therapist as buttock pain, headaches, back pain, and neck pain, the therapist take into account the entire person and not just the site of injury. Treatment may be primarily directed to helping the patients recognize the aggravating factors and allowing them to help identify solutions. The orthopaedic therapist has to be ready with a variety of tools: education, exercise, and specific treatment modalities such as ice, ultrasound, stretching techniques, or devices.

To prepare therapists for this challenge, the Orthopaedic Section of the APTA has sponsored numerous continuing education opportunities, study groups, and home study courses.[8] The *Journal of Orthopaedic and Sports Physical Therapy* publishes case reports and studies as well as review articles and original research that present new approaches and concerns. Many schools and programs that certify some level of expertise have been developed by various organizations. Programs vary from a very narrow focus to those with a general musculoskeletal approach. Book publications on associated subjects seem to have appeared at an accelerated rate. All physical therapists have been challenged to present studies that validate the effectiveness of what they do. The field is faced with the challenge of basing practice on evidence rather than on teachings of experts that may have more charismatic appeal than scientific rationale for treatment approaches. This movement is not only the function of becoming more scientific in our approaches but also stimulated by the need to justify to insurance companies, patients, and physicians (our consumers) that what we practice has a solid factual base. Therefore, the student and clinician need to approach new developments (and untested theories) with skeptical enthusiasm that seeks scientific validation. With this directed research effort and analysis, the field can continue to evolve in a credible fashion.

## REFERENCES

1. Murphy W. *Healing the Generations: A History of Physical Therapy and the American Physical Therapy Association.* Lyme, CT: Greenwich Publishing Group; 1995: 198–199.
2. Paris S, Santi D. History of the Orthopaedic Section: The 1970s. *Orthop Phys Ther Pract.* 1999;11(1):7–8.
3. Farrell JP, Jensen GM. Manual therapy; a critical assessment of role in the profession of physical therapy. *Phys Ther.* 1992;72:843–852.
4. White N. Growth 1985 through 1992. *Orthop Phys Ther Pract.* 1999; 11(3):8–10
5. Paris S. History; Present day schools of thought. In: Course Notes. . .The Spine. Stanley Z Paris; 1979:14–34.
6. Orthopaedic Physical Therapy Products (OPTP) Catalog. Vol. 13.
7. Farrell J. Partnerships for survival. *Orthop Phys Ther Pract.* 1999;11(4):7–10.
8. Wadsworth C. As dreams became realities: 1980 through 1985. *Orthop Phys Ther Pract.* 1999;11(2):10–12.

CHAPTER 6

# Clinical Practice: Geriatric Physical Therapy

JENNIFER M. BOTTOMLEY

Geriatric physical therapy encompasses prevention of disability, rehabilitation when the need arises, and maintenance of maximal function capabilities in an older adult population. It requires a comprehensive, interdisciplinary, and holistic approach to care. Physical therapy is often complicated by multisystem changes and disease. The principles and practices of geriatric physical therapy differ in many respects from those applied to younger populations. It is the intent of this chapter to provide the reader with the various philosophies that make geriatric physical therapy unique. Additionally, the purpose of this chapter is to provide physical therapy students with a knowledge of rehabilitation principles and practices for working with the aged so that therapists can apply interventions to provide high-quality care.

Normal aging is not necessarily burdened with disability; however, almost all conditions that cause disability are more frequently seen in the older population. As a result, the aged are more likely to require assessment for rehabilitative services. Functional assessment for needed rehabilitative services should be an essential part of routine examination and evaluation by all health care disciplines working with the aged population. Geriatrics teaches that maximal functional capabilities be attained; therefore, it can be argued that rehabilitation is the foundation of geriatric care. The basis of geriatric physical therapy is to assist healthy elders to maintain the highest level of functioning and the disabled aged to recover lost physical, psychological, or social skills so that they may become more independent, live in personally satisfying environments, and maintain meaningful social interactions. This may be done in any number of settings including acute and subacute care settings, rehabilitation centers, home and office settings, or in long-term care facilities such as nursing homes.

Because of the complexity of the interventions needed in dealing with the aged, an *interdisciplinary* team approach is required. The rehabilitation process also requires education of patients and their families. Finally, rehabilitation is more than a medical intervention: it is a philosophical approach that recognizes that diagnoses and chronological age are poor predictors of functional abilities, that interventions directed at enhancing function are important, and that the "team" should always include patients and their families.

## DISABILITY: A DEFINITION

The meaning of disability is key to an understanding of geriatric rehabilitation. When referring to alterations in people's function, three terms are often used interchangeably: impairment, disability, and handicap. A more distinct understanding of these concepts is valuable in geriatric rehabilitation, and a "systems approach" is most useful. In the systems approach, a problem at the organ level (e.g., an infarct in the right hemisphere) must be viewed not only in terms of its effects on the brain, but also in terms of what its effects are on the person, the family, the society, and, ultimately, the nation. It goes beyond the pure "medical model," in which only the current medical problem is assessed to determine rehabilitative goals.[1] From this perspective "impairment" refers to a loss of physical or physiologic function at the organ level. These could include alterations in heart function, nerve conduction velocity, or muscle strength. Impairments usually do not affect the ability to function. However, if an impairment is so severe that it inhibits the ability to function "normally," then it becomes a "disability." Geriatric physical therapy rehabilitation interventions are most often oriented toward adaptation to or recovery from disabilities.[1] Given the proper training or adaptive equipment, people with disabilities can purse independent lives. However, obstructions in the pursuit of independence can arise when people with disabilities confront inaccessible buildings or situations that limit rehabilitation interventions, such as low toilet seats, buttons on an elevator that are too high, or signs that are not readable. In these cases a disability becomes a "handicap." Society's environment creates the handicap.[1]

## DEMOGRAPHICS OF DISABILITY IN THE AGED

The aged are disproportionately affected by disabling conditions when compared to younger cohorts. According to Guccione, the "old-old" age group (85 plus years of age) comprises the highest percentage of disabled persons; indeed, 40% of all disabled persons are over the age of 65. Three fourths of all cerebrovascular accidents occur in persons over the age of 65; the highest incidence of amputations has been reported in the aged; and hip fractures, on the average, most often occur between the ages of 70 and 78. The Federal Council on Aging has reported that, of all those persons studied over the age of 65, 86% have at least one chronic condition, and 52% have limitations in their activities of daily living. It is the impact of these disabilities on the level of independence that needs to be considered rather than the presence of an impairment or disability.

Disabilities in old age are associated with a higher mortality rate, a decreased life span, greater chronic health problems (e.g., cardiovascular, musculoskeletal, neurological), and an increased expenditure for health care. Disabilities resulting in an inability to ambulate, feed oneself, or manage basic activities of daily living like toileting or self-hygiene (e.g., bathing) are very strong predictors of loss of functional independence and an increased burden on caregivers.[2–4] The greater the disability, the greater the risk of institutionalization. Rehabilitative measures can be cost effective by enhancing functional ability and attaining greater levels of independence. Higher functional capabilities and greater levels of independence have been associated with fewer hospitalizations and a lower mortality rate among the aged.[1]

Geriatric physical therapy includes both institutional and noninstitutional services for the aged with chronic medical conditions that are marked by deviation from the "normal" state of health and manifested in physical impairment. Unless treated, these conditions have the potential for causing substantial and frequently cumulative disability. The aged with disabilities need assistance with such daily functions as bathing, dressing, and walking. This increased need for help is often compounded when there is no spouse, nearby family, or able friends. With this social isolation, common in the aged, continuing professional medical care is required to ward off the debilitating affects of inactivity and depression.

## MULTISYSTEM CHANGES

It is rare that an older adult has only one diagnosis. The national statistic for individuals over the age of 65 is six diagnoses on average.[1,2] Physical therapy in the elderly often requires treating more than one major condition at a time. Thus, critical pathways are often complicated by coexisting diseases and physical changes. One unique component of geriatric physical therapy is the need for a holistic approach to intervention. For example, someone referred to physical therapy after a total knee replacement may have a compromised cardiovascular system with history of myocardial infarct and claudication in the lower extremities. The cardiac status will limit the application of a standard total knee physical therapy protocol. Often, the cardiac condition becomes the priority in treatment intervention, and the total knee secondary. You cannot treat just the knee, you have to treat the whole person. The physical therapist working with the elderly needs a higher level of clinical decision-making skills than in any other area of physical therapy practice.

## FUNCTIONAL ASSESSMENT OF THE AGED

The assessment of functional capabilities is the cornerstone of geriatric physical therapy. The ability to walk, transfer from bed to chair or chair to toilet, for example, and manage basic activities of daily living independently is often the determinant of whether hospitalized aged patients will be discharged home or to an extended-care facility. Functional assessment tools that are practical, reliable, and valid are necessary to assist all interdisciplinary team members in determining the need for rehabilitation or long-term care services. In the home care setting, precise assessment of patients' function can detect early deterioration and allow for immediate intervention.

Functional capacity is defined as three levels of activities of daily living: (1) basic activities of daily living (ADL), including such self-care activities as bathing, dressing, toileting, continence, and feeding; (2) instrumental activities of daily living (IADL), such as using the telephone, driving, shopping, housekeeping, cooking, laundry, managing money, and managing medications; and (3) mobility, described as a more complicated combination of IADL activities, such as leaving one's residence and moving from one location to another by using public transportation. IADL and mobility are more complex and are concerned with people's ability to cope with their environments. This classification of ADL, IADL, and mobility has become standard in most functional assessment tools.[1]

As a clinical tool, functional assessment scales are invaluable. Initial assessment identifies areas of functional deficit and can assist the physical therapists in developing treatment regimens that address specific needs. Subsequent assessments measure progress toward rehabilitation goals. On a broader scale, functional assessment can assist public policymakers in the provision of health care services by determining the levels of need in a population. Demographically, it is apparent that Americans are living longer; the question is, are these added years of life years of vigor and independence or years of frailty and dependence?

By design, functional assessment scales are meant to determine specific outcomes. Outcomes of interest to those working with the aged include mortality, hospitalization, institutionalization, special interventions, and declining physical function, to name a few. Numerous functional assessment tools are available to determine physical, emotional, cognitive, and social functioning in various care settings.

## FUNCTIONAL ABILITIES OF THE CAREGIVER: A REHABILITATIVE CONSIDERATION

A neglected area of examination and evaluation in geriatric physical therapy is the functional abilities of caregivers for the elderly. Aged patients, given a choice, would prefer to stay at home rather than recuperate and rehabilitate in a institutional setting. The aged have strong ties to their homes, and the help of their spouses, other relatives, and friends is a crucial component in making rehabilitation in their homes possible. Home care, by professionals, can protect the health of informal caregivers and maximize patients' ability to perform ADLs by including a systematic assessment of the living environment as a key part of care planning. Provision of such assistance openly acknowledges that caregivers, who are often aged themselves, have some decrease in physical ability that needs to be considered as it relates to caring for disabled relatives. It has been demonstrated that more than 90% of persons 75 to 84 years of age can manage without help to perform such tasks as grooming, bathing, dressing, eating, and other basic ADLs. The more complicated skills of transferring and ambulation are more compromised with greater than 50% of persons aged 75 to 84 years of age presenting with limitations in their capabilities of performing these activities without assistance.[5] These ADLs require greater assistive skills on the part of the caregiver. Assessment of the home environment needs to incorporate the abilities (or disabilities) of the individual(s) providing care. Adaptive equipment, such as a sliding board for transfers or a rolling walker for ambulation, is available to assist the caregiver in caring for his or her spouse, relative, or friend. Attention to the abilities of the caregiver can facilitate the ease of care and decrease the burden placed on the caregiver.[1] The provision of home health care services may be necessitated when safety is an issue. Thorough evaluation of the functional capabilities of the aged individual and the caregiver, in addition to assessment of the environmental obstacles that may be encountered, will increase the likelihood of a positive outcome.

## PRINCIPLES OF GERIATRIC REHABILITATION

Three major principles are important in the rehabilitation of the aged. First, variability of the aged must be considered. Variability of capabilities within an aged group is much more pronounced than within younger cohorts. What one 80 year old can do physically, cognitively, or motivationally, another may not be able to accomplish. Second, the concept of activity is key in rehabilitation of the aged. Many of the changes over time are attributable to disuse. Finally, optimum health is directly related to optimum functional ability. In acute situations rehabilitation must be directed toward (1) stabilizing the primary problem(s), (2) preventing secondary complications (such as bed sores, pneumonia, and contractures), and (3) restoring lost functions. In chronic situations rehabilitation is directed primarily toward restoring lost functions. This can best be accomplished by promoting maximum health so that the aged are best able to adapt to their care environment and to their disabilities. Each of these principles—variability, inactivity, and optimum health—will be discussed in greater detail in the following sections.

### Variability of the Aged

Unlike any other age group, the aged are more variable in their level of functional capabilities. In the clinic, we often see 65-year-old individuals who are severely physically disabled, yet sitting right alongside of that individual is a 65 year old who is still building houses and felling trees. Even in old old age, variability in physical and cognitive functioning is remarkable. An example of physical variability is John Kelly, who at the age of 89 was still running the Boston Marathon, compared to a frail bedridden 89-year-old person in a nursing home who is not responsive to his or her environment.[1] Cognitively, the differences can also be identified as remarkable. The spectrum spans from the demented institutionalized aged to those aged who are presidents and Supreme Court justices. Chronological age is a poor indicator of physical or cognitive function.

The impact of this variability is an important consideration in defining rehabilitation principles and practices of the aged. A wide range of rehabilitative services needs to be provided to address the varying needs of the aged population in different care settings. Awareness of this heterogeneity helps to combat the myths and stereotypes of aging and presents a foundation for developing creative rehabilitation programs for the aged. Older persons tend to be more different from themselves (as a collective group) than other segments of the population. Given this fact, interdisciplinary team members, policy makers, and planners in rehabilitation settings need to be prepared to design a wide range of services and treatment interventions. This becomes more difficult as the number of aged increases and the budget decreases; however, creating new and innovative rehabilitation programs could ultimately improve the functional capabilities and the resulting quality of life for many aged individuals.

## Activity Versus Inactivity

The most common reason for losses in functional capabilities in the aged is inactivity or immobility. There are numerous reasons for immobilizing the aged. "Acute" immobilization is often considered to be "accidental immobilization."[1] Acute catastrophic illnesses include severe blood loss, trauma, head injury, cerebral vascular accidents, burns, and hip fracture, to name only a few. Activity level is often severely curtailed until acute illnesses become medically stable. Chronic immobilization may result from longstanding problems that are undertreated or left untreated. Examples of chronic problems include cerebral vascular accidents (strokes), amputations, arthritis, Parkinson's disease, cardiac disease, pulmonary disease, and low back pain. Environmental barriers are a major cause of "accidental immobilization" in both the acute and chronic care settings. These include bedrails, the height of the bed, physical restraints, an inappropriate chair, no physical assistance available, fall precautions imposed by medical staff, or no orders in the chart for mobilization, social isolation, and environmental obstacles (stairs or doorway thresholds are examples). Cognitive impairments, CNS disorders such as cerebral vascular accidents, Parkinson's disease, multiple sclerosis, peripheral neuropathies resulting from diabetes, and pain with movement can also severely reduce mobility. Affective disorders such as depression, anxiety, or fear of falling may also lead to accidental immobilization. In addition, sensory changes, terminal illnesses such as cancer or cirrhosis of the liver, acute episodes of illness like pneumonia or cellulitis, or an attitude of "I'm too sick to get up" can negatively affect mobility.

The process of deconditioning involves changes in multiple organ systems including the neurological, cardiovascular, and musculoskeletal systems to varying degrees. Deconditioning is probably best defined as the multiple changes in organ system physiology that are induced by inactivity and reversed by activity (i.e., exercise).[1] The degree of deconditioning depends on the degree of superimposed inactivity and the prior level of physical fitness. The term *hypokinetics* has been coined to describe the physiology of inactivity.[6] Deconditioning can occur at many levels of inactivity. For simplicity and clarity, I will look at the two major categories of inactivity or hypokinetics. First, the acute hypokinetic effects of bed rest. Second, the chronic inactivity induced by a sedentary lifestyle or chronic disease–induced hypokinetics.

Looking at the aging process with one eye on the adverse affects of bed rest or hypokinetics as a possible concommitant of deconditioning and disability can lead us to discover more about the potential use of exercise as one of our primary rehabilitation modalities. The phrase "use it or lose it" is a concept with tremendous ramifications for aging, especially in geriatric rehabilitation. Exercise has not been viewed as an important factor in health until recently. Until the 1950s the rate-of-living theory was promoted. According to this theory, the body would be worn out faster and life shortened by expending energy exercising.[7] Conversely, studies in the past decade have shown that regular exercise does not shorten life span, and may, in fact, increase it. Exercise is becoming increasingly viewed as beneficial for both the primary and secondary prevention of disease.[8]

There are several challenges to understanding the interaction between inactivity and health in older persons. The first is that the process of aging itself causes some changes that parallel the consequences of hypokinetics or inactivity.[1,8] Several studies have provided strong evidence that separates the aging process from the sedentary lifestyle.[8,9] It has been found that aged individuals can improve their flexibility, strength, and aerobic capacity to the same extent as younger individuals. It is obvious that some effects of "aging" can be directly related to inactivity. The second challenge in studying inactivity is separating the effects of inactivity from those of disease.[1,9] Many aged individuals who are deconditioned may also have superimposition of acute or chronic disease. Recent studies on younger subjects have helped to clarify some of the effects of inactivity alone (i.e., bed rest on physiologic changes and functional performance).[8] Another challenge exists. That is the challenge of understanding the relationship between physiologic decline and functional loss. Is the inability to climb stairs in an 85-year-old primarily from cardiovascular deconditioning, muscle weakness, or impaired balance secondary to sensory losses or a sedentary lifestyle? Is there a new disease process beginning? Is this normal aging? Is it simply a lack of practice that leads to functional decline?[1] An important concept in geriatric rehabilitation is that "threshold" values of physiologic functioning may exist.[1] Below these thresholds an aged person may suddenly lose an essential functional skill. An understanding of the consequences of inactivity is particularly important in addressing rehabilitation needs of the aged individual.

Inactivity's effect on the nervous system has not been studied as intensely as other organ systems. Perhaps this is related to the complexity of the nervous system and the lack of assessment techniques. In younger individuals changes in the nervous system with inactivity are minimal. In the aged, however, especially those individuals with concurrent acute or chronic illnesses, the consequences of inactivity on the nervous system may be particularly extreme.[1] Bed rest has been compared to the experience of sensory deprivation. Zubek and Wilgosh,[10] in a classic study of prolonged immobilization (i.e., immobilized during the day followed by bed rest at night), showed that occipital lobe frequencies seen on an electroencephalogram were substantially decreased in awake subjects. Exercise prevented some of these changes.[18] In addition to physical changes, performance on several intellectual tests deteriorated including verbal fluency, color discrimination, and reversible figures. These consequences could have a significant impact on an aged individual's level of functioning and rehabilitation potential.

The neuropsychologic consequences of a chronic level of inactivity, as in a sedentary lifestyle, are not easy to determine. Shepard[11] found that a moderate level of physical activity makes a person feel better, leading to better intellectual and psychomotor development. The underlying mechanism may include increased arousal, improved self-esteem and body image, and a decreased level of anxiety, stress, and depression.

Chronic inactivity also negatively affects balance. Postural sway is known to increase with aging. Inactivity may contribute to the progression of this decline. Research indicates that balance is better in active compared to inactive older adults. Results are similar for different types of exercise (e.g., golf, walking, range-of-motion exercise, conditioning exercises). In a study by Wolf, standing balance on one foot was improved following implementation of an exercise program.[12] A sedentary lifestyle is also associated with prolonged reaction times.[13] A comparison between young compared with older persons revealed an 8% decline in reaction and movement times when age was considered alone. A 22% decrement was present when non-active young and old groups were compared. "Exercise prevents the cycle in which disuse increases brain metabolism leading to decreased blood flow and neuronal loss."[8]

The summary of the effects of inactivity on the nervous system is of great significance in geriatric rehabilitation. Acute bed rest induces some cognitive changes including distortion of time perception and decrements in some intellectual tests. Mood changes occur as well. Consequences on cognitive and emotional function of chronic inactivity may include a poorer sense of well-being. Balance is impaired after both acute and chronic inactivity. Prolonged reaction times are associated with chronic inactivity. Realizing the consequences of inactivity superimposed on the "normal" changes with aging should alert the rehabilitation team to the importance of maintaining activity and maximal functional capabilities in the aged person.

Changes in the cardiovascular system have been studied most in relation to inactivity versus activity. An aged individual in good physical condition responds to submaximal exercise levels without significant increases in heart rate or blood pressure. In contrast, a deconditioned person encountering minimal to moderate activity level experiences a marked increase in these vital signs. Maximal workloads elicit similar increases in heart rate and blood pressure in both deconditioned and conditioned individuals;

however, the recovery rate (i.e., the return to resting vital sign values) is slower in deconditioned individuals.

Within the first week of bed rest there is a noted increase in resting heart rate.[11] In other words, the work of the heart is increased despite the fact that the body remains at rest. In very early studies on the effects of bed rest on cardiovascular function, it was found that by the end of the third week of bed rest the morning heart rate increased by as much as 21% and the evening heart rate by 33%. This is an average increase in resting heart rate of approximately 1 beat for every 2 bed rest days. Other investigations showed approximately a 4-beat increase, documenting lesser increases in resting heart rate over a 1-week period.[8,9] In each of these studies, 6 weeks of submaximal exercise was necessary before the resting heart rate returned to its baseline value. Total blood volume has been found to decrease after several weeks of inactivity.[8] These findings were based on studies of astronauts in the aerospace program, a presumably healthy group of individuals. It was determined that plasma volume decrements were greater than red cell mass decrements. Such a change could have significant import for older persons. There is a strong possibility that a decrease in total blood volume could be correlated with orthostatic hypotension in the aged, although this has not been studied in an elderly population to date.

Orthostatic hypotension occurs within the first week of inactivity in young subjects. This, and other cardiovascular signs of deconditioning, occurs even with armchair rest.[1,8] Orthostasis resolves very slowly, even when the recovery period includes maximal exercise levels.

In addition to the deterioration of the cardiovascular system at rest, any level of activity above the resting level becomes more strenuous. At submaximal levels of exercise, heart rate increases of 10 to 20 beats are common in the deconditioned individual. In addition to an increase in the heart rate, the stroke volume tends to decrease, making the heart less efficient in delivering blood to the working muscles.[1] Delayed recovery rates also indicate an increased cardiac and metabolic stress. The return to baseline heart rate in the conditioned individuals occurs in less than 2 minutes and the systolic blood pressure returns to a resting level within 4 minutes. After 6 weeks of bed rest imposed on a healthy individual, it takes 3 to 6 minutes for the heart rate and 5 to 7 minutes for the systolic blood pressure to return to pre-exercise resting levels.[11]

The cardiovascular consequences of chronic inactivity are similar to those seen in acute bed rest. Resting heart rates are higher. At submaximal activity levels, heart rate and blood pressure are greater than in physically fit individuals performing at the same intensity of exercise. Maximal oxygen uptake is lower than in individuals who exercise aerobically. The well-documented decline in maximal oxygen uptake with age is half as great in physically active individuals compared to inactive persons. The recovery rate is prolonged. The biggest difference in acute versus chronic inactivity effects on the cardiovascular system are the cumulative effects of long-term inactivity. In other words, the longer an individual remains inactive, the more pronounced the aforementioned cardiovascular changes are, and the longer it takes to return to a "healthy" pre-deconditioned baseline.[1]

Alterations in skeletal muscle with aging and with inactivity resemble those observed with denervation. It is well known that decreases in muscle mass occur with old age, with proximal muscles of the lower extremity particularly affected. This decrease in muscle mass is due to a decrease in both fiber number and diameter. No change in the number of motor neural fibers has been found, but the size of the motor unit decreases due to the loss of muscle fibers.[1] With aging and with inactivity then, we see a loss of lean body mass. The same changes are also observed in younger subjects on bed rest and in astronauts in a gravity-free environment.[8,9,11] Exercise positively affects body composition. It is reported that a loss of approximately 1.5% of muscle mass per day during a 2-week period of inactivity occurs.[8] Most of the studies on bed-rest effects on skeletal muscle have been done on younger subjects. The amount of strength lost by aged persons during bed rest has not been extensively studied. However, inactivity superimposed on the normal aging process previously mentioned is likely to have significant disabling consequences. The decrement in strength with aging is likely to be due partially to inactivity. Exercise programs have been found to improve strength in all age groups.[11–14]

The skeletal system functions to support, protect, and shape the body. Additionally, bone has the metabolic functions of blood cell production, the storage of calcium, and a role in acid-base balance. The most commonly known age-related change involving bone is calcium-related loss of mass and density. This loss ultimately causes the pathologic condition of osteoporosis. Bone density is lost from within by a process termed *reabsorption*. As we grow older, an imbalance occurs between osteoblast activity (bone build up) and osteoclast activity (breaks down bone).[15] Bone mass and strength decline with age. Osteoporosis is a major bone mineral disorder in the older adult. Qualitatively, osteoporotic bone exhibits a reduction in bone mass with a resulting decrease in bone strength. This is exacerbated with inactivity.[8,15]

In the pulmonary system, age changes and changes associated with inactivity can be organized according to mechanical properties, changes in flow, changes in volume, alteration in gas exchange, and impairments of lung defense. Decreases in chest wall compliance and lung elastic recoil tendency are two mechanical properties that are altered with age. Increased calcification of the ribs, a decline in intercostal muscle strength, and changes in the spinal curvature (resulting from osteoporotic collapse of the thoracic vertebrae) all result in a lower compliance and increased work of breathing.

Ventilation, diffusion, and pulmonary circulation are the three major components of the respiratory system that lose efficiency with age. There is an increased thickening of the supporting membranes between the alveoli and the capillaries, a decline in total lung capacity, an increase in residual volume, a reduced vital capacity, and a decrease in the resiliency of the lungs. It is difficult to completely separate pulmonary changes resulting with age from those associated with the pathology of emphysema or chronic bronchitis. Throughout a lifetime, exposure to occupational and environmental inhalants as well as cigarette smoke may result in chronic pulmonary changes and lung disease. These disease states closely parallel those of the aging process and also increase in incidence with advancing age.[16] Normal pulmonary aging includes a loss of elastic tissue leading to expiratory collapse of the larger airways, difficulty with expiration, and dilatation of the terminal air passages.

Aging and inactivity also affect the diffusion efficiency of the peripheral vascular system. Starting with the pulmonary system, impairment of gas exchange is illustrated by a reduced diffusing capacity of carbon monoxide, a lower resting arterial oxygen tension, and an increased alveolar–arterial oxygen gradient. Alveolar surface area and pulmonary capillary blood volume diminish with age. As a result, the oxygen dissociation curve shifts to the left, which makes oxygen less available at the tissue level. The ability to provide oxygen to working tissues diminishes with inactivity. Normal aging affects the cardiopulmonary system in a variety of ways as already discussed; however, in the absence of disease, the heart and lungs can generally meet the body's needs. The most evident change in cardiovascular and cardiopulmonary functioning with bed rest is that the reserve capacities are diminished. In other words, with any challenge, the body's demand for oxygen and perfusion may exceed available supply.

Of importance clinically in an older person is that normal aging causes changes and a decreased level of mobility results in an impairment of pulmonary defenses. Cilia are reduced in number and those that remain become less strong. The "mucous escalator" and alveolar macrophages (the germ killers) are less effective in removing inhaled particulate matter. In the absence of physiologic challenges, the system maintains fairly adequate defenses. However, an older individual who is chronically exposed to particle-laden air in addition to inactivity (which in essence diminishes the efficiency of the lungs) will become at risk for pulmonary dysfunction.[16]

As previously mentioned in regard to bed rest, the postexercise recovery period following effort is prolonged. Among other factors, this reflects a greater relative work rate, an increased proportion of anaerobic metabolism, a slower heat elimination, and a lower level of physical fitness. Extremes of immobilization can lead to a decrease in joint range of motion secondary to connective tissue changes. As a person ages, there is an increased criss-crossing or cross-linkage of the fibers that results in more dense extracellular matrices. The collagen structure becomes more stiff as it becomes more dense. The increased density also impairs molecular movement of nutrients and wastes at the cellular level.[1,6,11] Structurally, elastin fibers also develop increased cross-linkage with age. Water and elasticity are lost. The elastin fibers become more rigid, may tend to fray and, in some cases, are replaced by collagen completely. The clinical significance of this increased cross-linking is seen in resultant collagenous contractures. Bonds between adjacent collagen strands can produce shortening and distortion of the collagen fibers. This shortening may result in contractures with a progressive restriction in tissue mobility. Fibrinous adhesions have great clinical implications in working with the elderly. Some decrements in flexibility can be reversed by exercise.[8,11] The most effective means of maintaining mobility is early intervention with bed exercises. What is not lost does not need to be regained. Prevention of contractures is of extreme importance in geriatric physical therapy, and the only way to accomplish this is to maintain activity (even if an aged person is on bed rest).

## Optimal Health

The last principle in geriatric rehabilitation is the principle of "optimal health." The great English statesman, Benjamin Disraeli, said, "The health of people is really the foundation upon which all their happiness and their powers as a state depend." The World Health Organization (WHO) defines health as a state of complete physical, mental, and social well-being, not merely the absence of disease or infirmity.[17] The existence of complete physical health refers to the absence of disease, impairment, or disability. Physical health is quite conceivable. Mental and social well-being are closely related, and possibly less obtainable today. Mental health as defined by WHO would include cognitive and intellectual intactness as well as emotional well-being. The social components of health would include living situation, social roles (e.g., mother, daughter, vocation), and economic status.

As seen in normal aging changes, there are some cumulative effects biologically, physiologically, and anatomically that may eventually lead to clinical symptoms. It has also been noted in the section on activity versus inactivity that some of these changes are associated with inactivity and not purely a result of progressive aging effects. In light of this, I would suggest that a preventive approach to physical health needs to be in the foreground when addressing the needs of the aged. Preventing impairment and disability is a key principle in geriatric rehabilitation. It is reasonable to assume that the health status of an individual in their 70s and subsequent decades of life are in a suboptimal range. Thus, the scope of health status for the aged should be focused toward preventing the complications that could result from that suboptimal health condition. In considering suboptimal health, the goal of geriatric physical therapy should be to strive for relative optimal health, i.e., the maximal functional and physical capabilities of the aged individual considering their current health status.[1]

In reviewing the importance of promoting relative optimal health in terms of the musculoskeletal, sensory, or cardiopulmonary system, an example of an aged woman with a hip fracture may help in illustrating the concept of optimal health. She may be in suboptimal health and suffering from osteoporosis, but we do not treat her until she fractures her hip. The resulting complications could include pneumonia, decubiti from bed rest, all of the changes previously noted in relation to inactivity, in addition to the possibility of death. We need to intervene at the suboptimal level rather than wait for illness or disability to occur. This intervention could include weight-bearing exercises to enhance the strength of the bone, strengthening exercises of the lower extremities to provide adequate stability and endurance, balance exercises to facilitate effective balance reactions and safety, education in nutrition, and modification of her living environment to ensure added safety in hopes of avoiding the "fall" that results in a hip fracture.[1] Another excellent example of preventive intervention to maintain optimal health is in the example of the case of the diabetic aged individual. It is known that sensory loss in the lower extremities resulting from diabetes mellitus often predisposes that individual to ulceration of the foot. An ill-fitting shoe or a wrinkle in the sock may go unnoticed and lead to friction, skin breakdown, and a resulting foot ulcer. If undetected, even the smallest ulcer may lead to amputation of a lower extremity. Screening of the foot during evaluation can prevent this devastating loss. Intervention could include education of the aged individual in foot inspection (or education of a family member or friend if the diabetic aged individual's eyesight is compromised), proper shoe fitting, and techniques for dealing with their sensory loss (i.e., as temperature sensation diminishes, the individual needs to test bath water temperature with a thermometer, or have the spouse test the water, before putting her or his insensitive feet into a steamy bath). With proper skin care and professional (podiatric) care of the nails and callouses, there is less likelihood that injury will occur.[18]

Encouraging healthy behaviors such as decreasing obesity, stress, and smoking, and increasing activity could be the elements necessary in maintaining health and striving for optimal health as defined by WHO.[17] As health care professionals involved in geriatric rehabilitation, we need to be good **evaluators** and **screeners**. Good investigative skills could detect a minor problem with the potential of developing into a major problem. A thorough assessment of physical, cognitive, social, and emotional needs could help us to modify rehabilitation programs accordingly to truly improve the health and functional ability of our aged clients.

## REHABILITATIVE MEASURES

Rehabilitation should be directed at preventing premature disability. A deconditioned aged individual is less capable of performing activities than a conditioned aged individual. For example, the speed of walking is positively correlated to the level of physical fitness in an aged person.[1] When cardiovascular capabilities are diminished (i.e., maximum aerobic capacity), walking speeds are adjusted by the aged person to levels of comfort. Himann[19] found that exercise programs geared for improving cardiovascular fitness improved the speed of walking. The more conditioned the individual, the faster the walking pace.

If disease and physical disability are superimposed on a hypokinetic sequelae, the functional consequences can be disastrous. Pain often prevents mobility. For instance, the pain experienced by an aged individual with an acute exacerbation of osteoarthritic knee pain accompanied by inflammation of the knee capsule may reflexively inhibit quadriceps' contraction. Although the quadriceps' strength may have been poor in the first place due to inactivity, the absence of pain still permitted this individual to rise from a chair or ascend shallow steps. Now, with the presence of acute pain, these activities cause severe discomfort and threaten the capability of maintaining an independent lifestyle. In this situation, rehabilitation efforts should focus medically on reducing the inflammation through drugs or ice (physician, nurse); maintaining the joint's mobility during the acute phases by joint mobilization techniques of oscillation and low-grade passive range in addition to modalities such as interferential current to assist in reducing the edema and decreasing the discomfort (physical therapy); joint protection techniques and prescription of adaptive equipment such as a walker to protect the joint (occupational and physical therapy); provision for proper nutrition in light of medications/nutrient (pharmacist/dietician) effects and evidence that vitamin C is a crucial component in health of the synovium[20]; and social and psychological support (e.g., social worker, psychologist, religious personnel) to provide emotional and motivational support. These interventions to prevent the debilitating effects of bed rest highlight the need for an interdisciplinary approach when addressing geriatric rehabilitation.

Rehabilitation of the aged individual should emphasize functional activity to maintain functional mobility and capability, improvement of balance through exercise and functional activity programs (i.e., weight-shifting exercises, ambulation with direction and elevation changes, and reaching activities, to name a few), good nutrition and good general care (including hygiene, hydration, bowel and bladder considerations, and rest) as well as social and emotional support. It is important to optimize overall health status by implementing the concept of "independence." The more individuals do for themselves, the more they are capable of doing independently. The more that is done for an aged individual, the less capable he or she becomes of functioning on an optimal independent level and the more likely the progression of a disability. The advancing stages of disabilities increase the individual's vulnerability to illness, emotional stress, and injury. Aged persons' subjective appraisal of their health status influences how they react to their symptoms, how vulnerable they consider themselves, and when they decide they can or cannot accomplish an activity. Often an aged person's self-appraisal of her or his health is a good predictor to rehabilitation clinician's evaluation of health and functional status, but such assessments may also differ in many ways. In older persons, perceptions of one's health may be determined in large part by one's level of psychological well-being and by whether one continues in rewarding roles and activities.[1]

Exercise programs have potential for improving physical fitness, agility, and speed of response.[11] They also serve to improve muscle strength, flexibility, bone health, cardiovascular and respiratory response, and tolerance to activity.[9,12] Evidence suggests that reaction time is better in elders who engage in physical exercise than in those who are sedentary.[12,14] In addition, exercise has been shown to provide social and psychological benefits affecting the quality of life and the sense of well-being in the elderly.[1] Intuitively, it would appear plausible that an aged individual who is in better physical condition will experience less functional decline and maintain a higher level of independence and a resulting improvement in his or her perceived quality of life. The risks of encouraging physical activity are small and can be minimized through careful examination and evaluation.

A general measure to ensure the highest functional capacity should encourage early resumption of daily activities following trauma or acute illness. Safety measures to prevent falls and avoid accidents should include reinforcing wearing properly fitted shoes with good soles, low broad heels, and heel cups or orthotics to stabilize the foot during ambulation; the importance of wearing prescription eye glasses needs to be stressed; and the staff and family should be educated in reducing potential hazards within the patient's living environment (i.e., decreasing the amount of furniture, fixing loose carpeting, obtaining a commode, installing handrails around the toilet and tub areas, and railings in the hallways as needed). These are just a few examples of safety-proofing the environment in which the elder lives so that the individual may function at his maximum level. Adaptive equipment to enhance the ease of activities of daily living is very helpful. Adapting the environment to improve safety is essential in geriatric rehabilitation.

Pain management is a very important factor in geriatric rehabilitation. Pain is one of the most difficult pathophysiologic phenomena to define. Pain is human perception or recognition of a noxious stimulus. In geriatric rehabilitation we deal with two basic types of pain: acute and chronic. Chronic pain can be broken down even further into two subcategories: acute-chronic and chronic-chronic. Treatment of acute pain may include medications to reduce inflammation, ice, heat, or compression (also to reduce edema when warranted), rest, and gentle mobility exercises. (Low-grade oscillation techniques of joint mobilization are very helpful in pain relief and maintenance of joint mobility.) Rarely are modalities such as ultrasound or electrical currents (high galvanic current reduces edema, interferential current neutralizes the tissue and assists in fluid removal) used in the acute pain situation in the aged individual, although they are widely used in acute sports-related injuries in younger populations. The reasons for this are not documented, although this author's clinical experience teaches that the more conservative approaches of rest, ice, compression or elevation, and gentle exercise in combination with nonnarcotic analgesics seem to be quite effective in treating acute pain in the older person.

Chronic pain is more frequently observed in the aged and is more difficult to control. Chronic pain may not always correspond with objective findings. It is well recognized that emotional and socioeconomic factors play a role in chronic pain. Tension and anxiety often lead to muscle tension and decreased activity. This can be a vicious cycle. Situational depression may exacerbate this type of pain. In management of acute-chronic pain (such as the example of an acute osteoarthritic condition), treatment is similar to the acute pain management with the exception of the inclusion of various modalities. For instance, ultrasound may be used to break up a tissue adhesion, interferential or high-galvanic electrical stimulation may be used to break up adhesions, reduce swelling, and enhance the circulation to the painful area. Joint mobilization techniques are often employed to improve and maintain mobility. Nonnarcotic analgesics can be prescribed, but the aged are more susceptible to the cumulative effects as well as side effects of these drugs.

Foot pain and discomfort from bony changes such as those induced by lifelong use of ill-fitting shoes, arthritic changes, or age-related shifting of the fat pads under the heel and the metatarsal heads can severely curtail the ambulatory abilities of the aged. Proper shoe gear and shock-absorbing orthotics that place the foot in a neutral position have been clinically observed to facilitate ambulation and prevent disability. Assistive devices such as a cane, a quad cane (a more stable 4-legged cane), or a walker can also be prescribed to improve stability during ambulation and reduce the stresses on painful joint.

Wheelchair prescription may be necessary for longer distances (usually recommended for use outside the home) or when ambulation is no longer possible (i.e., in the case of a bilateral amputation or severe diabetic neuropathy). Wheelchairs should be prescribed to meet the specific needs of the aged individual. For instance, removable arms may be needed to enhance the ease of transfers, or when severe cardiac disease results in lower extremity edema, elevating leg rests may be prescribed for lower extremity elevation. Likewise, if upper extremity capabilities are limited by advanced rheumatoid arthritis or quadriplegia, an electric wheelchair will greatly improve that individual's capabilities of locomotion. Other considerations may be a one-arm manual drive chair for a hemiplegic or a "weighted" chair to shift the center of gravity and improve the stability of the chair in transfers for the bilateral amputee. All of these considerations necessitate the team approach in obtaining the equipment that best suits the needs of the individual.

Proper positioning and seating for the aged individual that requires extended periods in sitting is required to decrease discomfort and keep pressures off of bony prominences, provide adequate postural support, facilitate feeding, and prevent progression of joint contractures and deformities. Many "geri-chairs" are on the market that address specific positioning needs. Arm chairs that assist in rising from a seated position include higher chairs that decrease the work of the lower extremities for standing or electric "ejection" chairs that actually extend to bring the individual to a near-standing position. Functional assessment of the aged person is vital in the prescription of these specialized devices.

## SPECIAL GERIATRIC REHABILITATION CONSIDERATIONS

### Nutrition

I review nutrition here only as it impacts on functional capabilities. A car needs gas in order to run; a human being needs adequate energy sources in order to function on an optimal level. Nutritional levels need close monitoring in relation to energy needs and functional activity levels. Increased feeding difficulties may be secondary to decreased appetite, poor oral status, visual or sensorimotor agnosia, cognitive declines (decreasing attentiveness), and physical limitations. Environmental cues and adaptive eating equipment can often be employed to facilitate feeding. Postural considerations need to be addressed as well. A poor sitting posture can further decrease the ease of feeding by preventing upper extremity movement or making chewing and swallowing difficult as a result of head position.

Specialized feeding programs may be necessitated if there is neuromuscular involvement. For instance, an aged person sustaining a cerebral vascular accident may have difficulty swallowing or may have mouth closure due to weakness in the muscles needed for these activities. In these cases, specialized muscle facilitation techniques can be employed to promote swallowing and facilitate mouth closure. Commonly termed a *dysphasia team*, made up of nursing, dietary, speech, physical, and occupational therapy, the feeding needs of a neurologically involved individual can be comprehensively addressed. This team in the geriatric rehabilitation setting is a vital component in obtaining maximal functional capabilities. They function to promote adequate nutrition through neuromuscular facilitation techniques, proper posturing and supportive seating, and adaptive eating utensils. Ultimately, the goal of this team is to permit independent feeding by the aged person.

## Falls

Falls are not part of the normal aging process. They are due to an interaction of underlying physical dysfunction, medications, and environmental hazards.[1] Poor health status, impaired mobility from inactivity or chronic illness, postural instability, and a history of previous falls are observable risk factors. The ultimate goals of rehabilitation are to combat the inactivity and loss of mobility that predisposes to falls. Some of the ad hoc measures currently used to prevent falls—physical restraints and medications to reduce activity—are now suspected of increasing the risk of falling.[21]

The fear of falling is often a cause for inactivity. This is commonly seen in an individual who has sustained a previous fall. The guarding patterns that aged individuals use as a result of this fear (i.e., grabbing furniture that may not be stable or supportive) may, in fact, lead to further danger. Intervention by a psychiatrist or psychologist is often necessary to diminish this fear.

Functionally, limitations of range of motion, decreased muscle strength, joint mobility, coordination problems, or gait deviations can predispose an aged individual to falling. Specific strengthening and gait training programs assist in preventing falls by improving overall strength and coordination, balance responses and reaction time, and awareness of safe ambulation practices (for example, freeing one hand for use of a handrail when carrying packages up the stairs). Some individuals will have inadequate strength and balance to ambulate without an assistive device. Assistive ambulatory devices may also provide a safer mode for locomotion. Walking aids such as canes and walkers are beneficial for prevention of falls in some cases, whereas, in other cases, they actually contribute to the cause of the fall.

Gait evaluation is one of the most important components in fall prevention. The "get-up-and-go" test is a method used often to test strength, balance, coordination, and safety during gait. The aged individual is asked to get up out of the chair without using her hands, walk approximately 20 feet down the hall, turn around and come back to the chair, and then stand still. While standing still with the eyes closed, a gentle push on the sternum can be given to test righting reflexes. Finally, the individual is directed to sit down without the use of her hands. Each component of the test is analyzed. For instance, the inability to arise from the chair without the assistance of the hands is indicative of hip extensor and/or quadriceps weakness. If step symmetry is absent (i.e., the individual is taking irregular steps), the cause can often be pinpointed just by observation. A leg length discrepancy may be present or the hip abductors may be weak. These alterations in anatomical structure or muscle status can easily be determined by close evaluation of the gait pattern. Lower extremity pain may also result in irregular steps as the individual attempts to avoid the painful extremity. A tendency to veer, lose balance, or hold on to surrounding objects may be indicative of dizziness, muscle weakness, or poor vision. While turning, loss of balance or a stiff, disjointed turn may alert the clinician to the possibility of neurological disorders such as Parkinson's disease or drug-induced muscle rigidity (often seen in aged individuals on psychotrophic drugs such as haloperidol).

With good basic patient and family education and modification of the environment to reduce hazards, it is possible to prevent falls through methods that do not undermine mobility or autonomy. It is important to identify and treat reversible medical conditions, as well as physical impairments in gait and balance. Many falls can be prevented through proper exercise to maintain strength, sensory integration techniques to promote all functional activities by improving balance and coordination, good shoes and orthotics to provide a proper base of support and gait training activities, and modifications to "safety-proof" the living environment.

Rehabilitation specialists have an important role in recommending interventions to prevent falls. When disease states and medications responses are stable, an individualized program of safety education, environmental adaptations, lower extremity strengthening exercises, balance exercises, and gait training should be implemented.

Safety education is an important first step in the prevention of falls. Many older individuals are not aware that they are at risk for falling. Often, simple instructions about environmental adaptations and encouraging a person to allow plenty of time for functional activities is all that is needed to facilitate their safety. Many aged people feel the need to rush to answer a phone or doorbell. They should be discouraged from rushing because that could result in a fall. Caretakers and visitors should also be a part of the safety education process. They are often able to remind the person who is at risk for falling of the need for added precaution.

Aged persons who complain of dizziness during changes of position should be evaluated for postural hypotension. These individuals should be taught to change positions slowly and to wait before moving to another position in order to allow the blood pressure to accommodate to the change.

The purpose of strengthening exercises to prevent falls is to provide adequate force production of the lower extremities and trunk muscles for support of posture and control of balance. Some aged individuals will tolerate a progressive resistive exercise program. Others will derive greater benefit from a more functional approach to strengthening exercises. For example, practicing sit-to-stand movements and the reverse is a functional means of strengthening extensors and flexors of the lower extremity. Going up and down stairs one stair at a time requires less strength, range of motion, and balance than walking step over step. A functional way to increase this activity is to begin with one stair at a time and progress to step over step. Marching in place while standing can also be a lower extremity flexor-strengthening activity. For further strengthening, this exercise can be increased by asking the individual to hold the leg in flexion for the count of 3. During this activity, isometric strengthening also occurs in the extensors, abductors of the stance leg. Aged individuals should hold on to the back of a chair or the rim of the kitchen counter during this exercise for safety.

No matter which approach is selected for strengthening, the following precautions are recommended:

1. Many aged individuals have osteoporosis. Resistance and unilateral weight-bearing exercises may be excessive for them. It is possible to fracture an osteoporotic bone during strengthening exercises.
2. Many aged individuals have osteoarthritis. Isometric exercise may be less painful for them. Prolonging the amount of time that the contraction is held is an effective way to increase strength without adding external resistance.
3. It is especially important for aged individuals to avoid holding their breath (Valsalva maneuver) during exercise. Counting out loud helps to avoid this problem.
4. The aged individual should be taught to monitor his or her heart rate during exercise.

Therapeutic exercises designed to improve balance are an important part of fall prevention. Balance exercises address three areas of posture control: response to perturbation, weight shifting, and anticipatory adjustments to limb movements. Individuals must be able to respond to an external perturbation such as a push to the shoulder or sternum with a postural adjustment that brings the center of gravity back over the base of support. The usual response to a lateral perturbation will be extension of the weight-bearing leg along with elongation of the trunk on the weight-bearing side. Flexion and abduction of the non–weight-bearing leg will also be seen. A small backward force would stimulate the reaction of the dorsiflexors at the ankles and flexion at the hips, whereas a small forward push should be followed by plantarflexion at the ankles and extension at the hips.[22] Weight-shifting movements of the entire body during standing involve muscular activity similar to that used in response to a perturbation; however, during weight shifting, the muscle activation occurs voluntarily. Balance must also be controlled when a limb movement occurs, such as reaching with the upper extremity or swinging with the lower extremity (Fig. 6-1). In this case, the postural adjustment actually occurs in anticipation of the limb movement in order to prevent the center of gravity from moving outside of the base of support. For example, a forward movement of the arm should be preceded by ankle plantarflexion and hip extension. In this way, a small backward

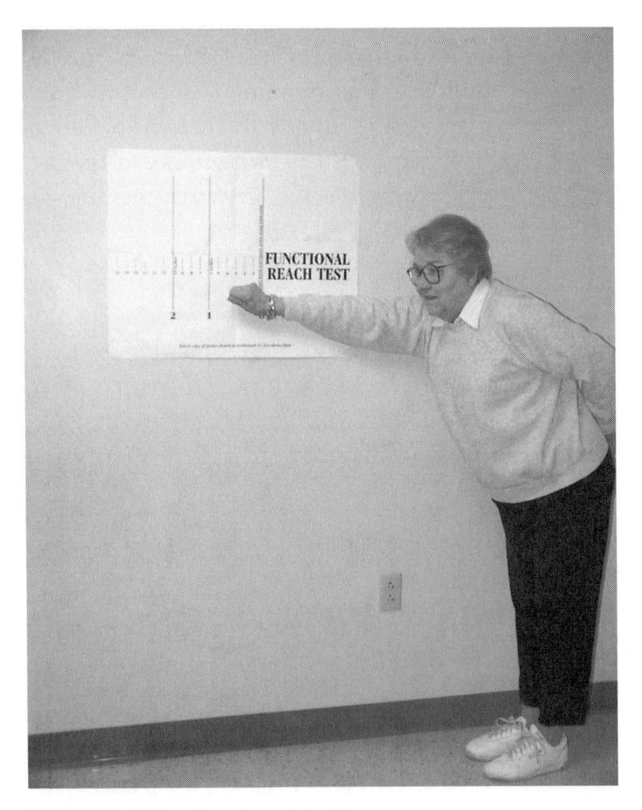


FIGURE 6-1 Functional reach testing.

movement of the center of gravity counteracts the forward displacement caused by the moving arm. Practicing each of these activities, that is, response to perturbation, voluntary weight shifting, and postural adjustments in anticipation of limb movement in standing, will help prepare the aged individual to use postural adjustment effectively during functional standing activities such as cooking, transfers, and ambulation. These activities are directed toward improvement of the motor component of balance (Figs. 6-2–6-4).

Altering the sensory conditions during balance activities encourages the aged person to attend to support surface or visual information selectively. Balancing in bare feet with eyes open or closed helps maximize the amount of somatosensory information that is available from the soles of the feet. On the other hand, balancing while standing on a piece of foam disrupts information from the sole of the foot and from stretch receptors in the ankle muscles and forces the individual to practice using visual input to stabilize posture. Maintaining balance while turning the head from side to side and while nodding the head is also important. Many aged people report falling

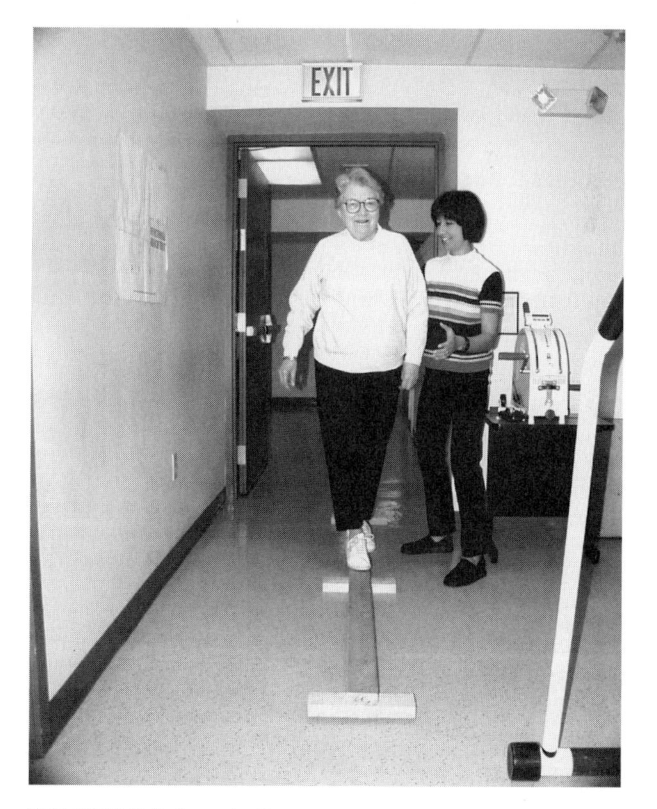


FIGURE 6-2 Balance testing.

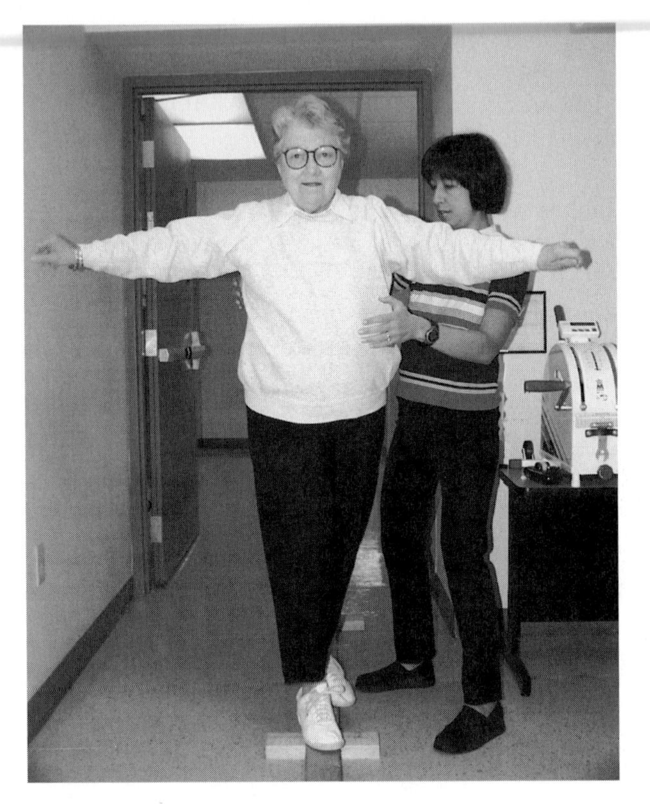

FIGURE 6-3 Balance activities: balance beam.

during head movements or while looking up to hang curtains or change a lightbulb. Aged individuals should be instructed to use caution during upward head movements.

When an individual is unable to control standing balance and is about to fall, the normal response is protective extension of the arms or legs. Protective reactions such as arm extension and the stepping response should also be practiced. Upper extremity protective extension can be practiced both forward and sideways against the wall in the standing position. Lower extremity protective reactions should be practiced in standing in forward, sideways, and backward directions. Brisk and accurately directed limb extension is the goal.

Balance exercises can be incorporated into functional activities for the aged. Moving from sit-to-stand and from stand-to-sit positions are examples of controlled voluntary weight shifting (Fig. 6-5). Shifting the trunk forward and back and from side to side while sitting are also examples of voluntary weight shifting. Voluntary weight shifting while standing with the individual's back to a wall is a safe way to facilitate control of balance.

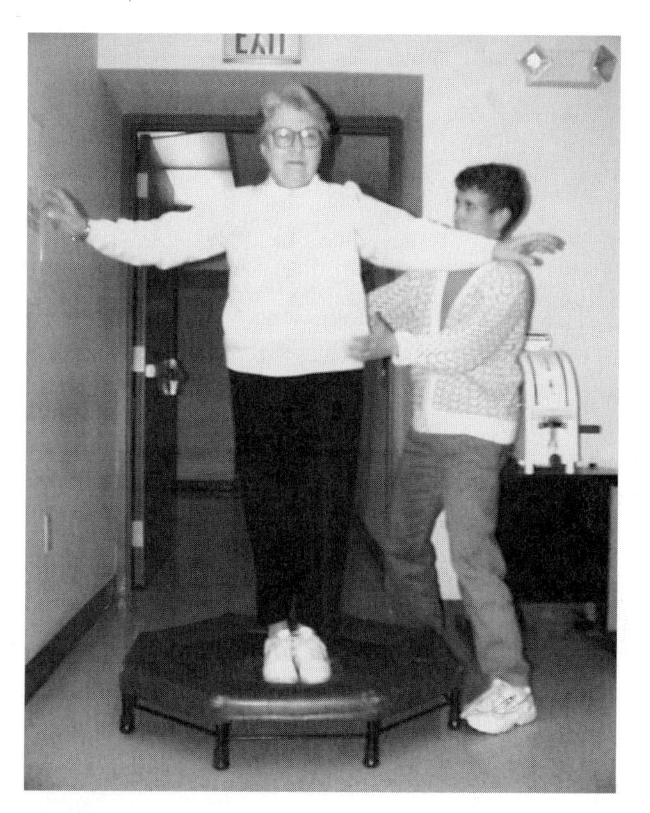

FIGURE 6-4 Balance activities: trampoline.

Dancing has also been recommended as a functional activity to improve balance for prevention of falls. Postural adjustments in anticipation of arm movements can be practiced during functional activities by standing and reaching for objects on the kitchen or closet shelves. Reaching should be practiced in a variety of directions.

Ambulation requires weight shifting. Manual guidance during ambulation helps organize the time and direction of weight shifting. Functional ambulation requires interaction with a variety of different support surfaces. Ambulation should be practiced on smooth as well as uneven surfaces and on levels as well as inclines, curbs, and stairs. Varying the amount of available light and background noise also simulates realistic environmental conditions. If step lengths are irregular, footprints on the floor make good targets for foot placement. Manual guidance is also useful for encouraging the individual to try a variety of speeds, for a variety of ambulatory speeds are necessary for function. Challenging activities like crossing a busy street can be made less threatening if the aged individual practices with the therapist or caregiver.

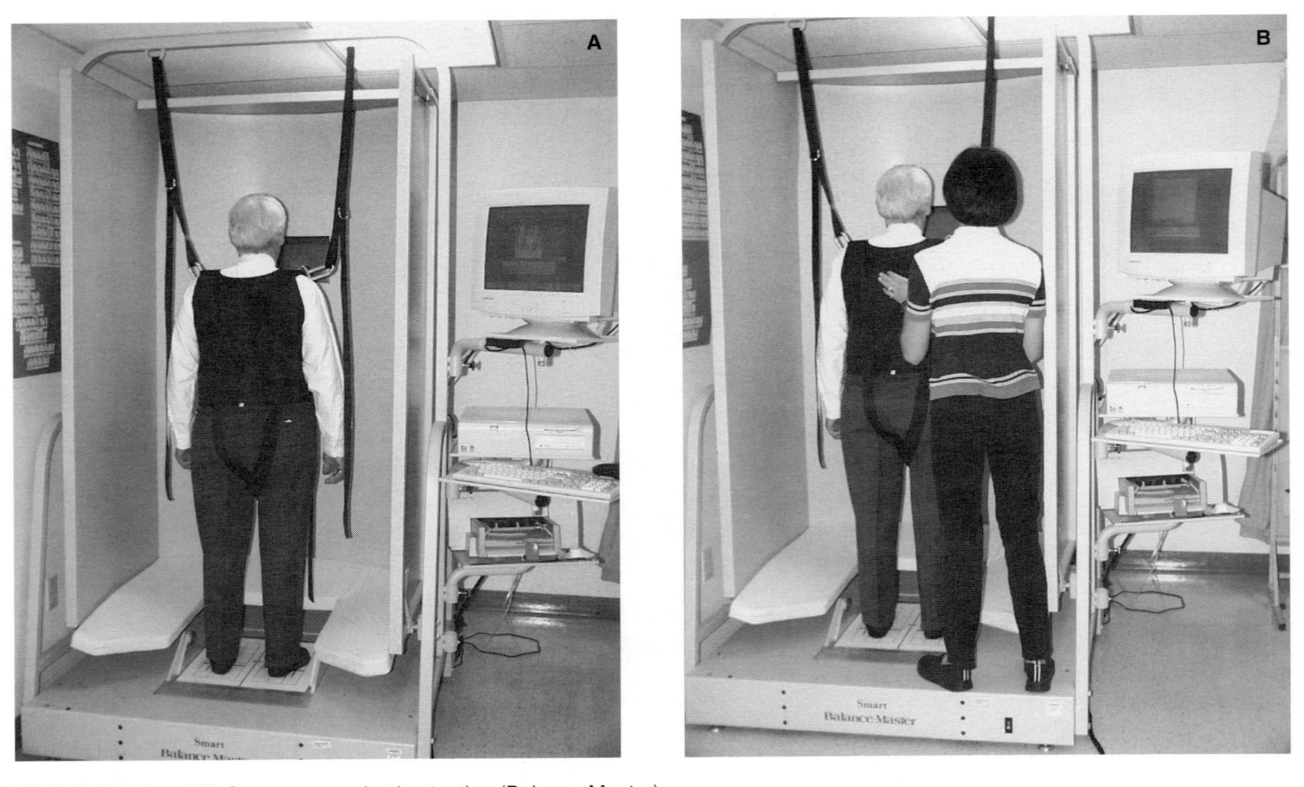


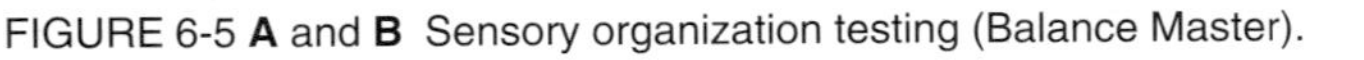
FIGURE 6-5 **A** and **B** Sensory organization testing (Balance Master).

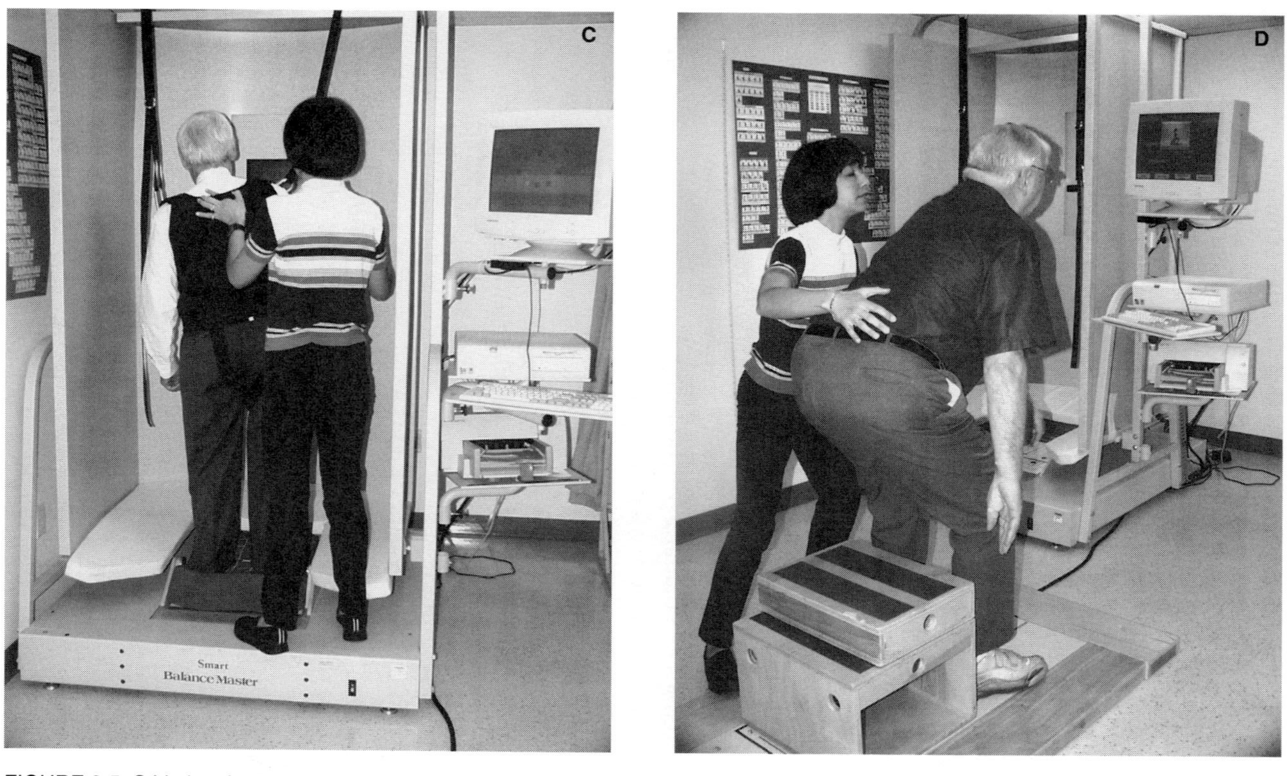


FIGURE 6-5 **C** Limits of stability testing. **D** Sit-to-stand testing.

Risk factors for falling among the aged suggest that falling should not be considered a normal concomitant of aging; rather, it should alert the health care professional to the possibility of underlying disease or accelerated sensory or neuromuscular degeneration secondary to disuse. Secondary or multiple diagnoses, use of multiple medications, especially diuretics and barbiturates, decreased vision and lower extremity somatosensation, and decreased lower extremity strength all appear to contribute to balance and gait deficits that, in turn, result in falling. Prevention of falling depends on addressing the specific problem area for each individual at risk. A team approach will be the most effective means to prevent falling by the aged.

### Adapting the Environment

The process of adapting to the environment, or of adapting the environment to the aged person, is especially important in geriatric rehabilitation. With decreased physiologic reserves, the aged person may not be able to continue an activity that is extremely demanding. For instance, an older person with a stroke and underlying cardiac insufficiency may need to learn wheelchair mobility skills. Therefore the environment will need significant modification. Doors may need to be widened, ramps installed, and counters lowered. Opportunities for obtaining new housing or adapting the present home may be restricted by financial concerns and personal preferences.

The interaction between the aged person and his or her environment becomes potentially precarious as one ages. These interactions are affected by the aged person's underlying physical status, living surroundings, and social systems. Of course, all persons interact with their environment. As one ages, however, the physiologic reserves, underlying medical problems, affective states, and a host of other factors complicate the relationship between the aged individual and his or her environment.

The response of rehabilitation providers is to manipulate the environment to make it safer. Assistive walking devices or modifications of the home may be recommended. But even these interventions are subject to differences when dealing with aging persons. The aged person with a disability may view such aids as unattractive or demeaning. Unlike eyeglasses, where the individual has a choice in enhancing his or her appearance, walkers or chrome-plated grab bars may project an image of illness and disability. The older person may have difficulty finding someone who can install home modifications. Some retired senior volunteer programs have carpenters available for this purpose, but many communities are without such support services.

Tasks are carried out within a physical and social context that has the potential for facilitating or hindering the use of functional capabilities. Push-button controls placed at the front of a range assist aged individuals with low vision, whereas dials situated at the back of the range handicap them. Similarly, caregivers can enhance functional independence by providing aged individuals with adaptive equipment, such as plate guards, bath brushes with elongated handles, and sock aids, or they can promote dependence by feeding, bathing, and dressing the individual. Evaluation of the environment is more difficult than task analysis because the environment of concern is the one in which the individual actually lives and has to function. Evaluation of physical space aims at ascertaining architectural barriers, safety and functional features, and the extent to which available equipment can be operated by the aged individual. Evaluation of the social context probes the availability of caregivers, their skills in rendering care and their need for training, their attitudes toward functional independence, and their experience of caregiver burden.

Those with disabilities or physiological or anatomical changes resulting from inactivity and aging may experience memory loss, disorientation, decreased ability to perform normal physical activity, a deteriorating ability to remember details, difficulty in verbal expression, and impairment in judgment. Each of these factors is important when modifying the physical and social environment to meet the rehabilitation needs of the aged. Social and organizational characteristics of institutions and the home setting could postpone the time when aged people become bedridden and require skilled nursing care.[1]

It is reasonable for the direct caregiver to seek advice about practical strategies that could reduce confusion or injury on the part of the disabled aged to prolong care at home. Environmental designs for aged patients have been studied, and several factors are consistently identified as environmental hazards, including poor illumination, inadequate color differentiation, cluttered furnishings and confusing layout (such as a table in a dimly lighted hallway), bland, nondistinct textiles, architectural features (such as split-level rooms) and climate control.[1] Certain environmental features are a threat to safety, can produce anxiety, and amplify cognitive deficits.

Visual limitations such as farsightedness, decreased ability to adapt to changes in lighting conditions requiring increased illumination to see, and an increased sensitivity to glare are not uncommon in the elderly patient. Several changes normally occur within the aging eye that affect safety within their environment and need to be considered when adapting that environment. The lens of the eye begins to thicken and yellow, and the muscles that control dilation of the pupil weaken. The thickening of the lens and delayed pupil dilation means that the glare and reflections often encountered in the environment cannot be tolerated.

Independence can be facilitated by bright and sharply contrasting colors. Considering the poorer differentiation of similar colors, if an aged individual is in a poorly lighted living room with a blue carpet, light blue walls, and lavender-and-blue-flowered furniture and draperies, they are in trouble. Contrasting colors or better lighting (which is economically more feasible) could positively facilitate safety in that room. Color coding of walls and corridors in hospitals and nursing homes using bright colors can aid aged persons in finding their own room, bathroom, sitting rooms, and so on. Contrast is extremely important. Contrasting colors can eliminate the difficulty of independently managing a stairwell or a poorly lighted hall where shadows can be hazards. Often this contrast can be accomplished through the use of fluorescent colors of tape (orange, lime green, or red).

Higher, reasonably firm, supportive comfortable chairs with high backs allow rising from a sitting position with minimal assistance. Wide arm rests, either wooden or metal, allow identification by touch when eyesight is poor or trunk rotation is limited. An aged individual should always be instructed to feel the chair seat with the back of their legs before attempting to sit down.

Human beings have a great propensity for adapting to less than ideal conditions. The aged, particularly those with a severe disability, have much more difficulty. Sensory stimulation should be incorporated into every aspect of rehabilitation. Repetitive visual cues using graphics, color, and lighting encourage independence, thereby increasing pride and self-esteem.

The relationship between physical condition and behavior is particularly important in patients with dementia. Changes in environmental design can accommodate the "normal" physiologic changes of aging and prevent the effects of disuse. If older persons cannot manage their environment safely, their independence, socialization, and activities of daily living are hindered.

## SUMMARY

Rehabilitation of the aged patients is one of the most challenging tasks for health care professionals. It is often difficult to separate the physiologic aspect of aging and disability from cognitive changes when designing a rehabilitation treatment program. With increased knowledge, we may eventually succeed in altering the natural history of "normal aging." Until then, rehabilitation of aged individuals needs to focus on obtaining the maximal functional capacity within the care environment by simplifying that environment and providing activity to ensure that disabilities do not result from disuse. To maintain the highest level of functional ability for the longest amount of time, decline in all sensory integration and physical functioning capabilities must be considered when providing rehabilitative care. One of the most salient aspects of geriatric rehabilitation is the simultaneous management of multiple conditions. For the rehabilitation specialist, these multiple diagnoses translate into multiple, and often multidimensional, impairments that complicate activities of daily living and prevent maximal functional capabilities.

Rehabilitation is a process that is not determined by a specific diagnosis or the care setting in which services are provided but by multidiagnostic circumstances and the aged individual's level of motivation. The primary goal of rehabilitation is to promote independent living, as defined by the aged themselves. When working with aged people, rehabilitation specialists need to be aware of the number of factors that make caring for them more complex, more challenging, and more fulfilling.

**Acknowledgments** The author conveys special thanks to Anita Alontc Roma, PT, MS, NCS, and Claudia C. Gazzi, PT, MHA; and Violent Johnson, Edgar Grove, and Bruce Musser, patient subjects.

## REFERENCES

1. Bottomley JM. Principles and practice in geriatric rehabilitation. In: Bottomley JM, Lewis CB. *Geriatric Physical Therapy: A Clinical Approach*. Norwalk, CT: Appleton & Lange; 1994:249–287.
2. Guccione AA. Implications of an aging population for rehabilitation: Demography, mortality, and morbidity in the elderly. In: Guccione AA (ed). *Geriatric Physical Therapy*, 2nd ed. St. Louis: Mosby; 2000:3–16.
3. Federal Council on the Aging. The need for long-term care. A chart book of the Federal Council on Aging. US Dept. of Health and Human Services publication No. (OHDS) 81-20704, 49. Washington, DC: Government Printing Office; 1999.
4. Bottomley JM. Understanding the demographics of an aging population. In: Bottomley JM, Lewis CB. *Geriatric Physical Therapy: A Clinical Approach*. Norwalk, CT: Appleton & Lange; 1994:3–22.
5. Branch L, Jette A. The Framingham Disability Study: Social disability among the aging. *Am J Public Health*. 1981; 71:1202–1207.
6. Lewis CB, Bottomley JM. Musculoskeletal changes with age: Clinical implications. In: Lewis CB. *Aging: The Health Care Challenge*, 2nd ed. Philadelphia: F.A. Davis; 1990:135–161.
7. Holloszy JO. Exercise, health, and aging: a need for more information. *Med Sci Sports Exerc*. 1983; 15(1):1–8.
8. Larson EB, Bruce RA: Health benefits of exercise in an aging society. *Arch Intern Med*. 1987; 147(2):353–359.
9. Thompson LV. Physiological changes associated with aging. In: Guccione AA (ed). *Geriatric Physical Therapy*, 2nd ed. St. Louis: Mosby; 2000:28–55.
10. Zubek JP, Wilgosh L. Prolonged immobilization of the body: Changes in performance and in the electroencephalogram. *Science*. 1963; 140:306–311.
11. Shepard RJ. *Physical Activity and Aging*, 2nd ed. Baltimore: Aspen; 1987.

12. Wolf SL et al. The effect of tai chi quan on postural stability in older subjects. *Phys Ther*. 1997; 77(4):371–384.

13. Rikli R, Busch S. Motor performance of women as a function of age and physical activity level. *J Gerontol*. 1986; 41:645–651.

14. Brown MB. Muscle fatigue and impaired muscle endurance in older adults. In: Guccione AA (ed). *Geriatric Physical Therapy*, 2nd ed. St. Louis: Mosby; 2000: 259–264.

15. Bottomley JM. Age-related bone health and pathophysiology of osteoporosis. *Ortho Phys Ther Clin North Am*. 1998; 7(2):117–132.

16. Bourgeois MC, Zadai CC. Impaired ventilation and respiration in the older adult. In: Guccione AA (ed). *Geriatric Physical Therapy*, 2nd ed. St. Louis: Mosby; 2000:226–244.

17. Bottomley JM. *Quick Reference Dictionary for Physical Therapy*. Thorofare, NJ: Charles B. Slack; 2000:322–323.

18. Birke JA et al. Methods of treating plantar ulcers. *Phys Ther*. 1991; 71(2):116–122.

19. Himann JE. Age-related changes in speed of walking. *Med Sci Sports Exerc*. 1988; 20(3):161–167.

20. Bottomley JM. Exploring nutritional needs of the elderly. In: Bottomley JM, Lewis CB. *Geriatric Physical Therapy: A Clinical Approach*. Norwalk, CT: Appleton & Lange; 1994:187–218.

21. Janelli LM. What nursing staff members really know about physical restraints. *Rehabil Nurs*. 1991; 16(6):345–348.

22. Woollacott MH et al. Aging and posture control: Changes in sensory organization and muscular coordination. *Int J Aging Hum Dev*. 1986; 23:97–114.

CHAPTER 7

# Clinical Practice: Pediatric Physical Therapy

DOLORES BERTOTI

## INTRODUCTION

Pediatric physical therapy offers unique challenges and rewards. Therapists and assistants working in pediatrics enjoy the opportunity to practice within many different environments: hospitals, outpatient centers, inpatient rehabilitation centers, homes, schools, and community centers. I have been a pediatric physical therapist for 25 years, continuing to find it as challenging and rewarding today as I did in my early years as a therapist. I hope that this chapter offers physical therapy students, physical therapist assistant students, and practicing therapists an insight, and perhaps an invitation to learn more about practicing physical therapy within a pediatric setting.

### History of Physical Therapy Services for Children

A discussion of pediatric physical therapy is best viewed within an historical framework of US history in conjunction with the history of the development of physical therapy as a profession. Physical therapy, especially as provided to children, has evolved over the past century because of the influence of several factors: medical advances affecting survival rates of children, legislative changes, changing societal perceptions, evolving community needs, and an increasing recognition of the rights of persons with disabilities.[1]

In the early years of physical therapy as a profession, most therapists served persons with musculoskeletal disorders, reflected by our early name "reconstruction aide," given to those therapists providing service to injured soldiers. A tremendous increase in physical therapy services occurred as a direct result of the polio epidemic in the 1920s, with this need continuing until the vaccine discovery in 1955. With other medical advances ensuring that children and adults with neurological impairment, such as spinal cord injury or stroke, could survive their actual injury and acute phases of rehabilitation, therapists became increasingly involved in the rehabilitation of children and adults with neurological impairment. During the 1940s and 1950s an interest in treating children with neurological problems led to the development of several still well-accepted neurophysiological and developmental approaches to treatment, such as neurodevelopmental treatment and sensory integration.

During the 1960s, the civil rights movement increased awareness of the rights of persons with disabilities and the concurrent responsibilities of medical providers, communities, and schools. In 1975, landmark legislation mandating education for children with disabilities was passed with physical therapy listed as one of several related services to be provided. Deinstitutionalization of the mentally handicapped during the 1970s further challenged communities to find better ways to improve the quality of life for persons with mental retardation, again opening up new venues of practice for pediatric physical therapists.

The practice arena for pediatric physical therapy has literally exploded and expanded to now include hospitals, outpatient centers, inpatient rehabilitation centers, homes, schools, and community centers. The Pediatric Section of the American Physical Therapy Association was formed in 1974, and the first pediatric specialists were certified in 1985.[1]

### Physical Therapy Practice and Pediatric Physical Therapy

Practice in any area of physical therapy (PT) requires a sound knowledge base in all the basic and specialized sciences that form the didactic background for any clinician. These basic PT skills can certainly be extrapolated to the unique requirements of any patient presenting within a specific period of the lifespan or with specific impairments. All therapists are best guided by a thorough knowledge of pathophysiology, sharpened by an understanding of primary impairments that frequently accompany that disease, and sensitized to a prophylactic approach to monitoring and preventing secondary impairments. The goal is always to maximize function for that unique individual within the constraints imposed by the disease, the impairments, and the environment within which that person functions.[2]

In the current health care environment, most physical therapists will have the opportunity to evaluate and treat individuals from the very young to the very old. Gone are the days of treating only within a specialty area, such as when all pediatric clients accessed health care through pediatric treatment facilities. However, there are some challenges unique to the area of pediatric physical therapy practice. Specialty practice in pediatrics certainly arises from generalist practice in physical therapy, but also requires expanded skills and addresses additional concerns indigenous to treating children who live within families. Expanded skills include a thorough understanding and appreciation of the development of functional motor skills, motor control and motor learning, age-related differences in musculoskeletal development, critical issues related to the management of common impairments, and a sensitivity to cultural diversity and family dynamics. Children are not simply "little adults." Pediatric physical therapists are unique in the level and quality of involvement with families as well as with personnel within the educational environment.

## DECISION MAKING IN PEDIATRIC PHYSICAL THERAPY

The conceptual basis for clinical practice in pediatric physical therapy is grounded in the disablement model and in the *Guide for Physical Therapy Practice*. The disablement model defines a variety of dimensions of disablement, including *impairments* of organ systems, such as deformities and limited strength, *functional limitations* in whole body segments, such as locomotion or hand function, and *disabilities* in the ability to perform age-appropriate activities, such as dressing, play, or work. The *Guide for Physical Therapy Practice*, a natural extension of the disablement model, is a consensus document developed in 1997 by the American Physical Therapy Association (APTA). This guide standardizes terminology and delineates practice guidelines to assist therapists in physical therapy diagnosis and the establishment of management strategies for commonly encountered diagnostic groups.[3] The *Guide's* second edition was published in 2001.[3]

All physical therapists, including pediatric practitioners, subscribe to the belief that the ultimate goal is to reduce disability by decreasing the negative impact of impairments and minimizing functional limitations. An example of a child with spastic diplegic cerebral palsy (CP) will be used to illustrate how pediatric therapists use the disablement model as a guide with which to plan intervention. In spastic diplegic CP, the child's impairments may include reduced muscular force, poor muscular endurance, and impaired balance. These impairments are thought to contribute to cause functional limitations, such as in moving around or engaging in movement activities. This child's specific movement limitations may involve moving around on uneven surfaces and climbing on playground equipment. As a result, this child may be limited in participation in physical education and recess. An appreciation of the dimensions of the disabling process can guide the therapist in elucidating which factors are contributing to limited function and help the therapist, family, and other members of the health or educational team to highlight goals and establish meaningfulness of these goals for the child.[4]

As in all areas of practice, clinical reasoning in pediatric physical therapy requires a strong knowledge base, and the ability to problem solve and make sound clinical judgments. Specific to pediatric practice, it has been suggested that pediatric therapists incorporate a minimum of five domains of knowledge into their thought processes:

1. understanding the child's motivation, commitment, and tolerances
2. assessing the environment within which the task is taking place
3. knowing the child's cognitive and physical capabilities and deficits
4. accurately perceiving the therapeutic relationship
5. being able to effectively establish both long- and short-term goals.

Pediatric physical therapists strive to base clinical practice decisions on available outcomes and evidence in an effort to be truly discerning and responsible in the delivery of optimum care.[4]

## THE SPECIAL VULNERABILITIES OF CHILDREN AND FAMILIES

Pediatric physical therapy is always family centered, tailored to address the priority concerns of the client and family. Families are respected for their primary role in nurturing their children. Family-centered care attempts to empower families to be equal partners in the relationship with service providers. This orientation creates a relationship of mutual respect between the therapist and family so that families can become advocates, exercise their rights to make choices, and receive the resource assistance required to meet their needs.

The National Center for Family-Centered Care (1990) proposes several key concepts that should guide therapists in provision of care to children and families:

- Recognition of the family as central and constant in a child's life
- Importance of family-to-family interaction, support, and networking
- Promotion of parent-professional collaboration at all levels
- Incorporation of the developmental needs of children into service delivery
- Implementation of policies and programs which provide emotional and financial support to meet family needs
- Respecting diversity
- Providing services which are accessible, flexible, and responsive to changing family needs.[5]

The following personal insight is a reflection on what is required of therapists who wish to work with families:

*RESPECT*

*Treat families with respect and dignity at all times. Try to realize the scrutiny that families and their children are often under by the countless service providers. Always try to give them the privacy and dignity they deserve. Remember to try to preserve, not challenge, family functioning. Although important, there is more to a child's life and the family's life than those specific therapy needs. Keep the therapy needs in focus. No one wants the child to succeed more than the family. Allow family members some creativity in trying to meet so many needs in limited hours. Be, at all times, honest. Parents deserve to know all that we know about their child. Allow families to make choices about intervention services. Be clear about what is available and what your recommendation is but this is ultimately the family's choice. Respect and support that choice. Don't be judgmental, however tempted. At all times, try to help preserve the integrity of the family and not interfere with it.*

*RECOGNIZE*

*Recognize the privileged position you are in—never underestimate how much parents rely on your empathy, honesty, and professionalism. You are privy to their intimate pains, sorrows, and joys. Honor that privilege. Families are often under a great deal of stress. Don't add to it! Be sensitive and flexible to the changing needs of families. Recognize the need, which we all have, for privacy. Know when to be vocal and when to be quiet.*

*RESPOND*

*Respond to the task at hand and to the needs of the families and children depending on you. Educate and empower the family to advocate for themselves. This is accomplished by effectively educating families so that they understand their child's needs more clearly than anyone else does. This should not threaten the professional, but, rather, creates a competent, educated partner—the parent. Inform parents of available resources and legislative changes. At all times, treat families as you would like to be treated. Remember that the therapist is a therapist for the whole family. Include grandparents and siblings in your educational approach. This will strengthen the family and prove invaluable for the child.*

## PROFESSIONAL ISSUES

### Collaboration with Other Disciplines

Because pediatric disorders are a developmental disability, they affect the "whole" child, including the child's movement, posture, perceptual skills, communication, cognition, and social-emotional growth. Therefore a coordinated effort among many disciplines and professionals is needed in the treatment of the child with motor impairment. In addition to the child and his family, other members of the team may include physicians, occupational therapists, speech pathologists, recreation therapists, orthotists, social workers, psychologists, and educational personnel. The child will best succeed through a concerted effort of all team members, working together to teach and support the child and family.

### Team Models

Regardless of the specific setting, pediatric physical therapy is provided as part of a coordinated team of individuals, including the child and members of the family. Several different team models exist that vary only in the way member roles are defined and interaction among members occurs. Team models include *intradisciplinary* (PT conducts evaluation and delivers therapy), *multidisciplinary* (PT conducts evaluation, seeks input from other disciplines, and delivers therapy), *interdisciplinary* (PT conducts evaluation and delivers therapy with incorporation of other discipline suggestions within the intervention), *transdisciplinary* (PT conducts evaluation in close collaboration with other professionals and intervention crosses boundary roles of related disciplines), and *collaborative* (combination of transdisciplinary and integrated approach). Within medical facilities, the multidisciplinary model is the most common. Within early intervention and preschool programs, models can be multidisciplinary, interdisciplinary, or transdisciplinary. The collaborative team model is the most often seen in school settings, where team members work closely together in a combination of a transdisciplinary and integrated approach to service provision.[1]

## SERVICE MODES FOR DELIVERY OF PEDIATRIC PHYSICAL THERAPY

### Level of Service and Treatment Frequency

All children with developmental disabilities will require the skills of a physical therapist throughout life. Service delivery can be through either direct or indirect service. Direct services include evaluation, treatment, and direct program planning. Indirect services may include screening, education, and consultation to others, including the family and educational and social service personnel. There will be times of increased frequency of treatment and times when physical therapy treatment is more consultative. During infancy and the preschool years, frequency is high in order to establish the child's maximum functional level. During the school years and adolescent years, therapy may be episodic with bursts of increased frequency during transitional times, periods of rapid growth, environmental change, or training in the use of new technology. It is conceivable that a person with a developmental disability will proceed through life with a constant but changing level of services by physical therapy.

Physical therapy for children can be offered in several settings and in several different modes of delivery. Settings include home-based, where PT is family centered, educational settings, where therapy takes on any number of different modes, both direct and indirect, as well as within the medical model. Wherever the specific setting, therapists need to remember to focus not only on the particular skill or immediate environment within which the child is attempting to function, but must constantly look forward and help the child and family to prepare for the future. It is essential that therapy goals be framed within an overall vision for the child. In most instances, the therapist subscribes to a lifespan approach and functions as a member of an interdisciplinary team.

### Family-Centered Therapy

The roles that families play in the management of children with disabilities has evolved, grown, and shifted dramatically over the past 20 years. Traditionally, medical intervention has been professional centered. Family-focused intervention styles have certainly attempted to include the family as collaborators with the professionals. Family-centered therapy, however, strives to have the family emerge as the **director** of the services and needed supports, which are set up to last even after the professionals are no longer involved. The focus, therefore, has shifted from the professional at the center to the family at the center. Therapists need to be educators and advocates for the family and child in order to empower families to succeed in their central role.[1,5]

### Integrated Therapy in the Educational Setting

In the past, physical therapy in the schools had traditionally been provided as a direct hands-on method of intervention. Children were typically pulled out of classrooms to receive therapy services and then reintroduced to the classroom at the end of the therapy session. This method of service delivery has not always been optimal in providing outcomes for children in educational environments. Currently, pediatric therapy can be identified to subscribe to any one of the following six different service delivery methods:

- Individual pullout: child is removed from class and the therapy session focuses on a specific concern
- Small group pullout: child and a small number of peers are removed from class and participate in a focused group activity
- One-on-one in the classroom: child is treated within the classroom, but in an area removed from peers and possibly working on an activity unrelated to the class routine
- Group activity: child and classmates are engaged in an activity addressing the physical needs of most of the children in the group
- Individual therapy during classroom routine: child is supported while engaging in a classroom routine in order to develop specific skills
- Consultation: therapist consults with teacher to exchange information and expertise relating to child's physical needs.

The last three methods are the most common, wherein physical therapy is delivered in an integrated manner. Education and physical therapy intervention occur simultaneously. Integration of services promotes closer team collaboration and allows children to master skills within the context of normal routines.[1]

## COMMON CLINICAL PROBLEMS

The spectrum of pediatric disorders encountered by the physical therapist is quite broad, and a child's diagnosis may encompass several body systems. In alphabetical order, the most common are amputations and limb deficiencies, cerebral palsy, congenital hip dislocation, cystic fibrosis, Down syndrome and other disorders associated with mental retardation, juvenile rheumatoid arthritis, multiple congenital contractures, muscular dystrophy, myopathies, osteogenesis imperfecta, and spina bifida including myelomeningocele. The three most common disorders are cerebral palsy, spina bifida, and mental retardation including Down syndrome. These will be briefly described to illustrate the role of the pediatric physical therapist.

### Cerebral Palsy

Cerebral palsy is a term of convenience applied to a group of motor disorders of central origin defined by clinical description. To apply the term *cerebral palsy*, there must be a motor impairment stemming from a malfunction of the brain that is nonprogressive and manifested early in life. Cerebral palsy (CP) as a clinical syndrome is a complex disorder that encompasses muscle tone abnormalities, sensory-motor disorganization, peripheral biomechanical alterations and, ultimately, varying degrees of impairment and/or disability. It is basically an umbrella term that describes a set of clinical conditions identified early in life. At least three related processes contribute to the functional disability of the child with CP. The first is the primary lesion in the central nervous system (CNS), affecting neural processing, neural maturation, and motor control. The second is a disturbance of muscle tone, muscle activation, and bone growth. Third is the learned response as the child develops movement patterns, often considered atypical, as a compensation for neural damage. By definition, therefore, CP is a comprehensive term used to designate a category of patients with a chronic but nonprogressive disorder of movement and posture with an onset during the developmental period and a wide range of associated deficits, including mental retardation (60%), visual impairment (50%), seizures (20–30%), and hearing impairment (6–16%). Additional related disorders include speech deficits, sensory impairments, visual-motor and perceptual disorders, oral-motor disorders, and behavioral disorders.[2]

The causes of CP are numerous and continue to be under ongoing discovery and investigation. Causes can be broadly categorized into prenatal, perinatal, and postnatal factors. Prenatal factors include environmental toxins, infection, drugs, placental ischemia, prenatal cerebral hemorrhage, anoxia or infection, and congenital brain abnormalities. Perinatal factors include anoxia from any cause, delivery trauma, and birth complications such as respiratory and hemolytic and electrolyte disturbances. Postnatal factors include head injury, vascular accidents, infections, and neoplasm. Contrary to widespread belief, birth asphyxia probably does not account for most cases of CP; rather, congenital brain abnormalities and infections are currently considered to be the leading causes. Additional risk factors include the risks associated with very low birth weight and prematurity.[2]

There are different clinical presentations of CP, classified according to either the clinical type or the parts of the body involved. The types of CP are spastic, hypotonic, athetoid, and ataxic. The distribution within the body can present clinically with a child with quadriplegia (total body), diplegia (trunk and lower extremities), or hemiplegia (one side involvement).

Cerebral palsy is primarily a movement disorder that uniquely presents during a period of tremendous organization, change, and development within the CNS. The development of normal motor control requires an integration of reflex or supporting systems for postural control into an emergent, adaptive postural control mechanism. This undoubtedly requires an undamaged CNS. In CP, the CNS is damaged, albeit plastic, early in life. Postural control, therefore, in the child with CP will develop secondary to the primary disease in the CNS and is limited more or less by all other simultaneous constraints, endogenous or environmental. Ultimately, the CNS will organize and reorganize in the young child and motor control will develop, although altered. The child, attempting to solve movement tasks, will present with disordered or abnormal movement.

Diagnostically, abnormal muscle tone can range anywhere along a continuum from high, defined as *hypertonus* or *spasticity*, to low, referred to as *hypotonia*, or may fluctuate from high to low. As with any patient with a neurological impairment, the child with CP will present with abnormal muscle tone as a symptom of disordered and altered motor control. The abnormal muscle tone seen in CP is also strongly influenced by body position and movement due to predominance of tonic reflexes. Since the emergence of normal postural control is delayed, altered or absent in the child with CP, tonic reflexes and abnormal muscle tone may be the characteristic expression of movement for this child. Children with CP also present with muscle weakness.

Children with CP basically present with impaired movement. In response to this, the secondary impairments are also somewhat predictable. Effective management strategies for children with CP, therefore, should attempt to impact on peripheral, central and compensatory mechanisms in order to effect any change in the child's functional abilities. Insightful management includes accurate assessment and treatment planning, including preventive or anticipatory care.[2]

### Spina Bifida

Spina bifida is a spinal cord and vertebral malformation, usually in the thoracic or lumbar region, as a result of a neural tube defect. This neutral tube defect occurs very early in the gestational age of the developing infant, at 3 to 4 weeks. The etiology is still uncertain. Associated defects include hydrocephalus, bowel and bladder dysfunction, and orthopedic problems such as clubfoot and hip dislocation. The most common type of spinal bifida is myelomeningocele, where a cyst is formed containing cerebrospinal fluid and herniated spinal cord.[6,7]

As a clinical syndrome, myelomeningocele causes variable functional limitations, depending on the location and severity of spinal cord involvement. Symptoms can range from minimal bowel and bladder incontinence with clubfeet to limited paralysis to complete paraplegia. Because of the involvement across multiple body systems, children with myelomeningocele require intervention from not only physical therapists, but also from orthopedists, urologists, neurosurgeons, and certified orthotists. The main goals of therapeutic intervention are to anticipate problems and develop proactive interventions in preventive management of the musculoskeletal system by use of orthoses, assistive devices, strengthening activities, and activities to maintain range of motion. Optimal trunk and lower extremity development and alignment are attained through the appropriate use of positioning, equipment, and supportive devices. The overall goal is to promote independence in daily care activities and locomotion, and to encourage the development of gross motor, fine motor, and cognitive skills.[7]

### Mental Retardation, Including Down Syndrome

The physical therapist plays a challenging and important, multifaceted role in the management of children with mental retardation. Mental retardation is characterized by significantly subaverage intellectual functioning, existing concurrently with related limitations in two or more of the following applicable adaptive skill areas: communication, self-care, home living, social skills, community use, self-direction, health and safety, functional academics, leisure, and work. About 3% of the population of the United States is assumed to have mental retardation, but only 1–1.5% are actually diagnosed with this condition. In 80% of the cases, the cause of the mental retardation is unknown. Of all the people with mental retardation 75% have a mild form, 20% a moderate form, and 5% have a severe or profound form. One of the most prevalent forms of mental retardation is Down syndrome with an incidence of one in 700 live births.[8]

In keeping with contemporary views of disablement, the key elements in the definition of mental retardation are *capabilities, environment, and function.* The previously used terms of mildly, moderately, severely, or profoundly mentally retarded are no longer used. Current classification carries with it an application of the new diagnostic criteria directly correlated to the child's need for support. Support services may come to the child with mental retardation from four sources: the individual child (e.g., ability to make choices), other people (e.g., parent, teacher), technology (e.g., assistive devices), or habilitation services (e.g., PT, OT, speech therapy).

Over 350 causes for mental retardation have been identified. These can be broadly categorized into prenatal, perinatal, and postnatal causes. Examples of prenatal causes include chromosome disorders, developmental disorders of brain formation, and environmental influences. Perinatal causes include neonatal and intrauterine disorders. Postnatal causes include examples such as head injuries, infections, and metabolic disorders. Movement disorders are associated with some causes more than others. Many children also present with a variety of associated disorders such as visual, hearing, or additional medical problems. The common impairment among all children with mental retardation is, most certainly, impaired cognitive functioning.[8]

Many types of mental retardation have associated neuromuscular, musculoskeletal, and cardiopulmonary impairments. Most neuromuscular impairments are present as a result of primary disease in the central nervous system. Secondary impairments then include deficits typically of concern to the physical therapist such as deficits in motor control, coordination, postural control, force production, flexibility, and balance. Physical therapy assessment and treatment of these impairments for children with mental retardation are similar to those procedures used in any pediatric setting. The mental retardation itself, viewed as an additional or confounding co-impairment, requires some adaptation in evaluation and treatment application because of the specific cognitive limitations presented by the child.[8]

Learning is impaired in children with mental retardation. Children with mental retardation demonstrate an impaired ability to handle advanced cognitive processes, simultaneous demands and organization of information, with subsequent effects on task performance as well as task mastery. Physical therapists must be able to adapt evaluation and treatment approaches to accommodate the co-impairment of deficient intellectual functioning. Clearly, the range of cognitive deficit and ability found in children with mental retardation is indicative of variant levels of performance, functioning, and potential. It is the task and the challenge of the therapist to assist the child to maximize his or her potential for optimum functioning across environments.[8]

## PEDIATRIC PHYSICAL THERAPY EVALUATION

In children with different clinical disorders, movement and postural control are attempting to be established within the constraints of a damaged but perhaps immature, plastic, and reorganizing CNS. These movement efforts may produce abnormal forces on a malleable, immature skeletal system. To accurately assess and treat children with movement disorders, therapists need to be able to sort out the primary movement disorder from its secondary effects and view the child as an active problem solver, solving a movement dilemma given the constraints of his or her environment, cognitive abilities, or neuromuscular system. Pediatric physical therapy evaluation consists of the following key elements.

### Assessment of Movement

Observation of the child's movement is simply that—observation without handling. A great deal of information can be gained through simple observation and analysis of the child's movement strategies. In a multitude of positions, several key questions can be answered regarding the child's alignment and mobility, functional antigravity control, and movement patterns. Functional movement can be assessed in all or any of the following positions: prone, supine, side lying, sitting, including noting any preferred sitting position and whether the child demonstrates only one sitting position choice or several choices, quadruped, kneeling and half kneeling, and standing.[9,10]

Movement patterns can also be observed during the child's transition from one position to another. If the child is not independently mobile, the same observations can be made regarding how the child responds to being moved or transferred by the caregiver. For the child with higher level motor skills, the therapist observes movement patterns during climbing onto furniture, ascending and descending stairs, negotiating ramps and uneven terrain, running, jumping, and unilateral stance. Assessment of movement through antigravity control also gives the therapist some insight into the child's functional strength.

### Assessment of Muscle Tone

Muscle tone is assessed by evaluating the amount of resistance to passive stretch and movement as well as by observing any evidence of visibly changing tone during movement or activity. The therapist notes the presence of abnormal tone, its severity and distribution. Tone is described as hypertonic, hypotonic or intermittent, and further described as mild, moderate or severe. Distribution of tone and its variations under different conditions is noted.

### Assessment of Postural Control

Postural control has historically been assessed by studying the observable evidence of the child's motor behaviors. In the past, reflex and equilibrium assessments were performed by the therapist to gain insight into the level of organization of the child's motor system. Current theories in motor control now indicate that it is more appropriate and meaningful to study the child's movements, noting the options or lack of movement options a child may have.

The presence of tonic or developmentally immature reflexes should be noted, more so as an indication of lack of alternative neural control choices rather than for the sake of actually testing for the reflexes themselves. Even more important to note is the influence of primitive or tonic reflexes on selective movement control and anticipatory mechanisms. The effects these reflexes have on positioning, handling, and functional movement needs to be described A delay in the acquisition of normal motor control, reflected as a persistent predominance of tonic reflexes, can have profound effects on the child with a movement disorder. Delay in the development of mature postural reactions can result in the inability to roll, sit up, play bimanually, reach, creep, and ambulate.[2]

### Assessment of Functional Movement

Functional evaluation includes an assessment of gross motor mobility skills through either observation or the administration of a standardized evaluation tool. Functional gross motor skills are possible because of the presence of several component elements: antigravity control, midline control, the ability to stabilize and bear weight, weight shifting, rotation, dissociation, and the ability to grade and refine selected muscular responses. When assessing functional movement, the examiner analyzes the ability and ease with which these component elements allow for smooth, efficient, and purposeful movement to occur.

Functional assessment can be performed informally by noting which skills the child can and cannot perform. A standardized evaluation instrument is used for assessment, and can be categorized as either a test of motor function, a comprehensive developmental scale, or an assessment of functional capabilities. Examples of standardized instruments that are tests of motor function include the Gross Motor Function Measure, the Alberta Infant Motor Scales, the Toddler and Infant Motor Evaluation, and the Peabody Developmental Motor Scales. An example of a comprehensive developmental scale is the Bayley Scales of Infant Development. An assessment of functional performance can be performed with an instrument such as the Pediatric Evaluation of Disability Inventory (PEDI), specifically for children with disabilities, or the WEE-Fim.[2]

### Assessment of Strength

In assessing strength, it is sometimes difficult to directly test the force-generating ability of individual muscles in the presence of spasticity, abnormal extensibility, and poor selective control. Functionally, identifying the child's ability to move against gravity (concentric control), stabilize a body part (isometric strength), or lower a body part resisting gravity's influence (eccentric control) can assess strength. If the child is able to isolate a voluntary contraction, manual muscle testing or measurement of isometric strength can be done. Formal strength testing can be safely and reliably performed for children using standardized isokinetic tests and equipment.[11]

### Assessment of Gait

An understanding of the development of gait, the characteristics of immature versus mature gait, and the determinants of gait offer the clinician a framework for understanding and evaluating gait dysfunction in children with motor impairment. Evaluation of gait in children is performed by carefully assessing each phase of gait and the ability of the child to meet the main three functional gait subtasks of limb loading, weight transfer, and limb advancement. Careful analysis of one joint at a time and one motion at a time will lead to a determination of contributing impairments.

### Musculoskeletal Assessment

Musculoskeletal assessment is a routine portion of any physical therapy evaluation. An underlying knowledge of developmental biomechanics and an understanding of the primary pathophysiology of the child being evaluated is crucial for an accurate and preventive management approach. The pathomechanics of abnormal force production, either inadequate, excessively strong, or unbalanced, puts the child with a movement disorder at risk for various secondary deformities. Goniometric assessment of the child with CP requires common sense modification of standard physical therapy goniometric assessment practice. Differences in age-related norms exist secondary to developmental biomechanic and locomotor abilities. Age-related norms for children are readily available in pediatric textbooks.[11,12]

## PHYSICAL THERAPY INTERVENTION IN PEDIATRICS

The following sections on treatment will focus on different issues and treatment priorities throughout the life span: infancy, preschool, school age, adolescence, and into adulthood. Physical therapy treatment for children is individualized, based on the child's specific degree of involvement, strengths, impairments, age, intelligence, family concerns, and functional capabilities. Level of family involvement is a main contributing issue. Treatment priorities change over time and there are most certainly age-related specific issues. Intervention is always family centered with treatment goals tailored to address the priority concerns of the client and family. Family-centered care creates a relationship of mutual respect between the therapist and families. Client and family education is a vital, ongoing role of the physical therapist so that the family and client can make effective choices throughout the life span for children with disabilities. Treatment goals and priorities are established with input from the child and family, based on a thorough evaluation of the child that identifies the child's strengths, problems, constraints, but, most important, functional goals. The core about which all treatment is centered is the desired functional outcome.

Physical therapy should be designed to engage active involvement and responses from the child. Whenever possible, movement should be initiated by the child. The therapist can best serve as a facilitator and assist the child with solving his or her unique challenges with movement. The therapist does this by carefully analyzing the barriers or constraints encountered by the child and assisting by either removing them or decreasing their influence so that functional success can be achieved. Repetition and practice are important aspects of motor learning. Carryover is ensured when skills are taught and applied in the actual setting and situation in which they will be used. Treatment is tailored to address the functional needs of the child as the child grows and develops.

From infancy through adulthood, physical therapy goals focus on the prevention of disability by maximizing function, minimizing impairments, and preventing or limiting secondary impairments. Achieving these goals involves the promotion and maintenance of musculoskeletal integrity, the prevention of deformity, and the enhancement of optimal postures and movement to promote functional independence. Furthermore, the therapist attempts to prevent environmental deprivation that could increase existing disabilities and attempts to provide support and education for families and agencies involved with the child.

### Approaches to Treatment

Most therapists currently ascribe to an eclectic approach to treatment. The main emphasis is on a functional approach. The tools therapists use come from several schools of thought, with neurodevelopmental treatment being the most widely accepted treatment approach. Neurodevelopmental treatment (NDT) concentrates on the effects of the disturbed postural control mechanism on movement. Therapists attempt to help a child experience active movement with correct alignment and more efficient movement patterns, as well as to anticipate changes in posture. Through experiencing active, appropriate movement repeatedly in several positions, the child may learn to move more effectively. NDT theory and treatment application has gone through many changes since its inception in the 1940s, continuing to evolve as knowledge of movement and motor control grows. Current NDT theory supports the following key concepts:

1. During the acquisition of functional motor skills, the child focuses on the goal rather than the specific movement components of the task. The moving child is composed of many subsystems that are interactive and independent but also plastic and adaptive to both internal and external changes.
2. A standard of reference for proficient human motor function is based on a study of motor control, motor development, and motor learning. Learning and adaptation of motor skills involves repetition, practice, and experience.
3. Children with motor control problems associated with CNS pathophysiology present with predictable primary and secondary impairments. It is these impairments that limit function.
4. Intervention begins with assessment of the child's functional performance. Analytical problem solving is used to develop a treatment plan. Treatment focuses on increasing function by building on the child's

strengths while addressing the impairments. Therapeutic handling or facilitation using NDT principles is one strategy that can be used.

5. Facilitation techniques are strategies used to assist the child in attaining his or her own functional movement goals. Through facilitation, the therapist communicates with the child through somatosensory cues to foster any one of the following movement responses: a gain in stability or mobility, synergistic recruitment and timing of muscular activation, improved muscular timing, grading of a movement, or variability of movement when solving a functional task.[10,13,14]

The sensory systems are crucial for the acquisition, monitoring, and regulation of movement. Children with movement disorders often have sensory processing difficulties as well as decreased proprioception and kinesthetic awareness secondary to diminished or altered movement experiences. During facilitation, the therapist monitors the child's use of sensory systems through their responses to sensory feedback and encourages the use of feedback to initiate and refine movements. The Sensory Integration theory (SI) focuses on sensory aspects and their impact on attention, arousal, motivation, and movement. The principles of SI include providing opportunities to experience sensory experiences and encouraging the production of adaptive responses including appropriate motor behaviors and interactive skills. Incorporation of some of these principles in treatment is evident through the use of proprioceptive, tactile, and vestibular input. The child is assisted to form adaptive responses spontaneously to integrate the sensations encountered through movement exploration.[10]

Therapeutic exercise programs are developed based on the assessment findings and the child's functional abilities. Progression is directed at increasing strength, endurance, and coordination. The therapist has two options for progressing therapeutic exercise: to progress the movement from a gravity-eliminated position to a movement that requires that the child work against gravity, or to alter the amount of assistance or facilitation given by the therapist so that the child has to develop more force or control. Therapeutic exercise is directed at dissociation of one extremity from the other and the extremities from the trunk in order to achieve improved patterns of postural control. The therapist uses manual assistance or equipment to provide additional external support. Support is given judiciously so that the child has the opportunity to experiment with and experience increased levels of independence in movement. Dynamic handling and smoothly graded transitions with brief opportunities for midline control is optimal.[2]

## Use of Therapeutic and Adaptive Equipment

Equipment is used in pediatrics to assist the therapist in meeting the therapeutic goals and to promote attainment of functional independence for the child. Use of therapeutic equipment can range from the very simple towel roll placed under the scapula to promote scapular protraction for reaching, to the very complex, such as powered mobility. It is beyond the scope of this chapter to delineate every type of equipment or adaptation and its use. There is a plethora of choices, with more choices entering the market daily. Therapists should align themselves with a local supplier who can keep the therapist apprised of new products.

The therapist may wish to use therapeutic equipment during therapy as an extra pair of hands. Such uses include using the equipment to place the child in a set position to enhance the opportunity for movement, increase the possibility of desirable responses, decrease the possibility of undesirable responses, control the instability and thereby limit the degrees of freedom of a given movement, or to introduce instability into the context of movement. Equipment commonly used to meet these requirements includes wedges, rolls, bolsters, benches, and gymnastic balls.

Adaptive equipment is often a necessary adjunct to treatment for children. Equipment is provided to offer postural support, promote alignment, or offer mobility. Examples include adapted tricycles, switch toys, seating inserts, toilet adaptations, standers, strollers, and wide ranges of pediatric wheelchairs. The reader is referred to pediatric therapy textbooks and local vendors for current products and uses.

## AGE-RELATED ISSUES IN PEDIATRIC PHYSICAL THERAPY

Most children requiring physical therapy have a developmental disability, requiring different levels of service throughout the life span. At different age stages, the main focus of physical therapy will address key issues as described below.[2,9,10]

### Infancy

Physical therapy assessment and treatment during infancy focuses on accurate identification and description of the child's movement disorder and close work with the family. Infant assessment provides a baseline for the monitoring of improvement or regression, and the emergence of the clinical picture of the child with a movement disorder. Physical therapy in infancy is focused on educating the family, facilitating care-giving, making appropriate referrals for diagnosis, baseline assessment and social agency support, and promoting optimal sensorimotor skills. Early treatment for children has been advocated to help infants organize potential abilities in the most normal ways for them. During infancy, the main physical therapy goals can be established as follows:

*Handling and Care.* Parents learn positioning, carrying, feeding, bathing, and dressing techniques so that symmetry is promoted, abnormal posturing and movement are limited, and motor activity is facilitated. Basic principles are to teach methods that use a variety of movements and postures to promote sensory variety, including positions that will promote functional, voluntary movement.

*Facilitation of Optimal Sensorimotor Development.* Therapy focuses on the development of well-aligned postural stability along with smooth mobility to allow for the emergence of motor skills such as reaching, rolling, sitting, floor mobility, transitional movements, standing, and walking. These skills promote the development of spatial perception, body awareness, and mobility, which will in turn facilitate play, social interaction, and exploration of the environment. Movements that include trunk rotation, dissociation, weight bearing, weight shifting, and selected isolated movements are incorporated into everyday activity. Activities or specialized equipment may be introduced to allow for the attainment of functional skills when impairment prevents the natural emergence of that skill. For example, the sitting position allows children to visually explore their world and begin developing upper extremity skills. Infants with motor difficulties who are unable to sit can be supported with adapted equipment. Toys can be modified to allow for these skills to emerge with support.

*Family-Centered Care.* Infancy is a crucial time to establish a trusting relationship with parents, maintain hope, and empower parents to be informed, effective advocates for their child. It is vitally important to involve parents as collaborative members of the team.

### The Preschool Years

During the preschool years, the child's locomotor, social, and communication abilities are allowing him to attain some level of functional independence. It is now possible to predict the child's attainable motor skill level with more accuracy because the influences of impairments on performance become more evident. A major area of concern and a major question for parents is the child's ability to achieve independent mobility. In addition, skills in other areas of gross motor function continue to be a main goal in therapy in an effort to minimize disabilities. The focus expands to include performance of self-care activities such as dressing, toileting, and feeding as well as play, communication, social interaction, and problem-solving behavior. Functional strength can be assessed more accurately in the preschool period and functional assessments include evaluation of gait, transfers, and the need for assistive devices/adaptive equipment. Treatment centers on reducing impairments and preventing secondary impairments within a functional context. Optimal postural alignment and movements that are conducive to musculoskeletal development, neurophysiologic control, and function through exercise, positioning, and equipment are the main aims of most interventions. During the preschool years, the main physical therapy goals can be established as follows:

*Increase Strength.* Muscle strength is evaluated within a functional context. Concentric and eccentric power are both important considerations, allowing for control within many positions, such as moving from sit to stand, or using stairs. Treatment activities focus on performing activities that increase force production eccentrically, concentrically, and isometrically through the use of transitional movements, ball gymnastics, and functional training.

*Management of Abnormal Muscle Tone.* Spasticity, if present, is best viewed as a symptom of disordered motor control. Functional strengthening, as discussed above, will result in a clinical reduction in the influence of spasticity on motor control. The diminishment of spasticity through pharmaceutical, neurosurgical, or orthopedic intervention may be appropriate at this age. All of these interventions reduce the deleterious effects of abnormal tone, but may then reveal profound weakness. It is during the preschool years when a team decision may be made to seek one of these interventions. The therapy goals then would focus on maximizing strength and improving function.

*Preservation of Range of Motion.* Various approaches are used to maintain joint range of motion and muscle extensibility. Active and passive stretching are routine tools available to therapists, including teaching these techniques to children and caregivers. Use of bivalved casts, splints, or orthoses has been shown to prevent the secondary impairment of contracture, especially during periods of rapid growth.

*Skeletal Alignment and Weight Bearing.* Alignment of the body is important and should be promoted in a variety of positions with and without adaptive equipment. The human body cannot function properly if each segment is not biomechanically aligned for function. Seating systems and floor positioning aids may be prescribed. Standing programs are routinely started at 12 to 15 months of age if children are not able to stand on their own. Hips should be routinely evaluated radiographically before imposing a standing program. The benefits of standing include mineralization and increasing bone density, as well as promoting normal skeletal modeling and joint formation.

*Mobility.* Ambulation is a major concern of physical therapy during these years. Treatment emphasis is initially on pre-ambulation skills such as attaining effective alignment and weight bearing, promoting dissociation and weight shifting, and practicing balance skills. Assistive devices such as crutches, walkers, or gait trainers may be used. All children will not be able to achieve independent, efficient ambulation. At this age, therapists need to provide alternative mobility means, for example, an adapted scooter, tricycle, or power mobility device. It has been demonstrated that offering a child some kind of independent mobility contributes to motivation, self-esteem, and even cognitive development. Powered mobility does not preclude a goal of ambulation in therapy; rather these goals are supportive of each other. Prediction of ambulation ability presents a troublesome dilemma for both parents and health care professionals. The earlier that gross motor skills are achieved, the better the prognosis for ambulation. Therapists are cautioned in offering predictions to parents.

*Attainment of Functional Skills.* Physical therapy for the treatment of functional limitations is often intensive during the preschool years. Optimal treatment frequency is unknown, but periods of increased frequency have shown improvements in the attainment of specific treatment goals when these skills were incorporated into daily functional activities. Therapy needs to be meaningful for the child so that the child can integrate newly acquired skills into daily life.

*Family Involvement.* Current approaches emphasize the need for therapeutic intervention to be family centered. Family-centered management suggests that the therapist and family communicate openly and listen carefully to each other so that the child's and family's unique needs can be most effectively met. Siblings, grandparents, and day-care providers all should be included as appropriate.

### The School-aged Child

Entrance into school is often a time of tremendous crisis for children with disabilities and their families. This may be the time when the extent of the functional limitations and differences becomes poignantly clear. Therapists must be supportive of children and their families while facilitating communication with school service providers. Goals and treatment concerns are an extension of those listed in the preschool period, with continued emphasis on maximizing functional independence and prevention of secondary impairment. This may be an age when orthopedic surgical procedures are performed, requiring an increase in frequency of physical therapy treatment. Growth spurts need to be monitored carefully so that secondary impairments such as limitations in range of motion do not contribute to decreased function. Therapy for school-aged children emphasizes independence with self-care, mobility, and communication, as well as preventing deformity as the child grows.

Physical therapy within the school system offers unique opportunities and challenges for therapists. The US Congress has passed several pieces of legislation supporting the educational rights of children with disabilities, beginning in 1975 with the Education for All Handicapped Children Act. This mandate was extended in 1986 to include all children from birth through 21 years of age. In 1991, the Individuals with Disabilities Education Act (IDEA) reauthorized these mandates and added further mandates regarding assistive technology for functional activities. Under IDEA, physical therapy is a related service to which children are entitled under the law. In the school setting, goals must relate to educational outcomes.

### Adolescence

The adolescent years are certainly years of challenge and change for all children, including children with disabilities. This period may be quite difficult, as adolescents struggle with the same self-esteem issues as their peers, complicated by an increasing awareness of their limitations and perhaps a realization of the impact that their disability may have on others.[15] Emphasis in physical therapy is on maintaining or improving level of function while considering the additional stresses of growth, maturation, and the additional demands in independent life skills. Adolescents should be involved in setting goals and determining involvement in physical therapy. It is extremely important that self-responsibility be part of the therapeutic approach as the young adult takes on responsibility for his or her own health, which includes an understanding of the need for life-long management of his or her disability. During the adolescent years, the main physical therapy goals can be established as follows:

*Reducing Primary Impairment and Preventing Secondary Impairment.* Growth spurts are expected during adolescence. Bones tend to grow more quickly than muscles and, therefore, muscle shortening, contractures, "growing pains," and deformities should be preventively managed. The maintenance of muscle extensibility and joint integrity are primary concerns for the therapist. Casting and splints are effective management options. In adolescence, changes in body dimensions can also affect upright posture and movement. The center of gravity is higher; shoulders may broaden in boys while hips broaden in girls, changing the demands placed on lower extremity biomechanics, trunk control, and energy expenditure.

*Maintaining Force Generation.* As body mass and lever length increase, strengthening is an important aspect of therapeutic management.

*Mobility and Endurance.* Compensatory and supportive strategies may be necessary to maintain function and prevent disability during the adolescent years. Adolescents who are ambulatory may need an alternative form of mobility such as a manual chair for intermittent use throughout the day. Children previously in a manual chair may require a power chair for increased access, speed, and function. Driver training needs to be explored, usually through a local rehabilitation agency.

### Adulthood

Because pediatric physical therapists work with children who have developmental disabilities, therapists must be attuned to long-range planning and prophylactic management, cognizant of the reality that all children grow into adults with chronic disabilities. The goal of adulthood is functional independence within the constraints imposed by the disability. The extent to which young adults with disabilities can realize this goal is dependent on severity of involvement, social and cognitive abilities, and the availability of resources. The major goal is to maximize abilities and minimize the effects of impairments on function. During the period of transition into adulthood, the main physical therapy goals can be established as follows:

*Reduce Primary Impairment and Prevent Secondary Impairment.* The impairments of decreased force production and hypoextensibility still respond to therapy. Although secondary impairments may appear to be static, there can still be deterioration and therapy can prevent a negative impact on function. Overuse syndromes, joint degeneration, osteoporosis, and pathologic fractures need preventive management strategies.

*Life Skills.* Opportunities for maintenance of fitness, recreational programs, and adaptive living support is becoming more widely available. Therapists can help young adults explore resources available within the community. Therapists can also offer unique consultation services to community agencies.[15,16]

## SUMMARY

Physical therapy for children requires a sound generalist background in the fundamentals of physical therapy, augmented by additional skills in understanding psychomotor development, developmental biomechanics, and the psychosocial aspects of working with children with disabilities and their families. The challenges are great, matched only by the bounty of the rewards.

## REFERENCES

1. Ratliffe KT. *Clinical Pediatric Physical Therapy*. St Louis: Mosby; 1998:163–217.
2. Bertoti DB. Cerebral palsy: Lifespan management. Home study course 10.2.4. In: *Orthopedic Interventions for the Pediatric Patient*. LaCrosse, Wis: Orthopaedic Section, APTA; 2000.
3. *Guide to Physical Therapist Practice*. Alexandria, VA: American Physical Therapy Association; 1997.
4. Palisano Rj, Campbell SK, Harris SR. Decision making in pediatric physical therapy. In: Campbell SK (ed). *Physical Therapy for Children*. Philadelphia: WB Saunders; 1995.
5. Kolobe TH, Sparling J, Daniels LE. Family centered intervention. In Campbell SK (ed). *Physical Therapy for Children*. Philadelphia: WB Saunders; 1995.
6. Long TM, Cintas H. *Handbook of Pediatric Physical Therapy*, Baltimore: Williams and Wilkins; 1995.
7. Adams R. Spina bifida: lifespan management. Home study course 10.2.2. In: *Orthopedic Interventions for the Pediatric Patient*. LaCrosse, Wis: Orthopaedic Section, APTA; 2000.
8. Bertoti DB. Mentally retardation: focus on Down syndrome. In: Tecklin JS (ed). *Pediatric Physical Therapy*. Philadelphia: JB Lippincott; 1999.
9. Olney SJ, Wright AJ. Cerebral palsy. In: Campbell SK (ed). *Physical Therapy for Children*. Philadelphia: WB Saunders; 1994.
10. Styer-Acevedo J. Physical therapy for the child with cerebral palsy. In: Tecklin JS (ed). *Pediatric Physical Therapy*, 3rd ed. Philadelphia: Lippincott-Raven; 1998:107–162.
11. Bertoti DB, Stanger M. Pediatric musculoskeletal assessment: the impact of developmental factors. *Orthop Phys Ther Clin North Am*. 1994;3:31–43.
12. Brenneman SK, Stanger M, Bertoti DB. Age-related considerations: pediatric. In: Myers RS (ed). *Saunders Manual of Physical Therapy Practice*. Philadelphia: WB Saunders; 1995.
13. Barry M. Physical therapy interventions for patients with movement disorders due to cerebral palsy. *J Child Neurol*. 1996;11:S51–S60.
14. Whiteside A. Clinical goals and application of NDT facilitation. *NDTA Network*. 1997; Sept/Oct: 2–14.
15. Campbell SK. Therapy programs for children that last a lifetime. *Phys Occup Ther Pediatr*. 1997;17:1–15.
16. *Consumer's Guide: Therapeutic Services for Children with Disabilities*. Cambridge, MA: United Cerebral Palsy Association; 1995.

CHAPTER 8

# Legal and Ethical Standards

RON SCOTT

## Key Words and Phrases

Administrative Agencies
Administrative Rules and Regulations
Age Discrimination in Employment Act
American Board of Physical Therapy Specialties
American Physical Therapy Association
Americans with Disabilities Act
Board of Directors
Business Ethics
Certification
Chapter Ethics Committee
Civil Rights Act of 1964
Commission on Accreditation in Physical Therapy Education
Constitution
Corporate Liability
Credentialing
Declaration Against (Self) Interest
Due Process
Emergency Doctrine
Equal Employment Opportunity Commission
Ethical Decision Making
Ethics
Ethics and Judicial Committee
Family and Medical Leave Act
Federation of State Boards of Physical Therapy
Fiduciary
*Guide for Professional Conduct*
*Guide for Conduct of the Affiliate Member*
*Guide to Physical Therapist Practice*
Health Care Malpractice
Health Professional Ethics
Hostile Work Environment Sexual Harassment
Informed Consent
Institutional Ethics Committee
Intentional Misconduct
Judge-Made Case Law
Jurisdiction
Legal Obligations
Licensing Boards
Licensing Laws
Licensure
Model Practice Act

Morals
Negligence
Optimal Therapeutic Result
Ordinary Negligence
Organizational Ethics
Patient Bill of Rights and Duties
Procedural Document on Disciplinary Action
Professional Ethics
Professional Negligence
*Quid pro quo* Sexual Harassment
Secondary Sources of Legal Obligation
Sexual Harassment
Statutes
Strict Liability
Strict Product Liability
Supremacy Clause
Systems Approach to Ethical Decision Making
Therapeutic Privilege
Vicarious Liability

*Physical therapists and physical therapist assistants in all practice domains face a formidable challenge to comply with legal practice mandates, including, but not limited to, licensure, conforming practice, and other official conduct, professional and organizational practice and ethical standards, universally obtaining patient informed consent prior to care delivery, and managing employees in accordance with governing legal standards. Physical therapists and physical therapist assistants are fiduciaries or professionals in a special position of trust vis-à-vis patients under their care. This means that they must place patients' best interests above all other competing interests, including their own financial and related interests, and those of their employers. Under cost-containment-focused managed care, this lofty responsibility is seemingly more difficult to fulfill. The* Guide for Professional Conduct *(governing physical therapists' professional ethical responsibilities) and the* Guide for Conduct of the Affiliate Member *(governing that of physical therapist assistants) offer road maps to ethical comportment for physical therapy professionals; however, these standards do not expressly address the conduct or duties of extender personnel or of professional students. These deficiencies should be remedied. The Model Practice Act, like the Model Rules of Professional Conduct for attorneys, serves as an excellent guide for creating uniformity among disparate state physical therapy licensing statutes. Patients, employees, students, and other participants in physical therapy settings possess legal rights and are encumbered with legal duties. For clinical physical therapists, the most important duty owed to patients is to care for them in accordance with legal practice standards. To fall below minimally acceptable practice is to commit health care malpractice, which may be legally actionable if a patient is injured as a result of substandard care delivery. The legal bases for imposition of health care malpractice liability also include intentional misconduct toward patients (such as the commission of sexual battery), nonfulfillment of a therapeutic promise made to a patient (breach of contract liability), and strict liability (without regard to fault) for patient injury from dangerously defective care-related products or equipment, or from utilization of abnormally dangerous care-related procedures (possibly including cervical manipulation, at the hands of unqualified therapists). Patient informed consent is both a legal and professional ethical prerequisite to physical therapy intervention. The minimal disclosure elements for legally sufficient patient informed consent include patient diagnosis, nature of the proposed course of care, goals of intervention, risks of serious harm or complication associated with a recommended intervention (if any), and reasonable alternatives to the recommended intervention (and their relative risks and benefits). Disciplinary action by the Ethics and Judicial Committee of the American Physical Therapy Association serves to protect public and professional interests alike, by affording due process (or fundamental fairness) to respondents, complainants, and witnesses, and by assuring, to the extent possible, public safety and confidence in the process and its outcome.*

## LICENSURE, CERTIFICATION, AND CREDENTIALING

Licensure, certification, and credentialing of physical therapy professionals denotes special professional and legal status for those so recognized. Licensure is public recognition of special professional status, typically granted by state licensing boards and authorities. Although physical therapists are required to be licensed in order to practice their profession in all 50 states, physical therapist assistants are licensed in many, but not all states.

Many or most states grant license by endorsement for physical therapy professionals licensed in other states, without the need to retake a licensing examination. However, before engaging in physical therapy practice in any state, physical therapists and assistants must be licensed in that state. Initial licensure in a gaining state may involve the issuance of a temporary license, which typically expires (or must be renewed) after a relatively short time.

There are several other issues surrounding health professional licensure that are of importance to physical therapy professionals. There has been, in public fora over the past few decades, a sense that licensing laws have become too pervasive. The principal purpose of health professional licensing laws is to protect the patient and public from unqualified and unsafe providers. State legislatures have come to believe that not all classes of health care professionals require licensure for public protection (and that it is too burdensome a system to administer), and for that reason, there has been a trend away from continued proliferation of health professional licensing laws.

Another licensing law issue concerns the requirement for federal systems and entities to respect state licensure and other administrative practice requirements. The Supremacy Clause in Article VI, Section 2 of the federal Constitution subordinates conflicting state law to governing federal laws and regulations. For that reason, military physical therapists practicing in any state may not be limited in their official military (federal) practice by that state's licensing laws and administrative rules and regulations, since they are governed principally to federal law pursuant to Article I, Section 8 [concerning Congress' plenary power to "raise, support, and maintain" military forces] and Article VI of the Constitution.

Another important licensure issue concerns practice across state lines. The Internet has created consultative health professional practice opportunities nation- and worldwide; however, such practice in states in which one is not licensed may give rise to criminal liability, adverse administrative actions affecting licensure, and ethics adjudications by professional association entities. Before engaging in such practice across state lines, physical therapy professionals must obtain legal advice on its propriety.

Certification of health professionals serves as a private sector analog to public sector licensure. Certification of health care professionals may be an alternative or a supplement to licensure, and, like licensure, serves to validate individual provider competence. Many physical therapists and assistants are dually credentialed as licensed physical therapy professionals and certified athletic trainers. Athletic trainer certification is administered by the National Athletic Training Association.

Physical therapists having extensive clinical experience may also become board certified by the American Board of Physical Therapy Specialties (ABPTS). Currently, the ABPTS offers certification through examination and portfolio review in the following clinical specialties:

- Cardiopulmonary physical therapy (CCS)
- Clinical electrophysiology (ECS)
- Geriatric physical therapy (GCS)
- Neurological physical therapy (NCS)
- Orthopaedic physical therapy (OCS)
- Pediatric physical therapy (PCS), and
- Sports physical therapy (SCS)

Board-certified physical therapist-clinical specialists are entitled (and required) to use the specialty designator listed above after their "PT" designation. Periodic recertification is required to maintain board-certification status. Requirements for recertification vary from specialty to specialty, and may be obtained from the ABPTS.

## BUSINESS; ORGANIZATIONAL AND PROFESSIONAL ETHICS

As health professionals and business persons working within organizations, physical therapists and physical therapist assistants have professional, business, and organizational ethical standards that guide their practices. Resultant practice problems, issues, and dilemmas may arise on a recurrent basis for these professionals when professional, business, and organizational ethical standards and mandates come into conflict.

What are "ethics"? Ethics are standards of conduct governing behavior. For health care professionals, the principal classification of behavior affected by ethical standards involves interpersonal behavior, i.e., how to interact with patients and clients, coworkers and consultants, third-party payers, and a multitude of others, on an ongoing basis.

How do ethics differ from morals? Although ethical standards are grounded in moral beliefs, they are different and more narrow than morals in general. Moral beliefs are personal beliefs about important life issues, such as religion, abortion, the death penalty, commitment to marriage and children, and similar matters. Ethics represent viewpoints on important matters related to one's official conduct, such as within a profession, occupation, or business organization.

Every individual has notions of what his or her professional conduct should be. These ideals form individual ethics. Groups of individual professionals and workers also formulate workplace standards of conduct. For business organizations and systems, these (usually written) standards constitute organizational ethics. An occupation or cluster of related occupations may also develop ethical standards of conduct, which make up business ethics. A limited number of professional disciplines even develop and constantly refine professional ethical standards of conduct, such as the two professions within physical therapy—physical therapists and physical therapist assistants—with their respective publications, *Guide for Professional Conduct* and *Guide for Conduct of the Affiliate Member* (see Appendices 8-1 and 8-2).

The differences in focus between and among business, organizational, and professional ethics result mainly from the nature and perception of duties owed by constituent members to clients served by the organization, business, or profession. Whereas businesses generally have business ethical codes requiring fair dealing with customers and high-quality product and/or service delivery, professions focus on the fiduciary duty owed by members of the professions to clients. A fiduciary duty involves a special duty, in fact, the highest possible duty undertaken by anyone on another's behalf. A fiduciary voluntarily agrees to subordinate personal interests in favor of the best interests of clients served.* A licensed or certified health professional fiduciary puts the interests of his or her patients above all

* A *fiduciary* is a person who stands in a special position of trust in relation to another person. The fiduciary is charged by legal and/or ethical standards to place the best interests of clients above all other interests, including the fiduciary's own personal interests. A fiduciary is the polar opposite of a narcissist. Physical therapy professionals, like all other health care professionals, are fiduciaries to the patients and clients they serve.

others, including those of employers, payers, and oneself. Physical therapists and physical therapist assistants are fiduciaries to their patients and clients.

How does a physical therapist or physical therapist assistant deal with professional ethical problems, issues, and dilemmas that arise in practice? Although there are many models described in the professional literature for ethics resolution, one simple one is the *systems approach* to professional ethical decision making.[†]

In terms of health professional ethical decision making, the first step in using the systems approach is to identify a problem, issue, or dilemma (in increasing order of severity and immediacy) having ethical dimensions. Next, inputs are identified. These consist of facts, unknowns, and assumptions about the problem, issue, or dilemma. After that, possible solutions to the problem, issue, or dilemma are identified ("outputs"), and what the person taking action (the "actor") believes to be the optimal solution is implemented.

What makes the systems approach different from other ethical decision-making models is the addition of a feedback loop, which means that the actor carefully monitors the chosen solution for effectiveness and acts to modify (or discard and replace) it as necessary.

## PROFESSIONAL ETHICAL STANDARDS

There are two primary written resources delineating the professional ethical duties owed by physical therapists and physical therapist assistants to patients, clients, professional colleagues, and others. Both are promulgated by the American Physical Therapy Association (APTA). These ethical guidelines are the *Guide for Professional Conduct* (governing the official conduct of licensed physical therapist-members of the APTA) and the *Guide for Conduct of the Affiliate Member* (governing the official conduct of physical therapist assistant-affiliate members of the APTA).

What written or unwritten professional ethical standards govern the conduct of physical therapists and physical therapist assistants who are not members of the APTA? Physical therapy licensure statutes in all states are modeled, at least in part, after the *Guide for Professional Conduct*. It may also be that the provisions of the *Guide for Professional Conduct* and the *Guide for Conduct of the Affiliate Member* are more than APTA private standards because they delineate universally applicable professional ethical standards for physical therapy professionals. As such, they might be used

[†] For more detailed information on this model, see Scott RW. *Professional Ethics: A Guide for Rehabilitation Professionals.* St. Louis: Mosby–Year Book; 1998.

by courts, licensure boards, and other administrative bodies to assess the conduct of even non–APTA members.

The *Guide for Professional Conduct* and the *Guide for Conduct of the Affiliate Member* share unique attributes among health professional codes of ethics. For example, it is rare to find separate ethics codes for licensed primary health care professionals and licensed assistants, as exists with these two codifications. One problem associated even with these two codes is that other extender personnel, including athletic trainers, physical therapy and rehabilitation aides, and health professional students, are not expressly included in the coverage of either code's provisions. At the time of the writing of this book, the Ethics and Judicial Committee of the APTA was working on revisions to both documents, which may remedy this defect.

Another special feature of the *Guide for Professional Conduct* is that it contains both directive and nondirective provisions. Directive provisions in a code of ethics are imperatives, or mandates, and are represented by words like "shall," "shall not," and "may not." Nondirective provisions may be either permissive (with action verbs like "may") or imploring in nature (with action verbs like "should").

Copies of the current editions of the *Guide for Professional Conduct* and the *Guide for Conduct of the Affiliate Member* are reprinted and appear at the end of this chapter. Physical therapy professionals and students are strongly encouraged to maintain current copies of these documents in their work places and in their clinical notebooks, and to update them on an ongoing basis.

## SOURCES OF LEGAL OBLIGATION FOR LICENSED HEALTH PROFESSIONALS

There are five categories of sources of legal obligation for licensed health care professionals. These include constitutional mandates, legal obligations emanating from statutory laws, judge-made (trial) case law pronouncements within the jurisdiction of the provider, administrative agencies, rules and regulations, and legal duties associated with secondary source authorities.

There exists a hierarchy of precedence for legal authorities that must be obeyed. At the pinnacle of this hierarchy is federal constitutional law. The federal Constitution is known as the "supreme law of the land." With few exceptions, the legal mandates spelled out in the Constitution apply only to federal, state, and local governmental entities. One notable exception to this principle is the 13th Amendment to the Constitution, which prohibits involuntary servitude of one person by another—whether imposed by a governmental entity or a private citizen or business entity.

An important federal constitutional personal right affecting physical therapy is the constitutional right of individual privacy. As important as this right may seem, it is not one of the enumerated personal liberties found in the Bill of Rights and body of, and amendments to, the Constitution. Rather, the constitutional right to privacy is an implied right of recent origin and the subject of ongoing controversy among legal scholars. The constitutional right to patient privacy affects what use governmental entities and officials may make of patient-related information, including medical and billing records, whether on paper or computerized.

State constitutions may afford greater rights to citizens and residents of particular states than does the federal Constitution. State constitutions may not, however, take away rights granted to individuals under federal law.

Statutes are laws enacted by Congress or by state legislatures. Examples of important federal and state statutes affecting physical therapy professionals and their patients include the Americans with Disabilities Act (prohibiting access and employment discrimination of disabled persons), the Civil Rights Act of 1964 (Title VII of which prohibits employment discrimination based on race, ethnicity, religion, gender, or national origin), the Family and Medical Leave Act (providing employee job security in the face of illness, injury, or pregnancy), the Occupational Safety and Health Act (promoting and enforcing workplace safety), the Social Security, Medicare and Medicaid Acts (promoting the general welfare [Preamble, Constitution] through medical and financial social safety nets), and state physical therapy practice acts (delineating the permissible scope of licensed physical therapy practice).

Judge-made case law consists of legal trial and appellate court opinions from specific civil and criminal legal cases. These judicial decisions have the force of law, and are, when issued by the highest-level state courts, precedent that must be followed by lower-level courts within the state. Important examples of judicial cases affecting physical therapy professionals include health care malpractice civil cases brought by patients against providers and/or institutions for alleged injuries and criminal cases brought against individuals and/or institutions by local, state, or federal prosecutors for alleged wrongdoing.

Physical therapy professionals in all practice settings—like citizens and business people generally—have the greatest exposure to the legal system through interactions with administrative agencies at local, state, and federal levels. Administrative agencies exercise power over business affairs that has been delegated to them by Congress and/or state legislatures. Examples of important administrative agencies impacting physical therapy include the Equal Employment Opportunity Commission (concerning the equal and fair treatment of employees and job applicants by employers), the Internal

Revenue Service (concerning federal tax law), and the Occupational Safety and Health Administration (concerning workplace safety).

Important secondary sources of legal duty and of the professional standard of care include accreditation standards, such as those issued by the Joint Commission on the Accreditation of Health Care Organizations, the Commission on Accreditation of Rehabilitation Facilities, and the Commission on Accreditation in Physical Therapy Education; written institutional and association practice standards and guidelines, including, for physical therapists, the *Guide to Physical Therapist Practice*; unwritten customary practice standards; and professional, organization, and business ethical standards, including, for physical therapy professionals, the *Guide for Professional Conduct* and the *Guide for Conduct of the Affiliate Member.*

## MODEL PRACTICE ACT

The Model Practice Act is a document issued by the Federation of State Boards of Physical Therapy, a private, nonprofit 506(c) [trade association] organization made up of representative state physical therapy licensing boards from the 50 states. The Federation of State Boards of Physical Therapy, established in 1986, has as its co-primary functions to: serve as a resource entity for member state physical therapy licensing boards; enhance public safety through effective physical therapy licensing processes and procedures; set practice standards and physical therapist and assistant competence through the National Examination Program (through which the Federation develops and administers the Physical Therapist Examination and the Physical Therapist Assistant Examination); and provide continuing education to members and physical therapy professionals.

The purpose of the Model Practice Act is to foster uniformity among state licensing laws governing the practice of physical therapy. Such uniformity serves simultaneously to protect public, patient, and client interests in safety and provider competence, and to simply the regulation by administrative agencies of physical therapy professionals within their jurisdictions.

The Model Practice Act consists of three substantive sections: (1) Key Areas, whose provisions are directed to state statutes exclusively; (2) Guidelines for Rules, addressing itself to administrative rules and regulations; and (3) Appendices, containing background resource material for decision and policy makers.

The specific substantive content for Section 1, Key Areas and Section 2, Guidelines for Rules, is identical, and includes:

- Legislative Intent
- Definitions

- Physical Therapy Licensing Boards
- Licensure and Examination
- Lawful Practice
- Use of Titles
- Patient Care Management
- Grounds for Disciplinary Action
- Disciplinary Actions and Procedures
- Unlawful Practice
- Consumer Advocacy

The Appendices include the following content:

- Model Practice Act (less commentary)
- Model Definition for "Physical Therapy"
- The Federation of State Boards of Physical Therapy Position Paper on Physical Therapist Assistant Regulation
- The Federation of State Boards of Physical Therapy Model Language Changes for Licensure of Physical Therapist Assistants
- The American Physical Therapy Association's Code of Ethics and Guide for Professional Conduct
- The Federation of State Boards of Physical Therapy Guidelines on English Proficiency Standards

As has occurred in the legal profession with the American Law Institute's Model Rules of Professional Conduct, it is expected that the states will adopt the Model Practice Act in whole or in part over time. A copy of the Model Practice Act is reprinted in Appendix II, which appears at the end of this book. A new revision of the Model Practice Act is pending at the time of publication of this text.

Internationally educated physical therapists must meet prescreening certification requirements by the Immigration and Naturalization Service (INS) of the federal government in order to be admitted into the United States with an appropriate visa to seek state licensure. Those requirements include: (1) a baccalaureate science degree (or equivalent) in physical therapy from an accredited educational institution; (2) certification of professional status from the international administrative agency regulating physical therapy practice and physical therapists; and (3) demonstrated competence in English, as reflected by examination scores on the Test of English as a Foreign Language, the Test of Spoken English, and the Test of Written English. Additional requirements of state licensure boards may also apply to practice by foreign-educated physical therapists.

## RIGHTS AND DUTIES OF PATIENTS, HEALTH PROFESSIONALS, AND HEALTH PROFESSIONAL STUDENTS

Under US federal and state law, individuals and business entities possess legal rights and are simultaneously encumbered with legal obligations. Rights and duties are the "heads" and "tails" of a two-sided coin.

What is the primary duty of a clinical health care professional toward his or her patients? Is it to effect a cure for a disease, or to reverse the adverse consequences of an injury or alleviate an impairment or impairments? No. Although these goals of intervention represent the hopes and aspirations of both providers and patients, they are not what is basically required of clinical health care providers. What clinical health care professionals must do, however, is utilize their best skills and exercise their best clinical judgment to attempt to effect an optimal therapeutic result for patients under their care.

Specific patient rights and responsibilities may be delineated in institutional literature, such as handouts, or in universal documents, such as patient bills of rights and duties (See Fig. 8–1), posted in virtually every

# Patient Bill of Rights and Duties

## Patient Rights

**Quality Care.** You have the right to quality care and treatment that are available and medically indicated, regardless of race, gender, national origin, or religion.

**Respect and Dignity.** You have the right to considerate and respectful care, with recognition of your family, religious, and cultural preferences.

**Privacy and Confidentiality.** You have the right to privacy and confidentiality concerning medical care. This includes expecting any discussion or consultation about your case to be conducted discreetly and privately, and having your medical record read only by people involved in your treatment or the monitoring of its quality, and by other individuals only by authorization by you or your legally authorized representative.

FIGURE 8-1 Patient Bill of Rights and Duties, Brooke Army Medical Center, San Antonio, Texas. (*continued*)

**Identity.** You have the right to know the name and professional status of the individuals who provide your care and which practitioner is primarily responsible for your care.

**Information.** You have the right to understand tests, medications, procedures and treatments, their risks, their benefits, their costs and their alternatives prior to consenting to the test, medication, procedure, or treatment. You have the right to complete and timely information regarding your illness and known prognosis (expected outcome). You have the right to see and obtain a copy of your medical record.

**Refusal of Treatment.** You may refuse medical treatment within the extent permitted by law, and you have the right to be informed of the consequences of refusing that treatment.

**Advance Directives.** You have the right to designate a representative to make health care decision if you become unable to do so. You have the right to formulate an advance directive (living will and/or medical durable power of attorney), and to take part in ethics discussions pertinent to your care.

**Research.** You have the right to be advised of research associated with your care. You have the right to refuse to participate in any research projects.

**Safe Environment.** You have the right to care and treatment in a safe environment and the right to protective services in cases of abuse.

**Clinical Rules and Regulations.** You have the right to be informed of the facility's rules and regulations that relate to your conduct as a patient and how patient complaints are initiated, reviewed, and resolved.

## Patient Responsibilities

**Maintain Positive Health Practices.** You have the responsibility to develop and maintain positive health practices: good nutrition, sleep and rest, exercise, positive relationships, and stress management.

FIGURE 8-1 *Continued.*

**Providing Information.** You have the responsibility to give your physician and health care providers accurate and complete information about your illness, medical history, and medications. You have the responsibility of communicating to your health care provider your understanding of your treatment and what is expected of you.

**Compliance with Medical Care.** You have the responsibility for following your physician's and health care provider's recommendations to the best of your ability, to ask questions if you have problems and concerns, and work out alternative plans. You are responsible for keeping appointments, filling prescriptions, following through on health care instructions, and adhering to guidelines of the clinic.

**Making Choices.** You have the responsibility to make choices in your own best interest based on a clear understanding of your medical care, its costs, risks, and alternatives. You have the responsibility to ask for information on your illness, to learn what you can and to do what you can to help maintain the best health possible.

**Respect and Consideration.** You are responsible for treating physicians, health care providers, and other patients with respect, including the control of noise and listening and responding to questions and concerns.

**Smoking Policy.** You will refrain from smoking while in the facility or within 50 feet of the building.

**Medical Records.** If you hand-carry your medical records, you are responsible for ensuring the records are promptly returned to the appropriate medical treatment facility. ALL MEDICAL RECORDS DOCUMENTING CARE PROVIDED BY ANY MILITARY MEDICAL TREATMENT FACILITY ARE THE PROPERTY OF THE U.S. GOVERNMENT.

**Reporting of Patient Complaints.** You are responsible for helping the commander of the Fort Meade MEDDAC and the commander/director of this medical treatment facility provide the best possible care to all beneficiaries. You should report any recommendations, questions, or complaints to the designated patient representative.

FIGURE 8-1 *Continued.*

clinical setting in the United States. Even without such written guidance, patients do have legal responsibilities toward their health care professionals. The principal duty of a patient is to pay for health care services rendered on their behalf, most commonly through a third-party intermediary or insurer.

Health care clinical professionals should also make an express (i.e., clearly stated) part of their care contracts with patients the patient duty to cooperate to the maximal extent that is feasible and safe with the agreed-to plan of intervention. As such, patients become, as they in fact are, stakeholders in their own health care and recovery.

Patients and their health care providers owe each other mutual respect and civility. This means, at a minimum, that they respect each other's physical space and human dignity. Just as it is never acceptable for physical therapy professionals to commit assault or battery upon patients, it is equally unacceptable for patients to physically strike or threaten their health care providers. Consider the following case example, derived from an actual practice situation:

P., a home health physical therapist, conducts an initial visit inpatient A.'s home, for the purpose of examining and evaluating A., a patient who is post-CVA, for home intervention. No one except P. and A. are in A.'s home at the time of the visit. After obtaining A.'s informed consent to examine A., P. carries out the examination without incident. While P. is writing the initial examination/evaluation note, A. reaches into a nearby nightstand drawer and retrieves a loaded handgun. A. points the gun at P. and orally threatens to shoot P. unless P. leaves immediately. What should P. do?

In addition to exiting safety and quickly, P. should immediately notify law enforcement authorities and the home health agency regarding the situation that has occurred. A. poses an imminent danger to himself and others, and may lack full cognitive control. It is a judgment call as to whether P. reenters A.'s home again, or is replaced, if and when it is safe to commence intervention, by another physical therapist. In any event, the agency should not attempt to coerce P. into resuming care responsibility for A. if P. does not voluntarily assume such responsibility. No health care provider, under these circumstances, has a legal or ethical duty to risk imminent serious bodily harm or death respective to caring for a patient.

## CIVIL RIGHTS LAWS

At federal, state, and even local or municipal levels, civil rights statutes, case law, and administrative rules and regulations are in force to protect the basic civil rights of all citizens and legal aliens within the territory of the United States. The most important of these protections at the federal level include: the Age Discrimination in Employment Act, the Americans with Disabilities Act, the Civil Rights Act of 1964, and the Family and Medical Leave Act. These federal statutes are briefly described below.

The Age Discrimination in Employment Act of 1967 (ADEA) protects older workers, age 40 or older, from employment-related discrimination based on their age. This law, like those described below, protect workers from discrimination at all stages of employment, from recruitment and application for employment through retirement or termination of employment. The Americans with Disabilities Act of 1990 (ADA) expands the scope of protected classes of persons for purposes of federal civil rights protection to include those customers and employees having physical or mental disabilities. Title I of the ADA is the analog of the ADEA and of Title VII of the Civil Rights Act of 1964, in that it protects disabled employees and job applicants from employment discrimination. Title II of the ADA extends civil rights protection to disabled persons utilizing public facilities, such as airports, government buildings, and public colleges and universities. Title II of the ADA mandates that "public accommodations," especially including physical therapy facilities, be accessible to disabled patients and clients.

Title VII of the Civil Rights Act of 1964 mandates that employers not discriminate in hiring or any other aspects of employment against any persons on the bases of race/ethnicity, religion, gender, or national origin. It is from the global concept of gender discrimination that laws and regulations prohibiting workplace sexual harassment emanated. Sexual harassment, although seemingly obviously a form of gender discrimination, was not recognized by the US Supreme Court for 15 years after its inclusion in Title VII. There are two basic types of workplace sexual harassment. One is *quid pro quo* sexual harassment, in which someone in a position of authority coerces a subordinate to engage in sexual activity in exchange for favorable employment considerations, such as a pay raise or permission to attend continuing education courses. The other basic type of workplace sexual harassment is "hostile work environment" sexual harassment, which does not necessarily involve a superior and subordinate as perpetrator and victim, respectively. Under this prong of sexual harassment, a perpetrator's conduct substantially and objectively interferes. Anyone in the workplace may be a perpetrator (including patients, for whose conduct management is legally responsible).

## CLINICAL AFFILIATION AGREEMENTS

Clinical affiliation agreements are formal contracts between education institutions and clinical facilities for the clinical placement of physical therapy professional students. In recent times, these contracts have become more and more difficult to draft, reach agreement on, and administer. These difficulties involve such issues as the assignment of vicarious liability for student conduct (even though all professional physical therapy students are covered by mandatory professional liability insurance policies), and the relative rights and duties of the educational and clinical institutions, respectively. They universally require legal oversight in their development and implementation. An optimal approach to their use would be to create them as multiparty contracts, with rights and duties attaching to education and clinical entities and to students as co-primary contractees.

In a few cases, physical therapy clinical affiliation agreements are triparty contracts, binding not only educational institutions and clinical sites to their provisions, but students as well. A clinical affiliation agreement that binds students to clear, express contractual obligations benefits educational institutions, clinical sites, and students alike, in that student rights and duties are clearly delineated. A generic example of such an agreement appears in Fig. 8–2, and may be freely modified for use by physical therapy educational institutions. Academic coordinators of clinical education are cautioned, however, that the exemplar is intended as informational, generic, and nonspecific, so that it must be adapted to state law requirements and reviewed by legal counsel before implementation.

## BASES FOR HEALTH CARE MALPRACTICE LIABILITY

*Health care malpractice* is civil liability of a health care professional for patient injuries (physical and/or mental), with a legal basis for liability imposition. The term health care malpractice is used herein instead of medical malpractice, which affects only physicians and surgeons. At present, a larger group of primary health care providers—including physical and occupational therapists, speech and hearing professionals, nurse practitioners, physician assistants, and others—may be claimed against or sued by patients in their own capacities for malpractice.

The recognized legal bases for health care malpractice liability imposition include the following:

- Professional negligence, or substandard care delivery (Note that non-care–related negligence, e.g., a patient "slip and fall" on a wet surface, is *not* health care malpractice, but rather *ordinary negligence*.)
- Intentional care-related misconduct, including, among other torts, *battery* (harmful or offensive patient contact) and *sexual battery* (conduct intended to arouse or gratify sexual desires of the provider or patient)
- Breach of a therapeutic contractual promise
- "Strict" (without regard to fault) liability for abnormally dangerous care-related activities or patient injury by dangerously defective care-related products or equipment [strict product liability].

# UNIVERSAL UNIVERSITY, ANYTOWN, USA
# PHYSICAL THERAPY DEPARTMENT
# CLINICAL AFFILIATION AGREEMENT

This agreement between Universal University (UU) and: ____________
____________________________________________ (clinical site)
is effective as of ________________ (date).

UU is a private Anystate higher education institution with a Master of Physical Therapy (MPT) graduate program, desiring clinical internship sites for its professional-phase students. The clinical site has the requisite facilities and professional personnel to provide clinical internships for UU physical therapy (PT) students. The parties agree to the following:

UU responsibilities:

1. Exercise exclusive responsibility for the graduate education program, including, but not limited to: administration, curriculum, grading and graduation, student discipline;
2. Ensure that all students have professional liability, health insurance, and current CPR certification and immunizations, and retain vicarious liability for program-related student conduct in the clinic;
3. Provide evaluation forms to clinical sites for student assessment;
4. Prepare students academically prior to clinical placement;
5. Coordinate numbers and scheduling of students with the clinical site.

Clinical site responsibilities:

1. Provide an organized clinical internship plan for UU students, under mentorship of designated qualified clinical instructors;
2. Allow students to practice only under the direct supervision of licensed physical therapist clinical instructors and in conformity with state licensure laws;
3. Provide upon arrival to the clinic orientation for students, including, but not limited to, review of applicable policies, procedures, and protocols;

FIGURE 8-2 A generic sample of a clinical affiliation agreement. (*continued on next page*)

4. Provide appropriate facilities and experiences for students at the site;
5. Regularly, fairly, and objectively evaluate student performance (cognition, psychomotor skills, and affect), and report results to UU's academic coordinator of clinical education (ACCE) in a timely manner.

Student responsibilities (All UU student affiliates expressly agree to the following. [To be executed before affiliation commences]):

1. Follow directions from clinical instructors and other clinical faculty and staff, as appropriate;
2. Work diligently to achieve agreed goals of the affiliation experience, as established among UU's ACCE, the site clinical coordinator of clinical education (CCCE) and clinical instructor (CI), and the student;
3. Follow the clinical schedule of the assigned CI, at the discretion of the clinical site;
4. Regularly and enthusiastically participate in the full complement of clinical processes, such as journal club, community outreach events, etc., as the clinical education program permits and at the discretion of the clinical site;
5. Expeditiously report to CI and ACCE any circumstance potentially adversely affecting the student's ability to fulfill clinical internship objectives (Confidentiality will be maintained within educational and clinical "need-to-know" channels, except as otherwise required by law);
6. Be bound by the APTA Code of Ethics and Guide for Professional Conduct.

Additional points: In consideration for the clinical site undertaking mentorship of UU MPT student affiliates, UU will:

1. Award departmental appointment certificates to CCCEs and CI's as Clinical Instructors;
2. Permit students' CI's and CCCE to attend UU PT Department continuing education events at-cost.

This affiliation agreement is effective upon signatures below, and remains in effect for a 3-year period, automatically renewed unless terminated by mutual agreement of the parties, or upon 90 days written notice by either UU or the clinical site. The agreement is to be governed by the law of the state in which the clinical site is located, or by federal law, as applicable, and may be modified in writing by mutual consent of the parties. UU and the clinical site agree that no

FIGURE 8-2 *Continued*

individual or entity may discriminate against any patient, student, educator, clinician, or other person, on the basis of race, ethnicity, age, gender, religion, national origin, or disability. Both UU and the clinical site agree to be bound by the APTA Code of Ethics and Guide for Professional Conduct.

Universal University, Anytown, USA

By:____________________ ____________________

President or designee Date
Clinical Site

By:____________________ ____________________

CCCE or designee Date

By:____________________ ____________________

Student Affiliate Date

FIGURE 8-2 *Continued*

The vast majority of health care malpractice claims and lawsuits involve allegations of professional negligence or substandard care delivery. To prevail in a professional negligence health care malpractice case, a patient must prove the existence of the following core elements by a preponderance, or greater weight, of evidence:

- A special duty owed by the defendant-provider toward the patient (This special duty becomes operational when the provider agrees to provide health professional services for the patient.)
- Violation of the special duty owed (by providing objectively substandard care delivery)
- "Causation" (proof that the substandard care delivery resulted in injury to the patient)
- "Damages" (proof that the patient's injuries warrant the award of money in order to restore the patient, to the extent feasible, to the *status quo ante*).

Whether a defendant-health care professional met or violated practice standards in a professional negligence legal case is established largely through expert witness testimony on the standard of care for the defendant's discipline and expert opinion on whether the defendant met or fell below minimally acceptable practice standards. Expert witness testimony on the standard of care may be supplemented by information in authoritative and reference texts and journals, and by written practice protocols and guidelines.

Health care malpractice liability is a form of *primary liability*, i.e., liability for the consequences of one's own conduct. Rehabilitation professionals and organizations may also be indirectly or *vicariously liable* for the official conduct of employees and volunteers, but not normally for the conduct of independent contractors and their staffs, so long as appropriate steps are taken to alert the public of the fact that such workers are contractors and not employees.

*Corporate liability* is another form of primary liability, under which a business entity, including rehabilitation clinics and other facilities, are legally responsible for certain administrative activities. These activities include, among possible others:

- Monitoring the quality of health care service delivery in the facility or facilities, whether rendered by employees, contractors, consultants, volunteers, or others
- Maintaining safe and secure premises for patients and others.

While a rehabilitation services administrator bears primary responsibility for implementing and executing clinical risk-management program initiatives, every professional and support team member bears personal responsibility for effecting liability risk management on behalf of the organization. Clinical risk-management initiatives include, among others:

- Safety programs designed to minimize injuries to patients, staff, licensees (business visitors), and others
- Equipment calibration and ongoing safety inspections
- Adverse incident reporting
- Peer review and related patient care quality management processes
- Liability awareness education processes, especially those involving institutional and/or consulting health law attorneys systematically in in-service education programs.

To date, there have been approximately 30 physical therapy malpractice civil cases reported in the legal literature since 1960. (One reported physical therapy–related civil case dealt, not with alleged physical therapist malpractice, but with legal *discovery* i.e., the turning over to a party in a legal case, of a physical therapist–initiated incident report by a product manufacturer in a case brought against it by a patient under the therapist's care.)

In virtually every reported physical therapy malpractice case, the charges lodged against physical therapists by patients were grounded exclusively in alleged professional negligence, to the exclusion of all other potential bases of liability. Appellate courts ruled in patients' favor in 15 (50% of these cases), either by affirming trial court judgments or by remanding cases to trial courts for further proceedings. No one knows precisely the total number of physical therapy malpractice legal cases because the vast majority are settled, not appealed, or abandoned by plaintiff-patients pre-trial, and therefore not disseminated to the general public.

The following section briefly summarizes three of the most recently reported physical therapy malpractice appellate cases, and offers commentary on suggested clinical risk-management strategies and tactics to limit malpractice exposure based on the case holdings.

### Case 1: *Moretto v. Samaritan Health Systems* (Arizona, 1997)

Mr Moretto, a postoperative knee surgery patient secondary to an industrial injury, fell from a wheeled stool while undergoing physical therapy. Mr Moretto's physical therapist had directed him to sit on the stool while the therapist applied a knee brace and shoe to Mr Moretto's involved leg. As a result of the fall, Moretto sustained a lumbar disc herniation, and filed suit, claiming professional negligence on the part of the physical therapist.

The therapist-employee's hospital attorney won dismissal of the case at the pretrial stage of adjudication, successfully arguing that Moretto failed to obtain **assignment** (ownership) of his potential claim against the therapist and hospital from his employer's workers' compensation insurance carrier (required because the back injury was incident to a compensable workers' compensation claim, i.e., the knee injury), and that Moretto also failed to file his lawsuit in a timely manner, violating Arizona's **statute of limitations.** Moretto appealed.

The appellate court reversed the award of summary judgment in favor of the physical therapist and hospital, concluding that a shortened statute of limitations for secondary injuries related to industrial injuries that are the subject of workers' compensation claims did not apply to this case. The shorter time clock was inapplicable, the court ruled, because the back injury did not aggravate the work-related knee injury, and Moretto did not need to obtain permission from his employer to sue the physical therapist and hospital for their independent alleged health care malpractice. The case was **remanded** (sent back) to the trial court for further proceedings.

### Case 2: *Greenberg v. Orthosport, Inc.* (Illinois, 1996)

In this case, a workers' compensation lumbar spine injury patient was undergoing a functional capacity evaluation for possible return to work, during which she claimed that she sustained a neck injury from the test, and sued her physical therapist for malpractice. The trial-level court awarded pre-trial summary judgment in favor of the physical therapist, on the grounds that the state workers' compensation system provided the exclusive remedy for patient-plaintiff's alleged evaluation-related neck injury. The patient appealed the adverse decision against her.

The appellate court reversed, opining that summary judgment is a drastic measure depriving a plaintiff of her right to redress at trial. The appeals court ruled that, because the alleged physical therapy malpractice was non–work-related, it could be pursued judicially by the plaintiff outside of the workers' compensation system.

### Case 3: *Hebebrand v. Arrien* (Florida, 1996)

In an unspecified health care malpractice action brought by a patient against multiple primary care providers, including a physical therapist, the patient-plaintiff sought **equitable** (nonmonetary) **relief** for the alleged failure on the part of the defendants in the case to respond to the plaintiff's notice of claim as required under state statutory provisions. The court refused to strike (invalidate) the defendants' defenses to the plaintiff's case, as requested, but did leave open the possibility of **striking** (eliminating) the defendants' responses to the plaintiff's notice of claim on appeal, if required.

Although the numbers of reported and nonreported physical therapy malpractice cases remains relatively small compared to medical malpractice cases involving physicians, and to civil litigation cases generally, it is still imperative for physical therapists' (and patients') physical, mental, and financial well-being that prudent clinical risk management be practiced to limit, to the degree feasible, malpractice exposure. Effective risk-management skills must be introduced during entry-level health professional education, and reinforced throughout clinicians' professional careers, through continuing legal education and other appropriate means.

### Malpractice Case Summaries

The Arizona case raises the following practice issues: the nature of workers' compensation claims and attendant risks of liability exposure associated with caring for such clients; health care malpractice legal procedures, especially concerning summary judgment; and the statute of limitations, or time-clock for initiating legal action against a physical therapist for alleged malpractice. The Illinois case similarly raises the concern that the management of a workers' compensation or other litigation patient may require the professional relationship to be more formal and meticulous, especially regarding documentation, including recordation of oral statements made by such patients to professional and support personnel. It may be a fair inference that a litigation or claim patient may be more likely to initiate further litigation, requiring this extra level of clinical risk management, or self-protection, on the part of physical therapy clinical staff. Finally, the Florida case illustrates the need to apprise attorneys immediately of possible legal claims and to be responsive to legal documents, as required by law.

These most recent reported physical therapy malpractice cases reinforce the need for physical therapist and physical therapist assistant clinicians and clinical managers and facility administrators to keep abreast of case law reports and changes in the legal status quo. In particular, it may be prudent for clinicians to maintain relatively formal professional relationships with claims and litigation patients and clients, especially including workers' compensation patients and clients. This includes the risk-management measure of always creating and maintaining accurate, comprehensive, objective, and timely patient intervention documentation, and noncare–related office memoranda or memoranda for record, as appropriate, to record **declarations against** (self) **interest** made by such patients or clients regarding their conditions. Similarly, physical therapist-malpractice defendants must respond appropriately, and in a timely manner, to **legal process** (e.g., summons, complaint) initiated by patients and others against them.

Through effective liability risk management, the best interests of providers, health care organizations and systems, and patients/clients are best served, as is the compelling societal interest in minimizing health care malpractice litigation, with all of its attendant costs.

## PATIENT INFORMED CONSENT TO HEALTH CARE INTERVENTION

Patient informed consent is both a legal and professional ethical prerequisite to patient examination and health care intervention. The duty to make relevant disclosure of care-related information to patients and obtain their express assent to examination and intervention is grounded in respect for patient self-determination, or autonomy over health care decision making. This paradigm of placing patient autonomy considerations above paternalism, or beneficence, is relatively new, and not one that health care professionals voluntarily adopted. It has been an activist judiciary in the United States during the 20th century that has progressively and firmly mandated patient control over health care decision making.

Although the precise informed consent disclosure requirements vary from state to state, the following core information must be conveyed to patients before a health-related examination or intervention:

- Information about the nature of the physical examination
- Examination and evaluative findings
- Patient diagnosis
- Information about any recommended intervention, especially including disclosure of material risks of serious harm or complications associated with the recommended intervention
- Benefits associated with a recommended intervention ("goals")
- Information about (i.e., relative benefits and risks) reasonable alternatives to a recommended intervention.

After such disclosure is made, a primary health care professional must also solicit and satisfactorily answer patient questions about the proposed examination or intervention. Finally, a provider must formally ask for and obtain patient consent to proceed. All of the communication above, between provider and patient (or surrogate decision maker, if the patient lacks legal capacity to consent), must take place both in a language that the patient understands and at the level of patient understanding.

Legally recognized exceptions to the normal requirement to always obtain patient informed consent exist, including the emergency doctrine, consent of minor and mentally and/or physically incapacitated patients, and therapeutic privilege.

Under the emergency doctrine, patients presenting for care in a life-threatening emergency are presumed to consent to necessary, life-saving interventions, unless there are valid indices (such as a patient advance directive indicating otherwise) that the patient refuses to accept such interventions. Thus, a patient experiencing a myocardial infarction during physical therapy treatment is normally presumed to desire and accept life-saving cardiopulmonary resuscitation.

Minors normally co-consent to their own health care delivery, but the consent of a parent or legal guardian is also required. Privacy considerations (some recognized by state or federal law) may obviate the need for parental consent to care of minors, or may disallow parental notification altogether, such as care for sexually transmitted diseases, drug or alcohol abuse, or abortion counseling. For patients lacking physical or mental capacity (e.g., comatose or catatonic patients), the informed consent process is carried out with a surrogate (substitute) decision maker, either chosen by the patient before his or her incapacitation or appointed by a court or otherwise by law.

Therapeutic privilege is a rarely utilized, and even more rarely accepted, exception to the law of patient informed consent. Under therapeutic privilege, a patient's primary or attending physician makes a professional judgment that a patient cannot psychologically handle diagnostic or prognostic information, and dictates to the patient's care team that such information will not be conveyed to the patient. Providers caring for such a patient may challenge such a determination through communication with the physician imposing the informational "gag rule," or through intervention by an institutional ethics committee (a multidisciplinary advisory committee charged with advising physicians and other primary health care professionals on ethical issues).

## DISCIPLINARY ACTIONS AND PROCESSES

The American Physical Therapy Association has ethics jurisdiction over approximately 67,000 physical therapists and physical therapist assistants who are members of the professional association. A written complaint of possible unethical conduct on the part of member physical therapists or physical therapist assistants is the starting point for initiation of investigatory and disciplinary action, pursuant to the Procedural Document on Disciplinary Action of the American Physical Therapy Association.

A complaint may be made by anyone having knowledge (first-hand or otherwise, e.g., hearsay) of a suspected ethical violation by an association member. The written, signed complaint is forwarded to the state chapter president, who (1) forwards an informational copy of the complaint to the national-level 5-member Ethics and Judicial Committee [for which APTA General Counsel Dr Jack Bennett is staff liaison and legal advisor], and (2) makes an initial subjective determination as to whether the complaint is actionable. Acknowledgment of the complaint must be returned to the complainant by the chapter president within 15 days of receipt. Along with acknowledgment, the chapter president is charged to advise the complainant that the respondent (professional charged) may have the right to learn the complainant's identity at some point in the process.

If an ethics complaint is nonactionable because an allegation does not involve a violation of the Code of Ethics or Standards of Ethical Conduct (i.e., lacks subject matter jurisdiction), or if, in the judgment of the chapter president, the allegation does not warrant judicial action, then the complaint is summarily dismissed by the chapter president. If the complaint is actionable, then the respondent association member is notified of the charge(s) and of the specific provisions of the Code or Standards allegedly violated.

A chapter president may initiate judicial action *sua sponte* (at his or her own initiative without a written complaint), based on public information. Proof of commission of a crime related to a member's professional status, or of a felony, or of revocation of professional licensure, is *prima facie* (presumptive) evidence of an actionable ethics violation and triggers mandatory interim suspension of membership until the Ethics and Judicial Committee takes follow-up action at its next regularly scheduled (semiannual) meeting.

In all other actionable ethics cases, the chapter president forwards the case file to the chapter ethics committee for processing. The chair of the state chapter ethics committee then appoints an impartial investigator (association member or other appropriate person) to conduct a comprehensive, unbiased investigation of the charges against the respondent. At the conclusion of this process, the investigator makes findings of fact (but neither conclusions nor recommendations), compiles the investigative file, and forwards it to the chapter ethics committee for further action.

If, after receipt and analysis of the investigative file, the chapter ethics committee determines that charges against a respondent are unsubstantiated, the chapter ethics committee may dismiss the complaint, under which option the respondent does not have the right to learn of the name of the complainant. Otherwise, the respondent is notified of his or her right to a copy of the investigative file and to a hearing on the charges.

With or without a hearing, the chapter ethics committee makes specific conclusions and recommendations on the charges against a respondent, which may (and must) include either a recommendation for dismissal of the charges or further disciplinary action by the Ethics and Judicial Committee. Disciplinary actions by the Ethics and Judicial Committee include no official action, written reprimands, membership probation (from 6 months to 2 years), suspension of membership (of 1 year's duration or longer, with or without conditions for reinstatement), and expulsion from membership in the American Physical Therapy Association.

Once properly notified of the chapter ethics committee recommendations, a respondent has the right to request a hearing before the Ethics and Judicial Committee at its next regularly scheduled semiannual meeting in Alexandria, Virginia. At this hearing, as at the state level, a respondent may be accompanied by legal counsel, who may serve only as a silent advisor to the respondent during the proceedings. (A nonattorney spokesperson, however, may present a defense on the respondent's behalf before the Ethics and Judicial Committee.)

With or without a hearing at the national level, the Ethics and Judicial Committee takes action on a complaint as follows: the Committee may adopt the recommendation of the state chapter ethics committee and award the appropriate sanction, award a less severe sanction, dismiss charges outright, or remand (return) the case to the chapter ethics committee for further action.

After final Ethics and Judicial Committee action, a respondent has the right to appeal their decision to the Board of Directors of the APTA within 30 days. The Board may affirm the prior decision, award a less severe disciplinary sanction, dismiss charges against a respondent, or remand the case to the Ethics and Judicial Committee for further specific action.

Once final, publication of disciplinary action takes place in association publications of general circulation. Published information is limited by policy to the name of the respondent, the disciplinary action taken, and the effective dates of the action. Beyond this summary information, the details of disciplinary action are confidential, and not disseminated to other entities without a court order compelling such disclosure.

A primary intent of the APTA's disciplinary processes is to ensure that the rights of all parties to disciplinary procedures are respected. Although private associations are not legally required to comply with constitutional **due process**, or fundamental fairness, requirements, as governmental entities (such as licensure boards) are, the APTA, through its disciplinary processes, attempts to achieve, and routinely does achieve, fundamental fairness for participants in its disciplinary processes.

The stigmatizing effect of suspension of membership or expulsion from the professional association are devastating and potentially career-ending, especially for prominent members and educational program faculty and administrators. A copy of the American Physical Therapy Association's Procedural Document on Grounds for Disciplinary Action appears in Appendix II at the end of the book.

## SUMMARY

Physical therapy legal and professional ethical responsibilities are complex as well as obligatory upon physical therapists and physical therapist assistants. These duties apply in all practice settings, from clinical to educational to school to patient or client home to long-term-care facility, among possible others.

Compliance with legal standards is made easier for physical therapists by the recent publication of the *Guide to Physical Therapist Practice* by the APTA. Although expressly not intended as a legal practice guide, it is so utilized by attorneys, judges, and legislators, who ultimately control the legal system and determine the legal standard of care for health professions and professionals.

Professional ethical duties for physical therapists and physical therapist assistants are made clearer by the *Guide for Professional Conduct* and the *Guide for Conduct of the Affiliate Member*, respectively. These ethical standards affect all physical therapy professionals, since their provisions are made part of state licensure statutes, rules, and regulations.

Physical therapy professionals acting as managers potentially have defined legal duties owed to patients and clients, staff employees, professional students, volunteers and observers, contractors and their staffs, the employing entity, visitors and licensees, and even trespassers. The highest duty owed by physical therapy professionals is toward patients under their care. Physical therapy professionals are fiduciaries to their patients, i.e., they are charged by law to place patient best interests above all others—even their own. Managed care, with its acute focus on cost containment, makes compliance with this sacred duty more difficult.

Health care malpractice involves patient injury coupled with a legal basis for imposing civil (monetary) liability for personal (patient) injury. The principal basis for imposition of health care malpractice liability is professional negligence, or objectively substandard care delivery. Whether physical therapy care retrospectively met or fell below minimally acceptable legal standards is determined by expert testimony of peers and qualified others, and by reference to authoritative texts and guidelines, such as the *Guide to Physical Therapist Practice*, whose prospective components will include minimal data sets for patient examination and evaluation, and possibly recommended interventions that are evidence-based.

Patient informed consent to physical therapy care is a legal and ethical prerequisite to physical therapy examination and intervention. The minimal disclosure elements for legally sufficient patient informed consent (which may vary from jurisdiction to jurisdiction) include: (1) patient diagnosis, (2) the nature of the proposed intervention, (3) short- and longer-term goals associated with the proposed intervention, (4) risks of serious harm or complication associated with the recommended intervention (if any), and (5) reasonable alternatives to the recommended intervention (and their relative risks and benefits). Patient questions should always be solicited and satisfactorily answered as part of the informed consent process, at the level of understanding of the patient and in a language that the patient comprehends.

Physical therapy professionals facing adverse action for their official conduct may face legal, professional association (ethical), and administrative action in multiple venues, and often simultaneously. The best approach to avoid such adverse actions is through professional practice that simultaneously optimizes quality patient care and minimizes personal liability risk (i.e., effective quality and risk management).

## Activities, Cases and Questions

1. **Activity**: Telephone the clerk of courts for your city, county, or federal district court. Inquire about any pending health care legal cases—criminal or civil. Obtain the public records related to one such case and study them. Attend the public legal proceedings associated with that case: preliminary hearing(s), trial, sentencing, and appeal. Keep a diary about the case and discuss it with professional colleagues (or fellow students) in an appropriate forum, e.g., district professional association meeting, clinical in-service session, or classroom.
2. **Case**: G., a board-certified orthopaedic physical therapist-clinician, receives from the hand of a county deputy sheriff a summons and complaint in which A., a recently discharged patient of G.'s, announces the filing of, and rationale for, her physical therapy malpractice lawsuit against G. What steps must G. take immediately?
3. **Question**: What steps, if any, do you take in your professional setting to include institutional or other attorneys in in-service or continuing education experiences for staff, faculty, or students (as appropriate)? If the answer is "none," then consider utilizing legal professionals in such education experiences, because their input is not only highly interesting and relevant to providers, but also may help to diminish liability exposure incident to physical therapy clinical practice, education, and research activities.

### ADDITIONAL READINGS


Dimond BC. *Legal Aspects of Physiotherapy*. Oxford: Blackwell Science; 1999.

Furrow BR et al. *Health Law: Cases, Materials and Problems*, 3rd ed. St. Paul, MN: West Publishing; 1997.

*Greenberg v Orthosport, Inc*, No. 1-93-3379 (App. C. Ill., June 12, 1996).

*Hebebrand v Arrien*, No. 95-3601 (Dist. C. App. Fla., May 15, 1996). *Law and Liability Professional Issues Learning Series (Part 1: Liability Issues; Part 2: Professional Issues)*. Alexandria, VA: American Physical Therapy Association; 1999.

Liang BA. *Health Law and Policy: A Survival Guide to Medicolegal Issues for Practitioners*. Woburn, MA: Butterworth-Heinemann; 2000.

*Moretto v Samaritan Health Systems*, No. 1 CA-CV 97-0079 (C. App. Arizona, Oct. 30, 1997).

Murphy SS. *Legal Handbook for Texas Nurses*. Austin: University of Texas Press; 1996.

Scott RW. Physical therapy malpractice update II. *PT: Magazine of Physical Therapy*. 2000;8(2): 50–52.

Scott RW. *Legal Aspects of Documenting Patient Care*, 2nd ed. Gaithersburg, MD: Aspen Publishers; 2000.

Scott RW. *Health Care Malpractice: A Primer on Legal Issues for Professionals*, 2nd ed. New York: McGraw-Hill; 1999.

Scott RW. *Professional Ethics: A Guide for Rehabilitation Professionals*. St. Louis: Mosby-Year Book; 1998.

Scott RW. *Promoting Legal Awareness in Physical and Occupational Therapy*. St. Louis: Mosby-Year Book; 1997.

Scott RW. Malpractice update. *PT: Magazine of Physical Therapy*. 1996;4(4): 69–70.

Scott RW. Malpractice update. *PT: Magazine of Physical Therapy*. 1993;1(12): 62–64.

Swisher LL, Brophy CK. *Legal and Ethical Issues in Physical Therapy*. Woburn, MA: Butterworth-Heinemann; 1998.

## APPENDIX 8-1

## AMERICAN PHYSICAL THERAPY ASSOCIATION GUIDE FOR PROFESSIONAL CONDUCT

### Purpose

This *Guide for Professional Conduct* (Guide) is intended to serve physical therapists in interpreting the *Code of Ethics* (Code) of the American Physical Therapy Association (Association), in matters of professional conduct. The Guide provides guidelines by which physical therapists may determine the propriety of their conduct. It is also intended to guide the professional development of physical therapist students. The Code and the Guide apply to all physical therapists. These guidelines are subject to changes as the dynamics of the profession change and as new patterns of health care delivery are developed and accepted by the professional community and the public. This Guide is subject to monitoring and timely revision by the Ethics and Judicial Committee of the Association.

### Interpreting Ethical Principles

The interpretations expressed in this Guide reflect the opinions, decisions, and advice of the Ethics and Judicial Committee. These interpretations are intended to assist a physical therapist in applying general ethical principles to specific situations. They should not be considered inclusive of all situations that could evolve.

### How to Use this Guide

### PRINCIPLE 1

**A physical therapist shall respect the rights and dignity of all individuals and shall provide compassionate care.**

### 1.1 Attitudes of a Physical Therapist

A. A physical therapist shall recognize individual differences and shall respect and be responsive to those differences.
B. A physical therapist shall be guided by concern for the physical, psychological, and socioeconomic welfare of patients/clients.
C. A physical therapist shall not harass, abuse, or discriminate against others.
D. A physical therapist shall be aware of the patient's health-related needs and act in a manner that facilitates meeting those needs.

## PRINCIPLE 2

**A physical therapist shall act in a trustworthy manner towards patients/clients, and in all other aspects of physical therapy practice.**

### 2.1 Patient/Physical Therapist Relationship

A. To act in a trustworthy manner the physical therapist shall act in the patient/client's best interest. Working in the patient/client's best interest requires knowledge of the patient/client's needs from the patient/client's perspective. Patients/clients often come to the physical therapist in a vulnerable state and normally will rely on the physical therapist's advice, which they perceive to be based on superior knowledge, skill, and experience. The trustworthy physical therapist acts to ameliorate the patient's/client's vulnerability, not to exploit it.
B. A physical therapist shall not exploit any aspect of the physical therapist/patient relationship.
C. A physical therapist shall not engage in any sexual relationship or activity, whether consensual or nonconsensual, with any patient while a physical therapist/patient relationship exists.
D. The physical therapist shall create an environment that encourages an open dialogue with the patient/client.
E. In the event the physical therapist or patient terminates the physical therapist/patient relationship while the patient continues to need physical therapy services, the physical therapist should take steps to transfer the care of the patient to another provider.

### 2.2 Truthfulness

A physical therapist shall not make statements that he/she knows or should know are false, deceptive, fraudulent, or unfair. See Section 8.2.D.

### 2.3 Confidential Information

A. Information relating to the physical therapist/patient relationship is confidential and may not be communicated to a third party not involved in that patient's care without the prior consent of the patient, subject to applicable law.
B. Information derived from peer review shall be held confidential by the reviewer unless the physical therapist who was reviewed consents to the release of the information.
C. A physical therapist may disclose information to appropriate authorities when it is necessary to protect the welfare of an individual or the community or when required by law. Such disclosure shall be in accordance with applicable law.

### 2.4 Patient Autonomy and Consent

A. A physical therapist shall not restrict patients' freedom to select their provider of physical therapy.
B. A physical therapist shall communicate to the patient/client the findings of his/her examination, evaluation, diagnosis, and prognosis.
C. A physical therapist shall collaborate with the patient/client to establish the goals of treatment and the plan of care.
D. A physical therapist shall inform the patient/client of the benefits, costs, and substantial risks (if any) of the recommended intervention and treatment alternatives.
E. A physical therapist shall respect the patient's/client's right to make decisions regarding the recommended plan of care, including consent, modification, or refusal.

## PRINCIPLE 3

**A physical therapist shall comply with laws and regulations governing physical therapy and shall strive to effect changes that benefit patients/clients.**

### 3.1 Professional Practice

A physical therapist shall provide examination, evaluation, diagnosis, prognosis, and intervention. A physical therapist shall not engage in any unlawful activity that substantially relates to the qualifications, functions, or duties of a physical therapist.

### 3.2 Just Laws and Regulations

A physical therapist shall advocate the adoption of laws, regulations, and policies by providers, employers, third party payers, legislatures, and regulatory agencies to provide and improve access to necessary health care services for all individuals.

### 3.3 Unjust Laws and Regulations

A physical therapist shall endeavor to change unjust laws, regulations, and policies that govern the practice of physical therapy. See Section 10.2.

## PRINCIPLE 4

**A physical therapist shall exercise sound professional judgment.**

### 4.1 Professional Responsibility

A. A physical therapist shall make professional judgments that are in the patient/client's best interests.

B. Regardless of practice setting, a physical therapist has primary responsibility for the physical therapy care of a patient and shall make independent judgments regarding that care consistent with accepted professional standards. See Section 2.4.
C. A physical therapist shall not provide physical therapy services to a patient/client while his/her ability to do so safely is impaired.
D. A physical therapist shall exercise sound professional judgment based upon his/her knowledge, skill, education, training, and experience.
E. Upon accepting a patient/client for physical therapy services, a physical therapist shall be responsible for: the examination, evaluation, and diagnosis of that individual; the prognosis and intervention; reexamination and modification of the plan of care; and the maintenance of adequate records, including progress reports. A physical therapist establishes the plan of care and provides and/or supervises and directs the appropriate interventions. See Section 2.4.
F. If the diagnostic process reveals findings that are outside the scope of the physical therapist's knowledge, experience, or expertise, the physical therapist shall so inform the patient/client and refer to an appropriate practitioner.
G. When the patient has been referred from another practitioner, the physical therapist shall communicate the findings of the examination and evaluation, the diagnosis, the proposed intervention, and reexamination findings (as indicated) to the referring practitioner.
H. A physical therapist shall determine when a patient/client will no longer benefit from physical therapy services.

### 4.2 Direction and Supervision

A. The supervising physical therapist has primary responsibility for the physical therapy care rendered to a patient/client.
B. A physical therapist shall not delegate to a less qualified person any activity that requires the unique skill, knowledge, and judgment of the physical therapist.

### 4.3 Practice Arrangements

A. Participation in a business, partnership, corporation, or other entity does not exempt physical therapists, whether employers, partners, or stockholders, either individually or collectively, from the obligation to promote, maintain and comply with the ethical principles of the Association.
B. A physical therapist shall advise his/her employer(s) of any employer practice that causes a physical therapist to be in conflict with the ethical principles of the Association. A physical therapist shall seek to elim-

inate aspects of his/her employment that are in conflict with the ethical principles of the Association.

### 4.4 Gifts and Other Consideration

A physical therapist shall not accept or offer gifts or other considerations that affect or give an appearance of affecting his/her professional judgment.

## PRINCIPLE 5

**A physical therapist shall achieve and maintain professional competence.**

### 5.1 Scope of Competence

A physical therapist shall practice within the scope of his/her competence and commensurate with his/her level of education, training and experience.

### 5.2 Self-assessment

A physical therapist shall engage in self-assessment, which is a lifelong professional responsibility for maintaining competence.

### 5.3 Professional Development

A physical therapist shall participate in educational activities that enhance his/her basic knowledge and skills.

## PRINCIPLE 6

**A physical therapist shall maintain and promote high standards for physical therapy practice, education and research.**

### 6.1 Professional Standards

A physical therapist shall know the accepted professional standards when engaging in physical therapy practice, education and/or research. A physical therapist shall continuously engage in assessment activities to determine compliance with these standards. If a physical therapist is not in compliance with these standards, he/she shall engage in activities designed to reach compliance with the standards. When a physical therapist is in compliance with these standards, he/she shall engage in activities designed to maintain those standards.

### 6.2 Practice

A. A physical therapist shall achieve and maintain professional competence. See Section 5.

B. A physical therapist shall demonstrate his/her commitment to quality improvement by engaging in peer and utilization review and other self-assessment activities.

### 6.3 Professional Education

A. A physical therapist shall support high-quality education in academic and clinical settings.
B. A physical therapist participating in the educational process is responsible to the students, the academic institutions, and the clinical settings for promoting ethical conduct. A physical therapist shall model ethical behavior and provide the student with information about the Code of Ethics, opportunities to discuss ethical conflicts, and procedures for reporting unresolved ethical conflicts. See Section 9.

### 6.4 Continuing Education

A. A physical therapist providing continuing education must be competent in the content area.
B. When a physical therapist provides continuing education, he/she shall ensure that course content, objectives, faculty credentials, and responsibilities of the instructional staff are accurately stated in the promotional and instructional course materials.
C. A physical therapist shall evaluate the efficacy and effectiveness of information and techniques presented in continuing education programs before integrating them into his or her practice.

### 6.5 Research

A. A physical therapist shall support research activities that contribute knowledge for improved patient care.
B. A physical therapist shall report to appropriate authorities any acts in the conduct or presentation of research that appear unethical or illegal. See Section 9.

## PRINCIPLE 7

**A physical therapist shall seek only such remuneration as is deserved and reasonable for physical therapy services.**

### 7.1 Business and Employment Practices

A. A physical therapist's business/employment practices shall be consistent with the ethical principles of the Association.
B. A physical therapist shall never place her/his own financial interest above the welfare of individuals under his/her care.

C. A physical therapist shall recognize that third-party payer contracts may limit, in one form or another, the provision of physical therapy services. Third-party limitations do not absolve the physical therapist from making sound professional judgments that are in the patient's best interest. A physical therapist shall avoid underutilization of physical therapy services.
D. When a physical therapist's judgment is that a patient will receive negligible benefit from physical therapy services, the physical therapist shall not provide or continue to provide such services if the primary reason for doing so is to further the financial self-interest of the physical therapist or his/her employer. A physical therapist shall avoid overutilization of physical therapy services.
E. Fees for physical therapy services should be reasonable for the service performed, considering the setting in which it is provided, practice costs in the geographic area, judgment of other organizations, and other relevant factors.
F. A physical therapist shall not directly or indirectly request, receive, or participate in the dividing, transferring, assigning, or rebating of an unearned fee.
G. A physical therapist shall not profit by means of a credit or other valuable consideration, such as an unearned commission, discount, or gratuity, in connection with the furnishing of physical therapy services.
H. Unless laws impose restrictions to the contrary, physical therapists who provide physical therapy services within a business entity may pool fees and monies received. Physical therapists may divide or apportion these fees and monies in accordance with the business agreement.
I. A physical therapist may enter into agreements with organizations to provide physical therapy services if such agreements do not violate the ethical principles of the Association or applicable laws.

### 7.2 Endorsement of Products or Services

A. A physical therapist shall not exert influence on individuals under his/her care or their families to use products or services based on the direct or indirect financial interest of the physical therapist in such products or services. Realizing that these individuals will normally rely on the physical therapist's advice, their best interest must always be maintained, as must their right of free choice relating to the use of any product or service.

Although it cannot be considered unethical for physical therapists to own or have a financial interest in the production, sale, or distribution of products/services, they must act in accordance with law and make full disclosure of their interest whenever individuals under their care use such products/services.

B. A physical therapist may receive remuneration for endorsement or advertisement of products or services to the public, physical therapists, or other health professionals provided he/she discloses any financial interest in the production, sale, or distribution of said products or services.

C. When endorsing or advertising products or services, a physical therapist shall use sound professional judgment and shall not give the appearance of Association endorsement unless the Association has formally endorsed the products or services.

### 7.3 Disclosure

A physical therapist shall disclose to the patient if the referring practitioner derives compensation from the provision of physical therapy.

## PRINCIPLE 8

**A physical therapist shall provide and make available accurate and relevant information to patients/clients about their care and to the public about physical therapy services.**

### 8.1 Accurate and Relevant Information to the Patient

A. A physical therapist shall provide the patient/client information about his/her condition and plan of care. See Section 2.4.

B. Upon the request of the patient, the physical therapist shall provide, or make available, the medical record to the patient or a patient-designated third party.

C. A physical therapist shall inform patients of any known financial limitations that may affect their care.

D. A physical therapist shall inform the patient when, in his/her judgment, the patient will receive negligible benefit from further care. See Section 7.1.C.

### 8.2 Accurate and Relevant Information to the Public

A. A physical therapist shall inform the public about the societal benefits of the profession and who is qualified to provide physical therapy services.

B. Information given to the public shall emphasize that individual problems cannot be treated without individualized examination and plans/programs of care.

C. A physical therapist may advertise his/her services to the public.
D. A physical therapist shall not use, or participate in the use of, any form of communication containing a false, plagiarized, fraudulent, deceptive, unfair, or sensational statement or claim.
E. A physical therapist who places a paid advertisement shall identify it as such unless it is apparent from the context that it is a paid advertisement.

## PRINCIPLE 9

**A physical therapist shall protect the public and the profession from unethical, incompetent, and illegal acts.**

### 9.1 Consumer Protection

A. A physical therapist shall provide care that is within the scope of practice as defined by the state practice act.
B. A physical therapist shall not engage in any conduct that is unethical, incompetent or illegal.
C. A physical therapist shall report any conduct that appears to be unethical, incompetent, or illegal.
D. A physical therapist may not participate in any arrangements in which patients are exploited due to the referring sources' enhancing their personal incomes as a result of referring for, prescribing, or recommending physical therapy. See Section 5.

## PRINCIPLE 10

**A physical therapist shall endeavor to address the health needs of society.**

### 10.1 Pro Bono Service

A physical therapist shall render pro bono publico (reduced or no fee) services to patients lacking the ability to pay for services, as each physical therapist's practice permits.

### 10.2 Community Health

A physical therapist shall endeavor to support activities that benefit the health status of the community. See Section 3.

## PRINCIPLE 11

**A physical therapist shall respect the rights, knowledge, and skills of colleagues and other healthcare professionals.**

### 11.1 Consultation

A physical therapist shall seek consultation whenever the welfare of the patient will be safeguarded or advanced by consulting those who have special skills, knowledge, and experience.

### 11.2 Patient/Provider Relationships

A physical therapist shall not undermine the relationship(s) between his/her patient and other healthcare professionals.

### 11.3 Disparagement

Physical therapists shall not disparage colleagues and other health care professionals. See Section 9 and Section 2.4.A.

Issued by Ethics and Judicial Committee
American Physical Therapy Association
October 1981
Last Amended January 2001

# APPENDIX 8-2

# AMERICAN PHYSICAL THERAPY ASSOCIATION GUIDE FOR CONDUCT OF THE AFFILIATE MEMBER

## PURPOSE

The Guide for Conduct of the Affiliate Member (the Guide) is intended to serve physical therapist assistants who are affiliate members of the American Physical Therapy Association (the Association) in the interpretation of the *Standards of Ethical Conduct for the Physical Therapist Assistant*, providing guidelines by which they may determine the propriety of their conduct. These guidelines are subject to change as new patterns of health care delivery are developed and accepted by the professional community and the public. This Guide is subject to monitoring and timely revision by the Ethics and Judicial Committee of the Association.

## INTERPRETING STANDARDS

The interpretations expressed in this Guide are not to be considered all inclusive of situations that could evolve under a specific standard of the *Standards of Ethical Conduct for the Physical Therapist Assistant* but reflect the opinions, decisions, and advice of the Ethics and Judicial Committee. Although the statements of ethical standards apply universally, specific circumstances determine their appropriate application. Input related to current interpretations, or situations requiring interpretation, is encouraged from APTA members.

## STANDARD 1

***Physical therapist assistants provide services under the supervision of a physical therapist.***

### 1.1 Supervisory Relationships

Physical therapist assistants shall work under the supervision and direction of a physical therapist who is properly credentialed in the jurisdiction in which the physical therapist assistant practices.

### 1.2 Performance of Service

A. Physical therapist assistants may not initiate or alter a treatment program without prior evaluation by and approval of the supervising physical therapist.

B. Physical therapist assistants may modify a specific treatment procedure in accordance with changes in patient status.
C. Physical therapist assistants may not interpret data beyond the scope of their physical therapist assistant education.
D. Physical therapist assistants may respond to inquiries regarding patient status to appropriate parties within the protocol established by a supervising physical therapist.
E. Physical therapist assistants shall refer inquiries regarding patient prognosis to a supervising physical therapist.

## STANDARD 2

***Physical therapist assistants respect the rights and dignity of all individuals.***

### 2.1 Attitudes of Physical Therapist Assistants

A. Physical therapist assistants shall recognize that each individual is different from all other individuals and respect and be responsive to those differences.
B. Physical therapist assistants shall be guided at all times by concern for the dignity and welfare of those patients entrusted to their care.
C. Physical therapist assistants shall not engage in conduct that constitutes harassment or abuse of, or discrimination against, colleagues, associates, or others.

### 2.2 Request for Release of Information

Physical therapist assistants shall refer all requests for release of confidential information to the supervising physical therapist.

### 2.3 Protection of Privacy

Physical therapist assistants must treat as confidential all information relating to the personal conditions and affairs of the persons whom they serve.

### 2.4 Patient Relations

Physical therapist assistants shall not engage in any sexual relationship or activity, whether consensual or nonconsensual, with any patient while a physical therapist assistant/patient relationship exists.

## STANDARD 3

***Physical therapist assistants maintain and promote high standards in the provision of services giving the welfare of patients their highest regard.***

### 3.1 Information About Services

A. Physical therapist assistants may provide consumers with information regarding provision of services within the protocol established by a supervising physical therapist.
B. Physical therapist assistants may not use, or participate in the use of, any form of communication containing a false, fraudulent, misleading, deceptive, unfair, or sensational statement or claim.

### 3.2 Organizational Employment

Physical therapist assistants shall advise their employer(s) of any employer practice that causes them to be in conflict with the *Standards of Ethical Conduct for the Physical Therapist Assistant.*

### 3.3 Endorsement of Equipment

Physical therapist assistants may not endorse equipment or exercise influence on patients or families to purchase or lease equipment except as directed by a physical therapist acting in accord with the stipulation in paragraph 5.3.A. of the *Guide for Professional Conduct.*

### 3.4 Financial Considerations

Physical therapist assistants shall never place their own financial interest above the welfare of their patients.

### 3.5 Exploitation of Patients

Physical therapist assistants shall not participate in any arrangements in which patients are exploited. Such arrangements include situations where referring sources enhance their personal incomes as a result of referring for, delegating, prescribing, or recommending physical therapy services.

## STANDARD 4

***Physical therapist assistants provide services within the limits of the law.***

### 4.1 Supervisory Relationships

Physical therapist assistants shall comply with all aspects of law. Regardless of the content of any law, physical therapist assistants shall provide services only under the supervision and direction of a physical therapist who is properly credentialed in the jurisdiction in which the physical therapist assistant practices.

### 4.2 Representation

Physical therapist assistants shall not hold themselves out as physical therapists.

## STANDARD 5

***Physical therapist assistants make those judgments that are commensurate with their qualifications as physical therapist assistants.***

### 5.1 Patient Treatment

Physical therapist assistants shall report all untoward patient responses to a supervising physical therapist.

### 5.2 Patient Safety

A. Physical therapist assistants may refuse to carry out treatment procedures that they believe are not in the best interest of the patient.
B. The physical therapist assistant shall not provide physical therapy services to a patient while under the influence of a substance that impairs his or her ability to do so safely.

### 5.3 Qualifications

Physical therapist assistants may not carry out any procedure that they are not qualified to provide.

### 5.4 Discontinuance of Treatment Program

Physical therapist assistants shall discontinue immediately any treatment procedures that, in their judgment, appear to be harmful to the patient.

### 5.5 Continued Education

Physical therapist assistants shall continue participation in various types of educational activities that enhance their skills and knowledge and provide new skills and knowledge.

## STANDARD 6

***Physical therapist assistants accept the responsibility to protect the public and the profession from unethical, incompetent, or illegal acts.***

### 6.1 Consumer Protection

Physical therapist assistants shall report any conduct that appears to be unethical or illegal.

Issued by Ethics and Judicial Committee
American Physical Therapy Association
October 1981
Last Amended January 1996

## Focus on a Leader

**JONATHAN COOPERMAN, JD, MS, PT**
**CLINICAL MANAGER, CRYSTAL CLINIC, AKRON, OHIO;**
**PAST CHAIR, ETHICS AND JUDICIAL COMMITTEE,**
**AMERICAN PHYSICAL THERAPY ASSOCIATION**

1. *Jonathan, please briefly capsulize for readers your credentials, professional chronology, and current and recent professional activities.*

I graduated from the University of Maryland with a Bachelor of Science in physical therapy in 1979. I attained a Master of Science in clinical orthopaedic physical therapy from the Medical College of Virginia in 1989. I then attended The University of Akron, School of Law where I received my Juris Doctor degree in 1993. I was admitted to the bar in Ohio and I am a member of the American Bar Association.

My current title is Clinical Services Manager, Rehabilitation and Health Center, Inc, Akron, Ohio. I am responsible for the daily operations of a moderate-sized outpatient orthopaedic clinic, with five physical therapists, two physical therapist assistants, and one athletic trainer. At the time of this writing, I am the Chair, Ethics and Judicial Committee of the American Physical Therapy Association. I am also the Reimbursement Specialist for the Ohio Physical Therapy Association. I served on the Ohio Occupational Therapy, Physical Therapy and Athletic Trainer's Board from 1997–1999.

2. *What are the salient legal and professional ethical problems, issues, and dilemmas facing the physical therapy profession?*

Easily, the most pressing ethical dilemmas we face today as physical therapists arise as a consequence of managed care. Under this paradigm, therapists, like physicians, have had to deal with various forms of economic risk sharing, e.g., the capitation of services. This strains the fiduciary duty, which we owe to our patients, and thereby drives a wedge between the therapist and patient. Business arrangements have placed significant pressures, both overt and covert, on today's physical therapist. For example, how does a physical therapist deal with third-party payer limitations on the number of visits allowed for any given patient? Are we to look at this as a contract issue and simply state that the patients have willingly chosen their coverage, thereby conveniently setting aside our duty of beneficence? Given these limitations, are we incurring a greater risk of claims of abandonment? Does a "business as usual'" approach distance us from the patient and as such put us more at risk for allegations of malpractice? Does corporate-driven health care force us to place the needs of the shareholders ahead of the needs of the individual patient?

The managed care milieu has forced us as a profession to confront the issue of underutilization. Somewhat paradoxically, we have been driven by the same forces to be more efficient and to continually justify our interventions.

3. *Where do you believe physical therapy will be in 2050? What needs to be accomplished to get the profession where you envision it being in 2050?*

The term *evidence-based practice* might actually be a reality in 2050. Therapists will be able to define what it is they do and substantiate our outcomes. All therapists will contribute to, and have access to, a large data pool, made accessible by even greater advances in information management and technology. The patient will carry an ambulatory health care record (contained on a credit card) that will allow physical therapists to instantly download all vital information such as current medications, prior physical therapy interventions, radiograph reports, etc. However, technical advances will *not* eliminate the need for physical therapy, which will be more involved with wellness and prevention than ever before. Our population will continue to work longer hours and suffer more musculoskeletal breakdowns. Individually owned private practices will re-emerge as the dominant business form in outpatient physical therapy. All physical therapists will be doctorally prepared and the physical therapist assistant will hold a baccalaureate degree.

To accomplish this, we need to refocus our professional education. Physical therapy programs need to graduate students who are not researchers, but who understand the value of, and critically read, current research. Physical therapists must be taught the importance of collecting data and sharing it with the appropriate research institutions. In addition, physical therapy education needs to be broadened to include more classes in business, marketing, and human resource management. Individual therapists need to much more active in the legislative arena.

CHAPTER 9

# Professional Associations and Responsibility

RON SCOTT

## Key Words and Phrases

Affiliate Member
Associate Member
American Board of Physical Therapy Specialties
American Physical Therapy Association
Board of Directors
Bylaws
Chapters
Code of Ethics
Commission on Accreditation of Physical Therapy Education
Component Activities
Districts
Ethics and Judicial Committee
Executive Committee
Federation of State Boards of Physical Therapy
Foundation for Physical Therapy
Governmental Affairs
Honorary Member
House of Delegates
Life Member
National Assembly of Physical Therapist Assistants
National Association of Physical Therapy
Nominating Committee
Policy
Political Action
Political Action Committee
Professional Association
Professional Discipline
Professional Liability Insurance
Professionalism
Professional Responsibility
Publications
Reference Committee
Resolution
Speaker of the House
(Specialty) Sections
Standing Committees
Task Force

*This chapter describes the fundamental activities of the American Physical Therapy Association and related professional groups. Professionalism, the hallmark of members of a learned professional discipline, is addressed, especially the ethical duty to support professional organizations through active involvement. The structure of the American Physical Therapy Association is outlined in brief, mirroring its unique upside-down organization chart that places members at the apex of the hierarchal pyramid. The Focus on a Leader segment highlights Jayne Snyder, APTA Vice President and President, Foundation for Physical Therapy.*

This chapter is devoted to a detailed description of the American Physical Therapy Association (APTA) as it exists today, and of related professional groups serving physical therapists, physical therapist assistants, and support professionals.

As an introductory point, it is critically important to restate that professionals engaged in physical therapy practice have a professional responsibility to be members of, and actively involved in the activities of, the professional association: physical therapists as professional members, physical therapist assistants as affiliate members, and related professionals as associate members. Professionalism, or the exercise of professional responsibility, is a hallmark of a true professional. A professional person cannot justly complain that she or he is powerless to influence political and related professional practice outcomes if that person is not involved in the association and its processes. And involvement starts with membership, from the time one is a pre-professional student through the pendency of active practice and beyond. As with the lottery, "you can't win if you don't play!"

No single member of the APTA (or any other political, religious, or social organization) fully agrees with all of the policies, procedures, or direction of that organization or association. Meaningful positive productive change, however, to the extent such is a desired outcome, is most efficaciously accomplished from within, not from without.

There is strength in numbers, if not in unity of purpose and direction. From the public's perspective, it must be a mark of strength and prestige that at least a majority of professionals within a discipline are active members of their professional association.

Recent phenomena, such as the advent of managed care and concomitant reimbursement reduction for physical rehabilitation services, have had a deleterious effect on professional association membership and active participation therein, employment opportunities, compensation for professional services, and professional and postprofessional educational pursuits, among other professional activities. Although health care delivery paradigms and governmental-political regimens at all levels may wax and wane, nothing should allow true professionals to waiver in their fiduciary duties owed to their patients and clients or to their very professional disciplines, as manifested by their representative professional associations. Similarly, in times of crisis, there is an inherent duty on the part of professionals and their associations to offer succor to members in need—through moral support and reduced or restructured fee arrangements, among other relief.

The perceived problem of declining involvement of physical therapy professionals in their association and profession is further addressed in Chapter 10.

## STRUCTURE OF THE AMERICAN PHYSICAL THERAPY ASSOCIATION

As of January 1, 2000, the APTA (see Fig. 1-5) boasted nearly 67,000 active, affiliate, professional and affiliate student, life, and associate members. The mission statement for the Association is to represent and promote the profession of physical therapy, to further the profession's role in the prevention, diagnosis, and treatment of movement dysfunction, and the enhancement of physical health and functional abilities of members of the public.

The operations of the APTA are governed by bylaws, which delineate its purpose, functions, membership categories, rights and privileges, and governance, subject to modification. Interestingly, the organizational chart for this nonprofit 503c organization displays members as the highest authority within the Association, evidencing the importance of lay members and their input into Association policies (See Appendix III). The three categories of members include those within the American College of Physical Therapists, the National Assembly of Physical Therapist Assistants, and Physical Therapist/Physical Therapist Assistant Students. Membership categories include active, affiliate, student, life, and honorary.

Components, including sections, chapters, and assemblies, appear next in descending order of authority along the flow diagram. There are 50 state chapters. Sections parallel, but are broader than, clinical specialties, e.g., there is a Section on Women's Health, among numerous others. The Representative Body of the National Assembly of Physical Therapist Assistants is represented by separate lateral box at this level. There is also an active Student Assembly within the Association.

The principal policy-making body, the House of Delegates, next in order of authority, is composed of officers (Speaker and Vice Speaker), committees (elections and tellers, minutes, nominating, and reference), elected and appointed voting and nonvoting delegates, consultants (e.g., Ethics and Judicial Committee), and student ushers.

Subordinate to the House is the 15-member policy-making Board of Directors, which includes the six officers of the American Physical Therapy Association (President, Vice President, Secretary, Treasurer, and Speaker and Vice Speaker of the House of Delegates) and nine elected active members who serve 3-year terms of service. Board members receive honoraria for their extensive service commitments.

The House of Delegate issue items are referred to by RC (Reference Committee) number, and its adopted (binding) policies and (nonbinding) positions and guidelines are referenced as HOD (MM)(YR)(Minutes Page Number)(Vote Number). For example, the House of Delegates Position on *Pro Bono* Physical Therapy Services, HOD 06-93-21-39, was adopted at the Association's June 1993 Annual Meeting. Board of Director policies are similarly references as BOD 00-00-00-00.

Committees of the APTA are of three categories: the policy-guiding Executive Committee, standing, and ad hoc committees. Standing committees include, among others of note, the American Board of Physical Therapy Specialties, the Commission on Accreditation in Physical Therapy Education, the Ethics and Judicial Committee, the Political Action Committee, various advisory panels, and the Awards Committee. APTA awards are categorized as education, practice/service, publication, and research awards. They include, among notable others, the Lucy Blair Service Award, Eugene Michels New Investigator Award, Golden Pen Award, Mary McMillan Scholarship Award, and Minority Achievement and Scholarship Awards. Two Association honors categories include Catherine Worthingham Fellows (entitling fellows to utilize the initials "F.A.P.T.A." after their names and credentials), and the Mary McMillan Lecture Award. The Foundation for Physical Therapy awards scholarships and grants to physical therapy students, clinicians, and educators to support basic science and clinical research, and the advancement of the profession and of humankind.

At the base of the APTA organization chart are the vital 150 headquarters staff.

## RELATED PROFESSIONAL ORGANIZATIONS AND ALLIANCES

The Federation of State Boards of Physical Therapy has already been introduced in Chapter 1. Headquartered in Alexandria, Virginia, within several blocks of the American Physical Therapy Association headquarters, the Federation has responsibility for developing the physical therapist and physical therapist assistant licensure examinations, and for promoting and revising its Model Practice Act to the states for adoption. The current edition of the Act is reprinted in Appendix II for the express purpose of permitting students and faculty to utilize it in classroom exercises as a model.

The World Confederation for Physical Therapy, headquartered in London, England, and whose president is currently Dr Brenda Myers, serves to coordinate and promote physiotherapy throughout the world. Virtually all nations are member-states of the World Confederation, whose first congress took place in New York City in 1949. Since then, the World Confederation has sponsored congresses every 5 years. The next sheduled congress is in May 2003, in Barcelona, Spain.

The Tri-Alliance of Health and Rehabilitation Professionals consists of representatives of the APTA, American Occupational Therapy Association, and American Speech-Language-Hearing Association. Together, these three allied health discipline associations combine intellectual and political strength to address common issues, such as reimbursement issues with the federal Health Care Financing Administration. The Tri-Alliance also co-sponsors professional and educational programming and colloquia at representative professional meetings.

Finally, organizations such as the National Physical Therapy Association address focused issues, such as the role and advancement of African-American physical therapy professionals and students.

## SUMMARY

Physical therapy as an autonomous health professional discipline is only as strong as its members and representative professional associations. The American Physical Therapy Association has been instrumental in political action and educative efforts to position physical therapy prominently as a co-primary health professional discipline alongside medicine, dentistry, and other complementary disciplines. Managed care, the Balanced Budget Act of 1997, the Vector Study, and other factors tend to adversely affect professional association (but not student) membership. Active involvement by all members of this profession in professional association affairs, processes, and decision making is crucial to continued successful advancement of the profession. It is also a requisite of professionalism and duty. Finally organizations such as the American Academy of Physical Therapy address focused issues such as the roles and advancement of African physical therapy professionals and students, and health promotion for disadvantaged persons.

## Activities, Cases, and Questions

1. **Activity**: As student physical therapists or physical therapist assistants, join or initiate and help form an urban or rural *pro bono publico* health services group, and actively participate in its successful outreach to socioeconomically disadvantaged patients and clients. Through and with mentors in your professional association district, state chapter, and/or national office, collect and analyze data on the program(s) and disseminate results.

2. **Case**: A., a physiotherapist educated in England, is newly licensed in state X. A.'s intervention mix includes therapies and techniques not common to customary local practice. What measures can and should A. and local professional colleagues take to share ideas and practices?
3. **Question**: As professional students and educators, what constructive steps can you initiate and execute to maximize membership and active participation of fellow students and professionals in the professional association and related associations and groups?

## ADDITIONAL READINGS

*Guide to Oral History*. Alexandria, VA: American Physical Therapy Association; 1995.

*House of Delegates: Standards, Policies, Positions and Guidelines*. Alexandria, VA: American Physical Therapy Association; 1998.

McGinty SM, Cicero MC, Cicero JME, Schultz-Janney L, Williams-Shipman KL. Reasons given by California Physical Therapists for Not Belonging to the APTA. *Phys Ther*. 2001; 81:1224–1232.

Murphy W. *Healing the Generations: A History of Physical Therapy and the American Physical Therapy Association*. Alexandria, VA: American Physical Therapy Association; 1995.

*Take a Look at Today's Physical Therapist*. Alexandria, VA: American Physical Therapy Association; 1995.

*Un Futuro en la Terapia Física*. Alexandria, VA: American Physical Therapy Association; 1990.

## Focus on a Leader

### Jayne Leigh Snyder, MA, PT
### Vice President, American Physical Therapy Association, and President, Foundation for Physical Therapy

*1. Jayne, please briefly capsulize for readers your credentials, professional chronology, and current and recent professional activities.*

I recently began my second elected term of office as Vice President of the American Physical Therapy Association. I am also currently President of the Foundation for Physical Therapy. I own Snyder Physical Therapy, a private practice orthopaedic and sports physical therapy center, located in Lincoln, Nebraska. I have been active with the American Physical Therapy Association (APTA) since 1972, serving as Nebraska Chapter committee member and President, Secretary of the Private Practice Section, member of the APTA Board of Directors, and Chair, Federal Government Affairs Committee, which was involved in having the $1,500 outpatient rehabilitation reimbursement cap lifted.

In addition to my Bachelor of Science degree in physical education from the University of Nebraska, Lincoln, in 1967, I received my Master of Arts in Physical Therapy from Stanford University, Palo Alto, California, in 1972. I am also a certified Physical Fitness Specialist of the Institute for Aerobics Research, Dallas, Texas. I was an assistant professor in the Division of Physical Therapy, University of Nebraska, College of Medicine, Omaha, from 1972–1975, where I taught clinical education, functional anatomy, and neuroscience.

My current community activities include: member, Board of Directors, Nebraska Trails Foundation, American Discovery Trails Committee, and Great Plains Trails Network. I am also the President of the University of Nebraska's Relay Club.

*2. From an elected APTA official's perspective, what are the salient problems, issues, and dilemmas affecting the profession of physical therapy, now and in the near future?*

One of the most critically important issues from my perspective is membership retention in the American Physical Therapy Association and its state chapters. We have suffered a membership loss in recent times, due to the Balanced Budget Act of 1997 and its negative impact on physical therapy employment. With the passage of the Balanced Budget Refinement Act of 1999, reimbursement caps on physical therapy services in skilled nursing facilities, home health, and outpatient clinics were lifted, which helped the employment situation.

We need to work politically to increase reimbursement for physical therapy services and to encourage members to stay active in the APTA. Measures to promote membership retention include, among others, dues deferral and quarterly payment of membership dues.

3. *Where do you believe physical therapy will be in the year 2050? What needs to be accomplished to get the profession where you envision it being in 2050?*

By 2050, we will have full-blown direct access physical therapy practice in all 50 states. Even earlier, by 2020, our vision of physical therapists being the primary direct care providers for patients with musculoskeletal conditions will be realized. Physical therapists will all have individual billing numbers in all settings, and will possess physician-like independence.

Also by 2050, the Doctor of Physical Therapy degree/credential will be the standard, and physical therapists will be referred to as "doctor." Physical therapist assistants will be the exclusive extenders for physical therapy services. Physical therapist assistant education will remain consolidated at the associate degree level.

CHAPTER 10

# Salient Issues

RON SCOTT

## Key Words and Phrases

Clinical Education Crisis
Direct Access Practice
Diversity
Doctor of Physical Therapy
Education Program Proliferation
Encroachment
Interdisciplinary Relations
Interstate Practice
Intradisciplinary Relations
Licensure
Managed Care
Military Model
Vector Workforce Study

*The range of salient, important issues confronting the profession of physical therapy is as broad as the scope of physical therapy itself. Managed care has dramatically altered the practice and education landscapes through stringent cost-containment measures that have diminished reimbursement for physical therapy services. Education issues include proliferation of professional (entry-level) education programs, class size, recruitment of qualified students (and faculty), and the degree level for program graduates. Practice issues include, among others, supply and demand for professional labor, intra- and interdisciplinary relations, and scope of professional practice.*

## MANAGED CARE

Managed care is a term that describes the current predominant health care delivery model in the United States. Managed care began in earnest in the United States in the 1970s, when federal laws such as the 1973 Health Maintenance Organization Act required employers to offer a lower-cost health maintenance organization option to employees covered by employer-sponsored group health insurance. The idea of health care cost containment advanced during the 1980s when prospective (lump sum reimbursement) payment for health services was initiated for Medicare-funded inpatient health care pursuant to diagnostic-related groups (DRGs). Managed care matured to a great degree during the mid-1900s after the collapse of the Clinton universal health care initiative in 1993, culminating in the year 2000 with near-universal implementation of prospective payment for all health services—inpatient and outpatient.

Under the managed care health care delivery paradigm, cost containment at the macro- and micro-levels is nearly as important as is the quality of health care delivered. Managed care organizations and systems, like Wal-Mart in the retail sales industry, seek to integrate the financing and delivery of health care, minimizing cost outlays through bulk purchases, limited care delivery provider networks, and preapproval for many services.

Yet under managed care, costs are not being contained in the long term. Aggregate health care costs continue to rise at rates comparable to the former fee-for-service system. As many persons and families in the United States are uninsured or underinsured (estimated to be 40 million people) as before. Compensation for health professional services has decreased. The United State ranks 12th of 13 major nations in terms of overall quality of health care delivery systems, principally because of a relative dearth of primary care facilities and a lack of emphasis (and reimbursement) for preventive care.[1] And the "emergency room, to many, remains the doctor's office."[2] (It is there that patients with life-threatening emergencies cannot be turned away, pursuant to the 1986 federal Emergency Medical Treatment and Active Labor Act, also commonly called the "anti-patient-dumping law.")

Many physical therapists have expressed disdain with the managed health care model. Yet health care cost containment, initiated and pursued with vigor, may be the best solution to the health care patient and provider access crisis. It is the province of newly graduated physical therapists and assistants, along with other health professionals, to fashion real solutions for the 21st century and to positively influence health care governmental policy so as to effect real distributive (macro-level) and comparative (micro-level) justice in the system.

A recent managed care liability judicial case is noteworthy. On June 12, 2000, the United States Supreme Court, in a 9-0 decision, ruled that patients cannot sue health maintenance organizations for medical care denial decisions under the federal Employee Retirement Income Security Act of 1974 (ERISA), a statute governing employee pension and benefit plans. The Supreme Court held that managed care organizations are not engaged in medical care, but rather exclusively in facilitating the care of plan subscribers, whose health care providers may still be claimed against or sued in state courts by patients for health care malpractice. The Supreme Court left open the issue of potential corporate managed care organization liability for limited breaches of fiduciary duties owed to patients as health benefit plan subscribers.

## EDUCATION ISSUES

Professional education of physical therapists and physical therapist assistants stands at a crossroads at the advent of the 21st century. Seemingly, there exists an oversupply of education programs, the product of a several-decades-long proliferation of new programs. Countering that trend are market-driven macro- and microeconomic forces that have caused a number of physical therapist and physical therapist education programs to close, and most programs to downsize substantially in the past several years.

Although physical therapy professional educational curricula are largely standardized to ensure entry-level clinical competence of graduates and public (patient and client) safety, new issues have come to the fore. These include, among others, the appropriate degree to be awarded to physical therapist education program graduates, qualifications of program directors and academic faculty, and the crisis in clinical education.

The American Physical Therapy Association is currently leading discussions of converting graduate physical therapist education programs to Doctor of Physical Therapy degree programs by some unspecified date. Additional talking points relate to converting some, most, or all current licensed physical therapists to Doctors of Physical Therapy.

The rationale for promoting the Doctor of Physical Therapy credential is multifaceted. It includes the fact that existing graduate physical therapy education programs require an approximate range of 80 to 140 graduate credits for completion, far in excess of any conventional master's degree. The argument is made that physical therapist education program graduates already earn a clinical doctoral degree in most cases, so they should be awarded that degree and recognized as legitimate clinical doctors. Similarly, professional education program content has advanced so far over time to universally include topics like differential (medical) diagnosis, pathology, pharmacology, clinical research, and legalities, among other diverse topics, so as to legitimize the push for doctoral status.

There are, however, factors countering this rationale for physical therapy doctoral designation. There is strong resistance among some physicians to referencing physical therapists as "doctors." This position is largely grounded on the belief that patients will be confused if multiple members of their health care delivery teams are called "doctor." Similar resistance may arise from senior physical therapist, non–doctorally-prepared clinicians, for a variety of reasons. Objectively, patients, who have been socialized into recognizing only their physicians and surgeons as "doctor," may be confused over the change in title for their physical therapists.

Whether physical therapist professional education programs exist at the master's or doctorate level, the reality of the current education *environment* [I refuse to refer to it as the "marketplace," just as I cannot, in good conscience, refer to health care as an "industry." Ed.] is that the demand for physical therapy education is waning. A study by the University of Iowa, released at the Academic Program Directors' Special Interest Group, Section on Education, American Physical Therapy Association meeting in Chicago on October 21, 2000, revealed that for 55 physical therapy education programs, a decline in applications of approximately two thirds ensued between 1994 and 1999. Relative cost, the lengthy time commitment, and alternative complementary career options, among other variables, factor into students' decisions to pursue, or not to pursue, a career in physical therapy.

Continuing education is another area of potential problems and of great promise. With declining continuing education budgets in clinical facilities nationwide in response to cost-containment measures, more and more physical therapists and physical therapist assistants are required to self-fund their continuing professional education, training, and development. These practitioners seek out lower-cost, geographically proximate education options to get the most education for their money. The proliferation of distance learning continuing education opportunities may address these needs and concerns.

Liability issues inherent in professional, clinical, and continuing education range from academic malpractice for failure to adequately prepare students to practice to ordinary and professional negligence for student/participant injury to breach of contract for failure to fulfill contractual promises made to students/participants. The author's article, "CIs and Liability," is reprinted from *PT: Magazine of Physical Therapy*, 1995, and appears in Appendix 10-1 at the end of the chapter.

## PRACTICE ISSUES

As with education, there are myriad physical therapy clinical practice issues confronting the profession at the advent of the new millennium. These issues include, among others, possible diminishing growth in employment opportunities relative to that of recent decades, intra- and interdisciplinary professional relations, and direct access/scope of practice. These three salient issues are addressed below.

## Employment Prospects for Physical Therapists and Physical Therapist Assistants

The hypothesis that a systemic shift from cost-plus-based, fee-for-service health care delivery to prospective payment managed care would lead to employment changes in physical therapy was confirmed by a research study commissioned by the American Physical Therapy Association (APTA) in 1996 and released in 1997. The Workforce Study, carried out under contract by Vector Research, Inc, Ann Arbor, Michigan, examined physical therapy professional and support labor supply and demand parameters, and made predictions for physical therapy employment trends through 2007.

The APTA commissioned the Vector Study in large part because of its concern that highly favorable federal governmental employment statistics and predictions might be incorrect in light of the downsized managed care clinical reality. For example, at the time of the commission of the study, the Bureau of Labor Statistics was still predicting an 88% growth in physical therapy positions by 2005, whereas, clearly, employment prospects were not truly as rosy.

The Vector Research group concluded that the prior physical therapy professional labor shortage, characterized by rapidly increasing compensation, signing and retention bonuses, multiple employment offers, and lucrative employer-funded continuing education, among other benefits, was rapidly diminishing. Vector predicted a balance in physical therapy labor supply and demand by 1998, characterized by a stable employment environment, level compensation, and continuing relatively lucrative benefits and perks. After 1998, and through 2007, the favorable employment picture for physical therapy was predicted by Vector to substantially deteriorate, to the point where there might be a 30% surplus of physical therapists and a 50% surplus of physical therapist assistants in the market.

Why? According to Vector, precipitating factors supporting the near demise of the profession include increasingly aggressive managed health care cost containment, flat population growth, a disproportionate emphasis on caring for older patients (whom the Vector group label "only a small proportion of the United States population"), increased and more intense competition from complementary health care providers, and the negligible productive effect of technology on demand for physical therapy services.

Physical therapists in all practice settings have challenged the Vector assumptions as flawed. An end-of-chapter question addresses this issue. The complete text of the Workforce Study appears in Appendix 10-2 at the end of this chapter.

## Intra- and Interdisciplinary Professional Relations

Professional relations within the disciplines of physical therapy, i.e., between and among physical therapists, physical therapist assistants, complementary professionals working within physical therapy practice settings (e.g., certified athletic trainers, exercise physiologists), other extenders and support, and clerical and administrative personnel, are critically important to successful clinical practice and to patient/client confidence, satisfaction, and loyalty to physical therapy providers. Similarly, relations between physical therapists and relevant co-professionals outside physical therapy—occupational therapists, physicians, chiropractors, dentists, podiatrists, social workers, speech–hearing professionals, third-party payers, administrators, attorneys, and others—are important to practice success and to comity in the professional workplace.

In the recent past, potentially divisive issues have arisen that threaten the comity among co-professionals. These include, among others, challenges by physicians and chiropractors to physical therapists' traditional scope of practice to carry out sharp wound debridement and spinal manipulation, respectively. Other similar issues include the broadening scope of athletic trainers' practice to include therapeutic intervention for recreational athletes, occupational therapists' utilization of modalities, and supervision and domain of practice of physical therapist assistants, all encroachment (on physical therapist practice domain) issues.

Seemingly, physical therapists, individually and collectively, are waging or defending multiple legal and administrative battles, which are extremely costly in terms of time, money, and personal well-being. To the extent that these disputes can be resolved through conciliation, mediation, and lastly arbitration, in lieu of resort to litigation, they should be. Although physical therapy professionals cannot idly permit unfair assaults on their domain of practice, they can and should address such problems and their proponents with the utmost civility and congeniality, looking always for mutual win-win outcomes through effective intergroup negotiations. Perhaps Rodney King made the most prophetic statement of the last (or any) millennium when he said rhetorically, "Can't we all just get along?"

Diversity among physical therapy professionals is another salient practice issue. Cultural diversity entails the presence and participation in practice and decision making of the broadest possible range of diverse groups of clinical and support professionals in the workplace. Diversity may be based on race, ethnicity, nationality, religion, gender, age, disability, sexual preference and orientation, and other personal and character traits. Seemingly, physical therapy is making relatively slow progress in achieving a satisfactory balance of racial and ethnic diversity in the professional workplace. As of October 2000, only 3.5% of physical therapists are Hispanic and approximately the same percentage are African American. The APTA, education programs, clinical facilities and systems, and governments at all levels must redouble their efforts to expand opportunities for underrepresented minorities in physical therapy practice.

The final practice issue to be addressed concerns the extension of direct access practice for physical therapists among the states. As was stated in Chapter 3, the military model for direct access physical therapy practice is the most open and expansive one, under which credentialed physical therapists serve as primary care gatekeepers for patients and clients presenting with minor neuromusculoskeletal conditions. Of the approximately 33 direct access states, most provide more restrictive direct access practice, ranging from requirements for prior physician diagnosis in order to intervene to regulatory qualifications for direct access physical therapy providers, among other provisions. Are entry-level Doctors of Physical Therapy more qualified through professional education to be direct access primary care providers? Should they be automatically be addressed as "Doctor"? These open questions are left for discussion, resolution, and accommodation.

The APTA position (HOD 06-00-30-36) is that direct exclusive PT interventions include spiral and peripheral joint mobilization/manipulation and sharp wound debridement.

## Activities, Cases, and Questions

1. **Activity**: In two groups, examine the assumptions underlying the conclusions made by Vector Research, Inc, in the Workforce Study. For one group, defend the assumptions and conclusions; for the other, challenge them. Support your positions with literature-based references and other data.
2. **Case**: Y. is a recent graduate physical therapist from a DPT program. The physicians at her employment facility, a large medical center, refuse to permit Y. to be referred to as "Doctor," even with a qualifier as to Y.'s status as a Doctor of Physical Therapy. The physical therapy staff, none of whom are DPTs, concur with the physicians' directive. Y. wants to be respected for her DPT credential through title recognition. What can she do to project her professional autonomy?
3. **Question**: What measures can, should, and must be undertaken at the state chapter-professional association level to promote racial and ethnic professional diversity and gender equality in physical therapy practice?

## REFERENCES

1. Starfield B. Is US health really the best in the world? *JAMA.* 2000; 284:483–485.
2. Steinhauer J. Emergency room, to many, remains the doctor's office. *New York Times.* October 25, 2000; Sect A1, A25.

## ADDITIONAL READINGS

*Commonalities and Differences Between the Professions of Physical Therapy and Occupational Therapy*. Alexandria, VA: American Physical Therapy Association; 1994.

Fisher R, Ury W, Patton B. *Getting to Yes: Negotiating Agreement Without Giving In*, 2nd ed. New York: Penguin Books; 1991.

*Pegram v. Herdrich*, 98-1949, 530 US (June 12, 2000).

Scott RW. CIs and Liability. *PT: Magazine of Physical Therapy*, 1995;3(2):30–31.

Scott RW. *Professional Ethics: A Guide for Rehabilitation Professionals*. St. Louis: Mosby-Year Book, Inc.; 1998.

Vector Research, Inc. Workforce Study. Alexandria, VA: American Physical Therapy Association; 1997.

## APPENDIX 10-1*

## CIS AND LIABILITY

### Who's responsible for student conduct—student, CI, site, school? What CIs need to know.

A number of factors are converging to change clinical education, such as the explosion in the number of professional education programs at different degree levels, governmental health care reform efforts, and managed care. With the use of innovative clinical education models such as the 2:1 collaborative model discussed by Zavadak et al (pages 46–55), in which students supervised by one clinical instructor (CI) may be working as a team to treat patients, now is the time for CIs to strengthen their understanding of liability issues.

### What are the basics of malpractice law as it relates to physical therapy?

Any physical therapist who has the legal duty to care for a patient is primarily liable (responsible) for physical or mental injury incurred by the patient as a result of (1) professional negligence (substandard delivery of care), (2) intentional (mis)conduct, (3) breach of a contractual promise made to the patient, or (4) use of a dangerously defective modality or piece of equipment. (Sources such as Prosser[1] and Scott[2] elaborate on these basics.)

The clinician who supervises the activities of physical therapist assistants, physical therapy aides, students, and others (eg, athletic trainers) may be vicariously (indirectly) liable for patient injury resulting from the liability-generating conduct of these persons when it occurs within the scope of their employment or affiliation.[3,4]

### When is the school liable, and when is the site liable?

The party vicariously liable for student conduct usually is the party who has accepted such responsibility under a clinical affiliation agreement, or contract. This contract should clearly delineate the scope of vicarious liability for both site and school and should be undertaken only in consultation with both parties' attorneys. As an additional protective measure for both site and school, the contract also can include language that "memorializes"

* Reprinted, with permission, from Scott RW. *PT: Magazine of Physical Therapy* 1995;3:30–31.

The information in this article should not be interpreted as specific advice for any particular practitioner. Personal advice can be given only by personal legal counsel, based on applicable state and federal law.

the mutual understanding that the school will send only those students who are prepared to participate in clinical experiences.

In addition to vicarious liability, sites and schools may incur primary liability for their own negligence in supervising or preparing students who injure patients. A school, for example, may incur primary liability for the negligent instruction or preparation of a student or for the negligent or intentional misrepresentation of a student's competency or status.

In the absence of clear language spelling out who (or whose insurer) is liable for student conduct, a court may rely on the common-law "borrowed servant rule" to assign responsibility, based on whose interests (site or school) the student primarily was serving at the time of an adverse patient incident.

## What is the CI's supervisory responsibility?

A CI (or site) may incur primary liability for the negligent failure to review a referral order, a patient's treatment records, or a student's evaluation note before allowing the student to treat a patient. CIs (or sites) also may be primarily liable for the negligent failure to provide on-site and, when appropriate, direct supervision of a student during patient intake, evaluation, and treatment. As Smith[5] noted, the supervisory responsibility defined in certain state practice acts "may subject clinical faculty to a potential role of liability." He cited the Georgia State Physical Therapy Practice Act, which states that physical therapist students "in approved education programs can only perform physical therapy if they are supervised by a licensed physical therapist." Whether the supervision should be "direct" also differs from state to state.

Failure-to-supervise liability often is couched in legal terms, such as "patient or student abandonment." A CI who allows a student to evaluate and treat patients without supervision may face criminal legal action for aiding and abetting physical therapy practice by an unlicensed practitioner in addition to adverse licensure and professional association action for practice and ethical violations.

Malpractice exposure also may occur if a CI gives negligent instruction or guidance to a student that results in patient injury or if there is "negligent failure" to include students in systematic quality monitoring and evaluation processes carried out in the clinic.[6]

Center coordinators of clinical education (CCCEs) and managers need to ensure that CIs understand the rules of appropriate supervision of students and that CIs exercise sound professional judgment when assigning patients to students, based on factors such as student competence and special considerations associated with particular patients.[7]

It is essential that CIs review all student evaluations and countersign their notes before students carry out initial treatment of patients. This precaution helps protect all participants in the treatment process: patient, student, CI, and site. Because students are not licensed health care providers, the "student note" is not legally binding. The CI adopts, or is deemed legally to have adopted, all of the student's patient evaluation and treatment notes as the CI's own. If a malpractice monetary settlement is paid or a court judgment is awarded to a patient, it would be the CI's name, and not that of the student, that would be reported to the National Practitioner Data Bank (a data bank that stores malpractice information on health care practitioner[8]).

CIs have not only an ethical responsibility but a legal duty to honestly and accurately evaluate and report a student's clinical performance to academic coordinators of clinical education (ACCEs). Any critical, candid comments should be accurate, fair, and well documented in prior written counseling statements given to the students, in which the student was afforded clear notice of deficient performance, an opportunity to respond in writing to the allegation(s), and an opportunity (reasonable time) to remedy any deficiencies. A CI who misrepresents a student's level of competence may be held legally accountable for patient injury that results from that student's conduct.

Remember: Both statutory (legislative) law and common (judge-made) law require that clinical site personnel and academicians handle information about students as confidential.[2,9] Everyone who has official knowledge about students and their performance should understand the gravity of this responsibility.

## What role does informed consent play?

As is supported by APTA's *Code of Ethics* and *Guide for Professional Conduct*, the basic rule of law is that all health professionals have the ethical and legal duty to gain a patient's informed consent before treatment.[10] Informed consent is based on the patient's inherent right to self-determination or autonomy. The disclosure elements (ie, the information that must be disclosed to the patient) required for legally sufficient patient informed consent to evaluation and treatment when students are involved include:

1. Type of treatment recommended or ordered.
2. Any material (decisional) risks associated with the proposed treatment.
3. The expected benefit(s) of treatment (ie, treatment-related goals).
4. Information about any reasonable alternatives to the proposed treatment.
5. *The role of a student or students in evaluation and treatment.*

CIs should remember that it is their personal legal responsibility—not the student's—to obtain patient informed consent to physical therapy treatment. (Similarly, this responsibility cannot legally be delegated to a PTA.)

## What is the student's responsibility?

A student may be *singularly* responsible for patient injury when that student was negligent and failed to follow a CI's instructions or when the student's injurious conduct was malicious.

As may licensed PTs, students may engage in intentional liability-generating conduct. A student, for example, may commit or be accused of battery (inappropriate or offensive touching of a patient); *defamation* (false assertions about a patient that damage the patient's good reputation); *invasion of (patient) privacy* and, in particular, public dissemination of confidential patient information; or sexual harassment.[1,11]

## What about liability in clinical education and the ADA?

The Americans with Disabilities Act may require that facilities make reasonable accommodation for students with disabilities. The burden typically is on the student to apprise the school or site of the disability and request accommodation.[12] Although facilities must show flexibility in providing necessary assistance and accommodation so that qualified students can reasonably meet clinical education requirements for graduation, the ADA does not say that quality and safety standards can be lowered to the point of risking injury to patients.

## What risk management strategies can sites use?

- Require students to wear name badges, and instruct and compel them to use identifying initials such as "SPT" after their signatures on patient treatment record entries.
- Assign only seasoned clinicians as CCEs and CIs.
- On their arrival in the clinic, orient all students to the physical facility and its written policies, protocols, treatment guidelines, and other standardized operating procedures before they begin to evaluate and treat patients.
- Orient students to the equipment they will be using in the treatment of patients.
- Have students sign in an appropriate place that they have read all applicable policies and guidelines.

As Smith[5] wrote in his overview of liability and clinical education, there are "no cases of a physical therapy student being named in a malpractice suit. . .[and] physical therapists have enjoyed relative freedom from malpractice suits." But CIs (and clinical sites and schools) still should take risk management seriously, both to protect the health interests of the patient and to protect their own professional and legal interests.

## REFERENCES

1. Prosser W. *Prosser on Torts, 4th ed.* St. Paul, Minn: West Publishing Co; 1971.
2. Scott R. *Health Care Malpractice.* Thorofare, NJ; SLACK Inc; 1990.
3. Scott R. *Legal Aspects of Documenting Patient Care.* Gaithersburg, MD: Aspen Publishing Co Inc; 1994.
4. Scott R. Vicarious liability. *Clinical Management,* 1991; 11(5):14–15.
5. Smith HG. Introduction to legal risks associated with clinical education. *Journal of Physical Therapy Education.* 1994; 8(2):67–70.
6. Kearney KA, McCord EL. Hospital management faces new liabilities. *The Health Lawyer.* 1992; 6(3):1,3–6.
7. Fosraught M. Evolution of a Position. *PT:Magazine of Physical Therapy.* 2001; 9(3):38–42.
8. Fraiche D. Peer review and the data bank. *Clinical Management.* 1992; 12(3):14–17.
9. Family Educational Rights and Privacy Act of 1974, 20 USC 1232f(a)(b).
10. Rozovsky FA. *Consent to Treatment, 2nd ed.* Boston, Mass: Little Brown & Co; 1990.
11. Finley C. What is sexual harassment? *PT—Magazine of Physical Therapy.* 1994; 2(12):17–18.
12. Mirone JA. Cases in higher education. ADA Case Law. *PT—Magazine of Physical Therapy.* 1994; 2(6):33.

# APPENDIX 10-2

## WORKFORCE STUDY*

### INTRODUCTION

Historically, physical therapists (PTs) and physical therapist assistants (PTAs) have been in short supply despite substantial increases in physical therapy education programs over the last ten years. Indicators of this shortage include: strong increases in salaries over time, high job placement rates and multiple job offers for new graduates, and hiring bonuses offered as employment incentives. Additionally, Federal Government employment analysts have identified physical therapy as one of the largest employment growth areas.[1]

However, following the demise of President Clinton's Health Security Act (HSA), managed care has continued its expansion, and most health professions (physicians, nurses, and allied health providers) have felt the effect. Additionally, the future of the health care industry holds many questions. In its quest to balance the budget, the Federal Government is targeting Medicare and Medicaid as two major entitlements to be controlled. Large US employers are also committed to controlling the cost of health benefits offered to their employees. In view of these issues, the outlook for the health professions is not what it used to be.

Considering this uncertain environment, the American Physical Therapy Association (APTA) commissioned a study of the supply of and demand for PTs and PTAs for the years 1995, 2000, and 2005. This document presents an overview of the results of this study.

### OVERVIEW OF METHODOLOGY

Our approach to this study consisted of an assessment of the current balance between supply and demand, as well as forecasts of supply and demand through the year 2020. The assessment of current balance was based on examination of available data on salaries and vacancy rates, combined with over 40 interviews with education program directors, recruiters, state APTA representatives, researchers, as well as PTs and PTAs in the field. The focus of these interviews was an assessment of the current employment situation. Participants were asked to comment on the ease of finding positions, salary levels, and future job market expectations.

* Prepared for American Physical Therapy Association (APTA) by Vector Research, Inc., Ann Arbor, Michigan, 1997, Executive Summary

[1] Silvestri, GS. 1995. Occupational employment to 2005. *Monthly Labor Review*, 118(11), 60–79.

Supply projections account for US and international new entrants, deaths, retirements, and part-time labor force participation. Demand forecasts used age-, sex-, and insurance-adjusted per capita staffing models that reflect the current paradigm of population-centered health care planning. Demand projections incorporated the aging of the population, long-term economic growth, increased health maintenance organization (HMO) penetration, and the expansion of "California model" managed care within HMOs and other managed care organizations. Increased competition from alternative providers such as chiropractors, athletic trainers, and occupational therapists was also considered when developing these forecasts. The parameters were estimated using a synthesis of information from a broad and comprehensive search of available survey data bases, published and unpublished reports, and phone interviews with those knowledgeable in the field.

**NOTE: We would emphasize that the assumptions noted throughout this report are derived from data, interviews, and analyses. The conclusions in this report are based on these assumptions materializing. Should these assumptions change or other factors intervene, the conclusions would change accordingly.**

## CONCLUSION 1

The report indicates that:

- There has been and currently continues to be a shortage of qualified physical therapists.
- That shortage is diminishing.
- By 1998, a balance between supply of and demand for physical therapists will be reached.
- A surplus of physical therapists on the order of 20–30% will exist by 2005–2007.

## SUPPLY ASSUMPTIONS

- A rather conservative estimate of new education program development will still yield average annual increases in the number of new entrants of slightly more than 5% for physical therapists and 12% for physical therapist assistants.
- The number of internationally educated physical therapists will remain level beyond 1997 through 2005.

## DEMAND ASSUMPTIONS

- The growth in the US population will increase by only 0.9% during the time frame of 1995–2005.

- Physical therapists and physical therapist assistants will treat an older patient population. This older population represents only a small proportion of the US population, thereby having a small effect on overall increased demand.
- The older population is the one that is reimbursed at the most favorable rates for the provision of physical therapy services.
- Many states will adopt a more "aggressive" approach to managed care, similar to the model currently used by California and hereafter referred to as the "California model." The increased propensity for health care organizations to decrease expenses may reduce the number of physical therapy visits permitted per patient. If the number of visits is decreased, this may also reduce the demand for services through 2005.
- Competitors for the provision of physical therapy services will maintain a market share that is similar to their current share.
- Technology will have a negligible effect on the demand for physical therapy services. Some increases in technology will increase the demand for services, such as increases in the survival rate among premature babies (BLS, 1995). Others will allow patients to recover faster and thereby may create less of a need for physical therapy services.
- Demand for PTs may decrease by 10% between 1995 and 2005 due to the increased use of PTAs to complement PT practice.

## DISCUSSION

Exhibit 1 provides a continuum showing our estimate of the national employment picture for PTs and PTAs from 1990 to 2005. The shortage of the early 1990s was characterized by rapidly increasing compensation, applicants receiving multiple job offers, and a high demand for physical

**Exhibit 1: Balance Between Supply and Demand—An Estimated Timeline**

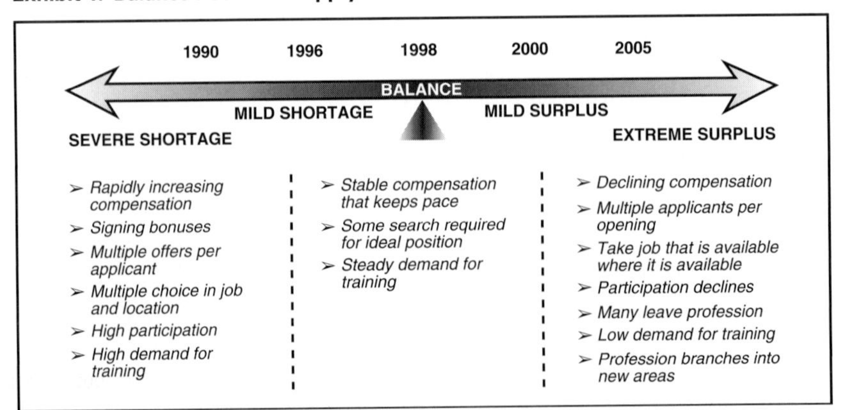

**Exhibit 2: Supply and Demand for Physical Therapists (1995–2005)**

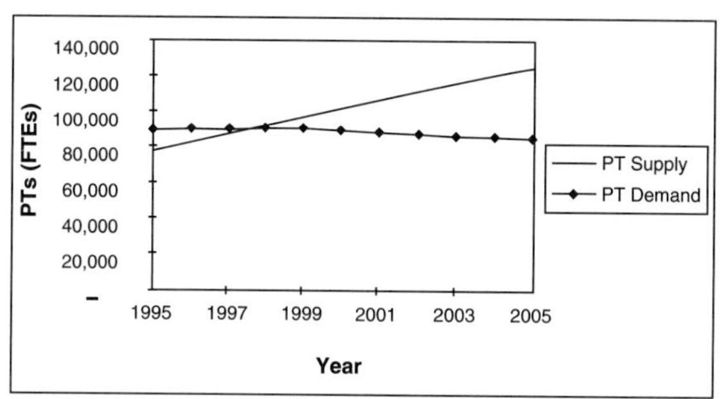


therapy academic and clinical education. By 1996, this shortage had largely abated due to rapid increases in the supply of PTs and PTAs and managed care cost controls.

By the end of 1998, we predict that the supply of and demand for PTs and PTAs will be in rough balance. In this "balanced" state, salaries will remain competitive but will not increase as they did under shortage conditions. In addition, job applicants may have to spend more time locating an ideal position. Because salary levels remain stable and competitive, we expect the demand for academic and clinical education to continue. However, during this time, growing reports of a softening of the job market will dissuade individuals from pursuing a physical therapy career, thereby lowering the demand for academic and clinical education.

By the year 2000, we predict a mild surplus, but it may not be considered a surplus by external observers.[2] PTs and PTAs will still find employment, but the positions may not be ideal either in setting or location. The year 2005 brings a larger surplus which may be accompanied by declining real compensation, lower rates of participation, and a decreased demand for academic and clinical education.

If no economic responses in addition to those we have assumed take place, in 2005 there will be a surplus of PTs in the range of 30 percent. This surplus may be mitigated, in part, by several market reactions that are discussed at the end of this report.

Exhibit 2 shows our best estimate of PT supply and demand for the years 1995-2005. Exhibit 3 plots the same data but focuses on the percent of excess demand.

The study's primary focus was the estimation of supply and demand in terms of full-time equivalents (FTEs). These estimates accounted for

[2] For example, the job market for RNs has worsened considerably in recent years, but it is not generally referred to as a surplus.

**Exhibit 3: Difference in Supply and Demand for Physical Therapists**

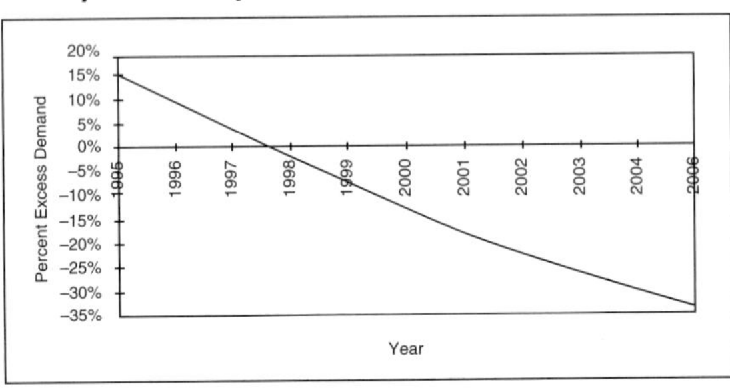


individuals practicing or working part-time. We translated FTEs into estimates of licensed individuals, as shown in Exhibits 4 and 5.

## CONCLUSION 2

The number of new PT and PTA entrants will continue to increase, due to the increasing numbers of education programs and, for PTs, the increasing numbers of internationally educated PTs entering the US. The number of PTAs per PT will almost double from 1995–2005.

## ASSUMPTIONS

### PT Supply:

- The best estimate of supply for base year 1995 for PTs is 99,249.
- New entrants to the profession for 1996 and beyond will increase. Increases stem from the estimated number of graduates from accredited and developing education programs.
- Supply losses due to mortality and loss of licensure reduce the number of licensed PTs each year.
- Based on entrance through the H-1B visa program and passing rates for the PT licensure exam, the number of internationally educated PTs will increase for 1996 and 1997 and then level off in the years beyond.

**Exhibit 4: Differences in Supply and Demand for Physical Therapists (Licensed Individuals)**

| Year | Supply | Demand | Difference |
|---|---|---|---|
| 1995 | 99,249 | 114,137 | −14,888 |
| 2000 | 199,941 | 113,703 | 16,238 |
| 2005 | 159,523 | 108,575 | 50,948 |

Source: VRI estimates

**Exhibit 5: Differences in Supply and Demand for Physical Therapist Assistants (Licensed Individuals)**

| Year | Supply | Demand | Difference |
|---|---|---|---|
| 1995 | 27,469 | 31,590 | –4,121 |
| 2000 | 53,267 | 46,611 | 6,656 |
| 2005 | 79,108 | 53,843 | 25,265 |

Source: VRI estimates

## PTA Supply:

- The best estimate of supply for base year 1995 for PTAs is 27,469.
- New PTA entrants for 1996 and beyond will increase. Increases stem from the estimated number of graduates from accredited and developing education programs.
- Supply losses due to mortality and loss of licensure reduce the number of PTAs each year.
- There are no internationally educated PTAs.

## DISCUSSION

Predicted annual new entrants for PTs and PTAs are presented in Exhibits 6 and 7. Graduates of currently accredited US programs are distinguished from those of known developing programs. Internationally educated new entrants are also identified. These estimates are conservative in the short term as they include only current accredited and known developing programs, rather than including trends in new program development. Note that these numbers represent licensed individuals rather than FTEs. The

**Exhibit 6: Annual Physical Therapist New Entrants**

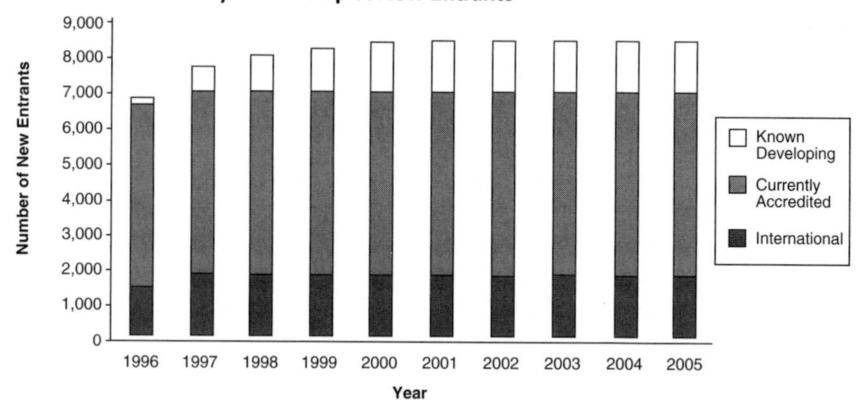

**Exhibit 7: Annual Physical Therapist Assistant New Entrants**

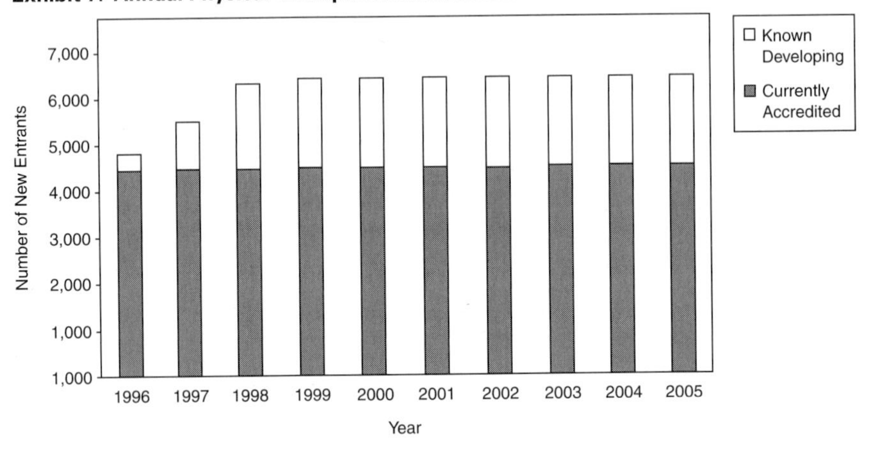


number of internationally educated PT new entrants has been increasing in recent years, and our forecasts were made with the assumption that this growth will continue for two more years and then remain at that level.[3] Given that internationally educated new entrants account for over 20 percent of PT new entrants, any increase or decrease in this population will have a substantial effect on supply in future years. The new entrants from PTA education programs increased nearly 13.5 percent per year.[4]

Using this information on new graduates, we estimate that the current PTA to PT ratio (0.28 in 1995) will increase to nearly 0.5 by the year 2005 and to over 0.6 by the year 2020. Exhibit 8 shows this increase at five-year intervals.

## CONCLUSION 3

Between now and 2005:

- The demand for PTs will be most affected by the growth of the population, long-term economic growth, the spread of the "California model" of managed care, and increases in the use of PTAs to complement PT practice.
- Such factors as the aging of the population, competition from other providers, and changes in medical technology will be of second-order importance. We expect the demand for PTs to decrease overall by 3% between 1995 and 2005.

[3] Federation of State Boards of Physical Therapy, *Foreign and US Examinees*, 1990–1995, May 29, 1996.

[4] American Physical Therapy Association. 1996. *PTA Fact Sheet 1996*. Alexandria, VA: American Physical Therapy Association.

**Exhibit 8: Physical Therapist Assistants Per Physical Therapist**

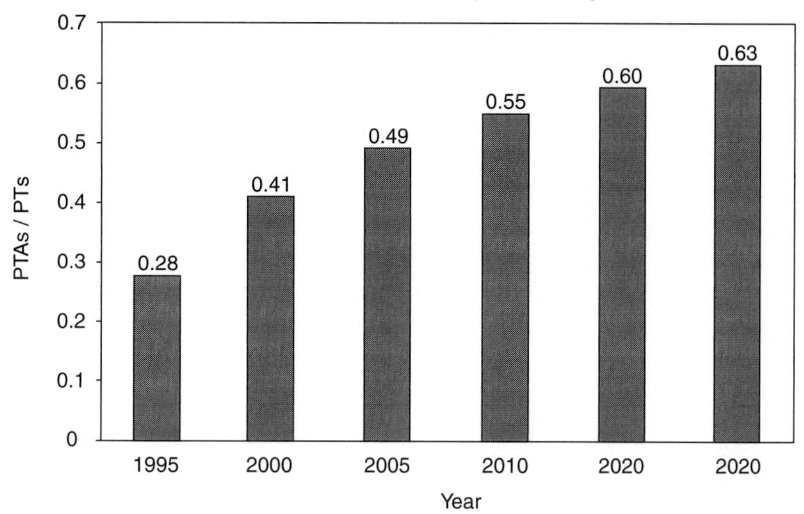


## ASSUMPTIONS

Current or baseline demand estimates form the basis from which to project future demand.

### Current Demand for Physical Therapists

- Total Baseline Demand for PTs = Supply of PTs + Unmet Demand.
- Unmet demand at the end of 1996 is estimated as 10% and is decreasing at a rate of about 5% per year. It is highest in rural areas and lowest or nonexistent in California.
- Recent data suggest growth in supply outstripped growth in demand by about 5% between 1995 and 1996.

### Current Demand for Physical Therapist Assistants

- Demand for PTAs = Supply of PTAs + Unmet Demand.
- Unmet demand for PTAs is similar to that for PTs.
- PTs can delegate a substantial part of service provision to PTAs.

### Future Demand

- The amount of delegation to PTAs will increase in the future and the differential growth rates relative to PTs will continue through 2005.
- Growth of the US population will increase at 0.9% per year. Although the elderly population uses a lot more PT services, this age group represents a small proportion of the total population, thereby having a small effect on overall increased demand.

- Each percentage increase in real per capita income can be expected to increase PT demand by 1%.
- The "California model" of managed care, which reduces the levels of PT services by 30–60%, will have the greatest effect on reducing PT demand.
- As traditional health care markets tighten, PTs have the incentive to retain their current market shares and will experience intensified competition from competitors.
- PTs will continue to outnumber chiropractors at a 2:1 ratio; anticipated growth of market share by chiropractors will result in a negligible reduced demand for PTs.
- Athletic trainers are not likely to gain share in the mainstream areas of PT practice.
- PTs overlap with occupational therapists primarily in the area of assistive technology.
- Technological improvements will both increase and reduce demand for PTs; the effects will cancel each other.

## DISCUSSION

Between now and 2005, the demand for PTs will be most affected by population growth, economic growth, the spread of the "California model" of managed care, and the dramatic increase in the number of PTAs. Factors such as population aging, competition from other providers, and advancing medical technology will be of second-order importance.

As shown in Exhibit 9, between 1995 and 2005, demand increases approximately 12 percent due to population growth and aging. When long-term economic growth is factored into this demand, growth doubles. Incorpora-

**Exhibit 9: Percent Change in Physical Therapist Demand (1995–2005)**

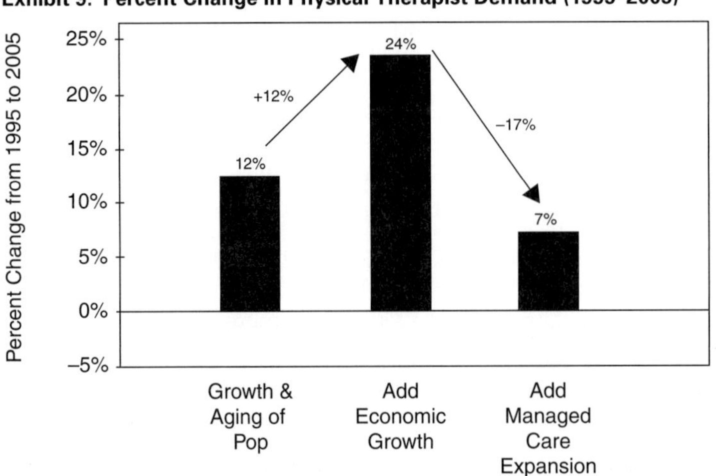


*Holding PTAs Per PT at 1995 Ratio

tion of the effects of the expansion of the "California model" of managed care, however, dampens the increase to only 7 percent.[5]

The impact of growth and aging of the population results in an increase in demand of slightly more than one percent per year. Most of this growth is due to the increased number of people (about 0.9 percent per year), with the remainder due to aging.

Additionally, the demand for PTs is significantly influenced by the national economic growth rate. Health care economists have demonstrated that the demand for health care increases with personal income, basically on a proportional basis. That is, when income increases by 1 percent, the demand for health care also increases by 1 percent. To test this relationship for applicability to PTs, we compared the 50 US states in terms of the number of PTs per capita and their average per capita income. Our estimates were close to this proportional relationship and were not statistically significantly different. Thus, we concluded that over extended periods of time, each percentage increase in real per capita income can be expected to increase PT demand by 1 percent.

As the "California model" of managed care expands, PT demand will be reduced but will nonetheless rise between 1995 and 2000. It then will level off through 2005. These results reflect our assumptions that the "California model" of managed care will spread to workers' compensation, automobile liability, and personal health insurance plans in the next several years. We assumed that Medicare will not begin implementing the "California model" of managed care until the year 2000.

The final factor that may substantially affect demand for PTs is the growth in numbers of PTAs. The projection of a 7 percent increase in demand for PTs shown in Exhibit 9 is based upon the 1995 ratio of PTAs per PT, which is .28 (i.e., slightly more than 1 PTA per 4 PTs). At this constant ratio, the demand for PTAs also increases by 7 percent. However, our supply projections imply that the ratio of PTAs per PT will increase to .49 (i.e., about 2 PTAs per 4 PTs) by 2005 because of the greater growth of PTAs relative to PTs. While there are clearly limits to what PTs can delegate effectively to PTAs, this ratio appears to be within the acceptable range of delegation when considered from the perspective of a national average across all patients and settings. Moving to this new higher ratio has a significant impact on the demand for PTs and PTAs. Instead of increasing by 7 percent, the demand for PTs declines by 3 percent.

[5] For this study, "aggressive" managed care is defined as the type of managed care that results when there is intense price competition such as in California. Using information from empirical studies and the field, we estimated reductions in PT demand due to aggressive managed care when compared with the current national norm and estimated the rate at which aggressive managed care will spread.

Compared with the factors mentioned above, our study found that the effects of demand due to the aging of the population, competition from other providers, and changes in medical technology were not as remarkable. Competition from other providers was not expected to significantly decrease demand for PTs; however, discussions with experts indicated that chiropractors have the greatest potential to make inroads into PT practice due to their increasing numbers and entrepreneurial outlook. We investigated the impact of changes in medical technology and found that, overall, technological advancements will not obviously increase demand for physical therapy (except those that improve life span). As our projections captured the effects of longer life span, no additional adjustments for technology were incorporated in the study.

## CONCLUSION 4

In future years the market will react to the growth of supply relative to demand. Major reactions most likely will include:

- Declines in real compensation;
- Less flexibility in choice of position (geographic location and practice setting); and
- A decreased demand for physical therapy education programs.

## ASSUMPTIONS

- Data on earned incomes of physical therapists indicate increases in income are declining.
- Based on interview data, PTs are experiencing more difficulty in obtaining the "most attractive" positions.
- Reports from educators indicated a decline in the physical therapy applicant pool size. Higher education administrators do not develop academic programs in areas of study that are not attractive to potential students.
- Supply projections assumed that all known developing programs would receive accreditation but that none of the "interested" institutions would actually develop programs.

## DISCUSSION

In future years, the market will react to the growth of supply relative to demand. Major reactions most likely will include: declines in real compensation, less flexibility in choice of position (geographic location and practice setting), and a decreased demand for physical therapy education programs.

The proper interpretation of the study's projections requires consideration of the various reactions that will occur in the job market as it moves from its historical shortage situation into a surplus. For example, the 11 percent surplus predicted at the end of the year 2000 does not mean that we expect there to be 11 percent unemployment among PTs and PTAs at that time. It does mean that we expect the market to adapt in ways that reflect supply growing faster than demand.

As one of the first market reactions, compensation will grow less quickly and eventually decline in real terms.[6] In considering compensation, it is useful to expand the notion to include non-monetary aspects of a position, such as setting, geographic location, and flexibility in hours. Over time, these non-monetary aspects of compensation will fall along with the monetary component.

A direct consequence of this reduction in compensation is that employers and consumers who previously could not effectively "demand" physical therapy services will enter the marketplace and push demand upward. This new demand will be concentrated in what might be called "second-choice" settings, locations, and arrangements. There will be more demand in the home health and long-term care settings because these settings will now be able to compete for physical therapy providers. Likewise, there will be more demand in rural areas and inner cities. And there will be more demand for PTs in positions that offer more flexibility to employers, such as temporary pools. This increase in demand is why we do not expect there to be 11 percent unemployment in the year 2000. There will be jobs but the positions will not, on average, be as well-compensated as the jobs available today.[7]

As compensation and flexibility in choice of location and setting are lessened, the increase in demand for PTs described above will be accompanied by a decrease in supply. Some PTs will change careers or leave the labor force altogether because they cannot obtain the job they want where they want it. A recent study of registered nurses (RNs) showed that female RNs significantly reduced their participation and hours worked when salaries fell.[8] This means that the 11 percent surplus projected for 2000 will be alleviated in part by a reduction in the amount of services offered by existing PTs.

[6] A decline in real terms means that compensation does not keep pace with inflation.

[7] This relates to the discrepancy between the number of PT jobs being projected by the Bureau of Labor Statistics (BLS) and the level of demand projected in this study. Our demand projections presented earlier are for jobs that have compensation levels comparable to today. We expect the number of jobs to exceed these projections of demand but compensation levels will not be up to today's standards. Thus, the BLS projections could be correct, but the jobs will not be comparable to current jobs. Of course, PTs will have some control over the outcome. The more successful PTs are at demonstrating the value of their services and expanding interest in their services to new areas, the more attractive the new jobs will be.

[8] Brewer, CS. 1996. The roller coaster supply of registered nurses: lessons from the eighties. *Research in Nursing and Health*, 19, 345–357.

We also expect the market for PT education to react to the changing market conditions. As the job market softens, there will be a decline in the number of qualified applicants to PT schools and a reduction in enrollment class sizes and numbers of programs. The number of US enrollments may begin to fall below our projections by the year 2000 due to market reactions. Reductions in the number of internationally trained new entrants are also likely. These expected market reactions will dampen the effects of the surplus but will not eliminate them.

### American Physical Therapy Association Workforce Study Predicts Surplus of Physical Therapists by the Year 2000

ALEXANDRIA, VA, May 19, 1997—An 11 percent surplus of physical therapists is predicted by the year 2000, and a 20–30 percent surplus is predicted by 2005–2007, according to a workforce study commissioned by the American Physical Therapy Association (APTA).

"The outlook for physical therapy is not what it used to be," said APTA President Marilyn Moffat, PT, PhD, FAPTA. "We expect that the employment market for physical therapy will become more competitive, salaries may level off, recent graduates may not get their first choice of location or practice opportunity, and physical therapists may seek or develop opportunities in nontraditional settings."

"Physical therapists have historically enjoyed high demand and 'hot career' status," Moffat said. "Now that we are facing a surplus situation, there will be a reallocation of physical therapy resources. The good news for consumers is that physical therapists may move into more underserved areas; those who have not had access to physical therapy in the past may be able to receive these necessary services."

Physical therapists may expand their practices more in preventive aspects of physical therapy, such as wellness and fitness; in home health and long-term care facilities; in areas such as women's health, oncology, and industrial physical therapy and ergonomics; and in rural and inner city locations. They may also become more available to provide physical therapy utilization review within the insurance industry.

The workforce study, conducted by Vector Research Inc., a private health care studies and analysis consulting firm, focused on an assessment of the current relationship between supply and demand and a forecast of the supply of and demand for physical therapists and physical therapist assistants through the year 2020. The study found that while the shortage continues, it is diminishing. By 1998, balance between supply and demand is expected, and a surplus of 20–30 percent is predicted by 2005–2007.

Future demand will be most affected by population growth, economic growth, and the spread of the "California model" of managed care. The projected increase in the number and utilization of physical therapist assistants may also have an effect upon the demand for physical therapists through the year 2005.

On the supply side, the study predicted that the number of physical therapists and physical therapist assistants will continue to grow at annual average rates of 5 and 11 percent respectively, and the number of internationally educated physical therapists will grow until 1997 and then remain level through 2005.

For many years, APTA has worked to increase the supply of qualified licensed physical therapists by helping to develop physical therapist and physical therapist assistant education programs; supporting the accreditation process; increasing public understanding of physical therapy as a career; and supporting doctoral scholarships to increase the number of qualified faculty members available to educate larger numbers of students.

Physical therapists, like many other health care professionals, are feeling the effects of the Federal Government's targeting of Medicare and Medicaid entitlements, managed care, and reductions in employees' health benefits.

The American Physical Therapy Association is a national professional organization representing more than 72,000 physical therapists, physical therapist assistants, and students of physical therapy throughout the United States. Its goal is to foster improvements in physical therapy education, practice, and research.

## American Physical Therapy Association Workforce Study

### Questions And Answers

Q. *Why did APTA commission Vector Research Inc. to conduct the workforce study?*

A. This is an uncertain environment for the health care industry. After the demise of President Clinton's Health Security Act, managed care has continued to expand and most health professions have felt the effect. The Federal Government is targeting Medicare and Medicaid as two major entitlements to be controlled, and large U.S. employers are committed to controlling the cost of health benefits offered to their employees. Considering that the outlook for the health professions is not what it used to be, the American Physical Therapy Association (APTA) commissioned the study to look at the supply of and demand and need for physical therapists and physical therapist assistants for the years 1995, 2000, and 2005. The Association's effort was also motivated by continued anecdotal reports that the often-publicized shortage of physical therapists was, in reality, diminishing. Vector Research, Inc., is a well-established and well-respected private consultant firm that specializes in health care studies and analysis.

Q. ***How do the study's findings correspond to the U.S. Department of Labor's Bureau of Labor Statistics predictions for the physical therapy profession?***

A. The Bureau of Labor Statistics (BLS) and Vector Research, Inc.'s (VRI) workforce study measure different entities. The BLS predictions estimate the number of physical therapist positions, while VRI projections estimate demand for personnel. BLS's 1994 prediction forecasts a healthy job outlook for physical therapists. They project substantial increases in the number of jobs between now and the year 2005. In a recent publication (*Dietetics, Nursing, Pharmacy, and Therapy Occupations*, 1996). BLS noted that the anecdotal reports about shortages of physical therapists are no longer commonplace. Thus, the BLS language describing the future number of positions is less optimistic than previously reported. In meetings between APTA staff and BLS, APTA was advised that information contained in the Vector workforce study will be referenced in future BLS reports.

Q. ***How does the expansion of managed care affect the demand for physical therapists?***

A. The simple increase in numbers of enrollees in HMOs will not have a substantial impact on the demand for physical therapists. Instead, a particular kind of managed care, like that being seen in California, will have a major effect on demand. As the "California model" of managed care expands, demand for physical therapists is predicted to be reduced by 17 percent in the future. This assumes that the "California model" of managed care will spread to workers' compensation, automobile liability, and personal health insurance plans over the next several years and that Medicare will not be implementing the "California model" of managed care until the year 2000.

Q. ***Will there also be a surplus of physical therapist assistants?***

A. The workforce study predicts changes in the supply of and demand for physical therapists and physical therapist assistants. Like physical therapists, physical therapist assistants will experience changes between supply and demand. In 1995, the study's base year, there was a physical therapist assistant shortage of approximately 15%. Balance between supply and demand was predicted to occur by the end of 1996. By 2005, physical therapist assistant supply will exceed demand by approximately 50%. This surplus will continue to increase through 2020.

Q. ***Will there be more utilization of physical therapist assistants under managed care?***

A. The answer to this question must be addressed in the aggregate and it will not apply to each individual physical therapist in practice or to each physical therapy service in existence. Currently, the ratio of physical therapist assistants to physical therapists is .28 (i.e., slightly more than 1 physical therapist assistant per 4 physical therapists); this ratio reflects the different numbers in each group and that physical therapists supervise and delegate tasks to physical therapist assistants. Due to the differential in growth rates between physical therapists and physical therapist assistants, this ratio is predicted to increase to .49 (i.e., about 2 physical therapist assistants per 4 physical therapists) by 2005. As the "California model" of managed care continues to expand, and because physical therapist assistants are less expensive to employ, it is projected that more physical therapist assistants relative to physical therapists may be hired. While there are clearly limits to what physical therapists can delegate effectively to physical therapist assistants, this ratio appears to be within the feasible range when considered from the perspective of a national average across all patient groups and settings.

Q. ***How will the surplus affect the number of entrants into the physical therapy profession?***

A. The manner and degree of any change in interest in the physical therapy profession cannot be predicted with certainty. However, if prospective physical therapists or physical therapist assistants are primarily motivated by factors such as job security, higher salaries, or a wide range of job opportunities, the profession's considerable appeal could be moderated by a supply/demand balance or a significant oversupply of professional or paraprofessional personnel. Also, the number of available visas for foreign-educated physical therapists could be reduced. Finally, while certain practice settings may be negatively affected by a surplus of physical therapists or physical therapist assistants, other settings may expand and thereby accommodate new graduates.

Q. ***How will the surplus affect the developing physical therapist and physical therapist assistant education programs? What is APTA's message to these programs? How many programs are there now?***

A. Programs that are currently under development might wish to consider reducing class size or altering projected enrollment patterns (e.g., enrolling a class every other year). For institutions considering a new program, a surplus of physical therapists or physical therapist assistants could make it considerably more difficult to justify development. In determining a new program's feasibility, marketplace realities (fewer jobs, lower salaries, scarcity of clinical facilities for clinical education, faculty shortages, etc.) can adversely affect the prospects for success. Although in the past these realities could be ignored if limited to only a few geographical areas, a more pervasive supply/demand imbalance would likely exacerbate their effects. In light of the workforce study,

APTA would encourage any institution to seriously consider the implications of the study's conclusions before initiating the application process for candidacy and accreditation of a new program.

Q. *What is APTA's strategy for addressing the surplus?*

A.
- APTA will promote an enhanced role for physical therapists in primary care;
- APTA will promote federal and state incentives to attract physical therapists to underserved areas;
- APTA will offer continuing education courses on marketing physical therapy services and developing necessary skills for expanding practices into new areas;
- APTA will monitor the status of physical therapist and physical therapist assistant supply and demand and the environment affecting both.

## 1998 GOALS AND OBJECTIVES OF THE ASSOCIATION

**Goal I:** **Participate actively in shaping the current and emerging health care environment to promote the development of high-quality, cost-effective health care services and to further the recognition of and support for the profession of physical therapy and the role of physical therapists.**

Objective A: Increase Public awareness of physical therapy and the selection of physical therapists for the treatment and prevention of injury, impairment, functional limitation, and disability and for the promotion and maintenance of health, fitness, and optimum quality of life.

Objective B: Improve coverage and reimbursement by public and private payers for physical therapy provided by or under the direction of physical therapists.

Objective C: Advocate for national health policy, federal and state laws, and federal and state regulations that appropriately govern physical therapy practice, education, and research.

Objective D: Promote the role of physical therapists as primary care providers of diagnostic and treatment services and integral members of primary care teams in health care delivery systems.

Objective E: Develop collaborative arrangements and/or activities with professional associations and organizations for the purpose of advancing common goals related to the provision of services.

**Goal II:** **Stimulate innovation in the practice of physical therapy that supports physical therapists and physical therapist assistants.**

Objective A: Address current patterns of practice affecting physical therapists, including the following: eliminate referral for profit in the provision of physical therapy services; educate managed care primary care providers as to the appropriate utilization of physical therapy services; and ensure high-quality care in the best interests of patients.

Objective B: Identify and promote high-quality, cost-effective models of physical therapy practice that include physical therapy personnel, ensuring the congruence of education and training.

Objective C: Promote the physical therapist as a key health care practitioner in the promotion of wellness, fitness, and preventive care.

**Goal III:** **Quantify and interpret the demand for, the need for, and the access to physical therapy services.**

Objective A: Determine the availability and distribution of physical therapy personnel on an ongoing basis.

**Goal IV:** **Stimulate innovation in physical therapy education and professional development at all levels to ensure currency with the changing environments in health care and education and with student and professional needs.**

Objective A: Design, promote, and continually reevaluate consensus-based standards for physical therapy education and educational models that are consistent with the mission of physical therapy education and responsive to changes in the educational, professional, and health care environments.

Objective B: Identify, design, and implement strategies that strengthen the linkage between accreditation and the profession of physical therapy, enhance efficiency and effectiveness of the accreditation process.

Objective C: Promote and expand Association and member involvement in educational issues and the development of policies and programs at institutional, state, and national levels.

Objective D: Design, implement, and evaluate programs and activities for career development and continuing education of physical therapists and physical therapist assistants.

**Goal V:** **Stimulate research to further the science of physical therapy, to influence current and emerging health care trends, and to advance the profession.**

Objective A: Promote research on physical therapy outcomes/effectiveness.

Objective B: Promote research that validates, formulates, or redirects APTA positions on relevant policy-related issues.

Objective C: Encourage interdisciplinary and collaborative research and promote Association involvement in research agencies.

Objective D: Develop, integrate, and disseminate the theoretical and empirical bases of physical therapy.

**Goal VI:** **Increase APTA's responsiveness to the needs of current and future members.**

Objective A: Increase total membership by 5.5%, physical therapist membership by 3.5%, physical therapist assistant membership by 14%, and student membership by 12%.

Objective B: Enhance collaborative communications across and among all elements of the Association.

Objective C: Provide for leadership development and training of individuals for elected and appointed positions at national and component levels.

Objective D: Foster association involvement by members in leadership positions through the development of mentorship activities.

Objective E: Continuously improve the effectiveness and efficiency of APTA's structure, programs, and services to carry out the mission.

Objective F: Develop and maintain a record of the Association's history.

Objective G: Strengthen the profession as a whole by eliminating gender inequities in physical therapy practice, research, and education.

## Focus on a Leader

**TED YANCHULEFF, MPA, PT**
**TEAM LEADER, THE PHYSICAL REHABILITATION & AQUATICS CENTER, LANCASTER HEALTH ALLIANCE, LANCASTER, PENNSYLVANIA**

1. *Ted, please briefly capsulize for readers your credentials, professional chronology, and current and recent professional activities.*

Over the course of 22 years as a physical therapist, athletic trainer, and rehabilitation administrator, I have been blessed to witness the growth of the rehabilitation field in an ever-changing health care model. As we approach the new millennium, I look back at my career, which has support by colleagues, physicians, friends, and most important, my family. To this end, many of the health care decisions I have made have had their origin in the following educational foundations: Harrisburg Area Community College, Associate Degree of Arts, 1975; University of Pittsburgh, Bachelor of Science in Physical Therapy, 1977; Pennsylvania State University, Masters in Public Administration, 1994; and National Certification as an Athletic Trainer, 1978.

Politically, I have served the Commonwealth of Pennsylvania as a board member and then progressed to the chairmanship of the State Board of Physical Therapy in the early 90s. My current professional societies consist of membership in the American Physical Therapy Association, including the sections of administration, aquatics and sports physical therapy, as well as the National Athletic Trainers Association with corresponding state affiliations to these organizations. At the time of this writing, I am serving as the South Central District Chairman of the Pennsylvania Physical Therapy Association.

2. *From a clinical manager's perspective, what are the salient problems, issues, and dilemmas affecting the profession of physical therapy, now and in the near future?*

From a clinical manager's perspective, the salient problems that affect the physical therapy profession have their "root cause" in the core areas of "tradition" and "change." In recent decades the physical therapy profession traditionally has shown tremendous linear growth in demand, opportunities, and salaries. Demand for Physical Therapy (PT) services was high, and the supply of physical therapists and physical therapist assistants lagged behind the opportunities provided by multiple health care settings and case mixes. However, the recent Vector Study indicates that supply has now exceeded demand, and corresponding changes in reimbursement provided in the Balanced Budget Act has caused a "white water" period in the physical therapy field.

The turbulence caused by these events has resulted in loss of jobs, lower salaries, and a reduction in opportunities for the PT profession to expand despite a graying of the American population. It is my contention that the current environment exists secondary to the profession's slow response to adapt to change in the clinical, outcomes, political, and research arenas.

Many of the keystone pathways used by physical therapists and physical therapist assistants alike need enhanced empirical data to supplement existing plans of care for many of the case mixes serviced. Lack of outcome data to support cost versus benefit of the charge, and the time frame of services rendered (more time required for functional benefit), need to be fully developed and promoted. Apathy, at times, with the political process has allowed for empowerment of laws and practice acts that have limited the scope of practice of the profession and allowed the development and use of many "health care extenders" to provide many of services once exclusively provided in the physical therapy profession's domain.

As the physical therapy profession continues to evolve, respect for the positive traditions of the past need to be recognized, but it will be our ability to change and create a mutual desired future with the consumers of services that will eventually provide long-term growth and survival of the profession.

3. *Where do you believe physical therapy will be in the year 2050? What needs to be accomplished to get the profession where you envision it being in 2050?*

In the year 2050, the "yin and yang" of the PT profession will have come full circle. The current emphasis on "illness" will be replaced with enhanced concepts of "wellness." Computer and high-technology information systems will provide the research foundation to provide design systems for the paralyzed to walk while providing "global pathways" to many of the neurological and orthopaedic diseases of the new millennium.

Physical therapy will play a significant role in developing a proactive healthy quality of life case-mix versus a post-event illness/disease model. The professional of tomorrow will be computer, pathway, and outcome literate, as well as fiscally competent. The paradigm of treating illness will be replaced by services that enable wellness over the course of one's life.

My year 2050 predictions that will have a direct effect on physical therapy professionals are: single source third-party payer for universal coverage for all Americans; average life expectancy exceeding 100 years; direct access in all 50 states; increased need for ethnic diversity secondary to whites becoming a minority in some areas of the United States; a cure for AIDS and most other fatal diseases; and therapy provided via Intranet-type medium in the home.

Many of the concepts once thought of as futuristic in the Star Trek movies will be common place in the year 2050, and the role of the physical therapy profession will be to supplement the medical model, enabling a more leisure lifestyle. To all therapists of this new era: "Live long and prosper."

APPENDIX I

# Developmental Timeline, Physical Therapy Profession in the United States, 1881–1995*

**1881** Sargent School, Boston, founded by Dudley Allen Sargent. Elliott Brackett and Robert Lovett join faculty.

**1887** Forerunner of the National Institutes of Health born at Marine Hospital, Staten Island, New York.

**1889** MIT hosts first national conference on physical training, Boston Normal School of Gymnastics founded by Amy Homans.

**1893** The Cotting School, the first free day school for children with disabilities founded in Boston.

**1894** First polio epidemic in U.S. recorded in Rutland, Vermont.

**1905** Mary McMillan receives degree in physical education and goes on to take post-grad courses in electrotherapy, therapeutic exercise, massage and anatomy in London.

**1910** McMillan takes her first professional position in Liverpool, England, working with Sir Robert Jones.

**1913** First formal government survey of injuries from industrial accidents.

**1913** Pennsylvania becomes first state to license physical therapists.

**1914** R.W. Lovett, known for his novel approach to polio treatment, creates the "Vermont Plan" to treat epidemic in state. Wilhelmine Wright, his assistant trains cadre of assistants in her system of "manual muscle testing." This work becomes basis of treating patients with polio and postural deformities.

**1914** Marjorie Bouvé, Marguerite Sanderson, and others found Boston School of Physical Education (future Bouvé-Boston).

**1916** McMillan returns to U.S. to work at children's Hospital Portland, Maine. Severe polio epidemic in New York and elsewhere.

**1917** United States declares war on Germany. Division of Special Hospitals and Physical Reconstruction authorized within the Army Medical Department. Marguerite Sanderson hired as director of Reconstruction Aide program.

**1917** J.B. Mennell publishes seminal text on scientific massage, Physical Treatment by Movement, Manipulation and Massage.

**1918** First Reconstruction Aides mobilized and trained. McMillan becomes second "re-aide." Walter Reed General Hospital's program is soon joined by those at Reed College and 13 other schools. Armistice declared in November.

**1919** Sanderson retires and McMillan takes over. "Re-aides" are demobilized. Charles Lowman founds Los Angeles Orthopedic Hospital and pioneers "hydrogymnastics."

**1920** McMillan resigns to return to private practice in Boston and to complete *Massage and Therapeutic Exercise* published 1921.

**1920** Organizational meeting for American Women's, Physiotherapeutic Association held at Keen's Chop House, New York. Mary McMillan elected first President by ballot. Bimonthly *P.T. Review* makes its debut in March.

**1922** First Annual Conference held in Boston. AWPA changes name to American Physiotherapy Association.

**1923** McMillan retires and Inga Lohne elected President.

*Source: Murphy W. *Healing the Generations: A History of Physical Therapy and The American Physical Therapy Association* 1995; Alexandria, VA: APTA, pp. 248–249. Used with permission of the APTA.

**1924** F.D. Roosevelt stricken with polio, establishes Warm Springs Foundation in Georgia.
**1926** *P.T. Review* renamed *Physiotherapy Review* and becomes monthly soon after.
**1927** NYU inaugurates first 4-year bachelor of science program to physical therapists.
**1927** Debate over what to call physical therapists arises with physicians and surgeons.
**1928** Standards for accreditation are developed with guidance of John Stanley Catilter, MD. Most accredited institutions are hospital-based and award post-baccalaureate certificates.
**1929** The Great Depression begins with the crash of the stock market.
**1933** Basil O'Connor organizes first "Birthday Ball" to raise money for polio programs.
**1933** APA asks AMA to assist with accreditation.
**1934** APA hires first paid staff member.
**1935** Social Security Act passed as part of "New Deal" package of social legislation. APA adopts first "Code of Ethics and Discipline" and American Congress of Physical Medicine and creates the American Registry for the purpose of conferring "registered" title to physical therapists who pass test.
**1937** National Foundation of infantile paralysis established.
**1938** "March of Dimes" coin collection inaugurated, and NFIP began injecting funds for various local programs related to polio.
**1938** APA gets first permanent address when office is rented in Chicago.
**1940** Educational programs shifted from hospital to university setting.
**1940** Sister Kenny arrives from Australia and is invited to Minneapolis General Hospital. NFIP asks APA to send observer team, including Florence and Henry Kendall.
**1940** Catherine Worthingham becomes wartime president of APA.
**1941** McMillan taken prisoner by Japanese at Manila's Santa Tomás prison camp.
**1941** First special-interest "Sections" meet at Annual conference in Palo Alto, California. Schools Section survives to become permanent fixture. Coincident with Conference, first continuing education programs held at Stanford.
**1941** Emma Vogel sets up war emergency training course at WRGH.
**1942** Allied Council, consisting of 39 organizations interested in welfare of injured and disabled, organizes. APA takes leadership role.
**1942** Public Law 828 recognizes women PTs as wartime members of the Army Medical, Department with "relative" rank of 2nd Lieutenant.
**1942** Paul Campbell becomes first male physical therapist to be elected to APA national office.
**1942** NFIP begins funding APA scholarship fund.
**1943** Special Women's Medical Service Corps program for African-Americans set up at Fort Huachuca, Arizona.
**1944** House of Delegates created as legislative body within APA. APA moves into its first national office at 1790 Broadway, New York, with Mildred Elson its first salaried Executive Director. Barbara White becomes first staff Education Secretary with underwriting by NFIP.
**1944** Bolton Bill (PL 78-350) insures permanent commissioned status to women professionals serving in Army Medical Corps.
**1944** Catherine Worthingham leaves Stanford to become NFIP's Director of Professional Education.
**1946** Ida May Hazenhyer writes first formal history of the American Physical Therapy Association, which appears in four issues of the *Review.*
**1946** Council on Physical Medicine selects the term "physiatrist" to designate physicians within its specialty. APA seizes the opportunity to change its name to the American Physical Therapy Association.
**1946** Schools Section begins to meet regularly.
**1946** Hill-Burton Act passed in Congress sets off a burst of hospital construction and expansion.
**1946** Kabat-Knott collaboration begins, leading to development of their theory of proprioceptive neuromuscular facilitation (PNF).
**1947** Institute of Rehabilitation Medicine opens as an adjunct to NYU with Howard Rusk as senior director and George Deaver as medical director of physical therapy.
**1948** National Institute of Health expands to become a multidisciplinary research agency.
**1949** *Physical Therapy Review* goes from bimonthly to monthly publication.
**1949** Florence and Henry Kendall publish *Muscles, Testing and Function.*

**1949** Army Air Corps becomes separate Air Force with its own independent physical therapy program.
**1950** School of Allied Medical Professions (SAMP) becomes first full-fledged school of allied health in the U.S.
**1950** Korean War begins.
**1950** Lucy Blair joins APTA as senior consultant to the Department of Professional Services.
**1951** World Congress on Physical Therapy holds its first formal planning session in Copenhagen. Mildred Elson is elected organization's first president.
**1952** Janc Carlin becomes editor of *Physical Therapy Review.*
**1953** Allied Health Professional Training Act passed.
**1953** Section on Self-Employed (Private Practice) formed.
**1954** APTA develops seven-hour-long professional competency examination with help of Professional Examination Service and makes it available to state licensing boards.
**1955** PL 84–294 passes, giving men physical therapists equal status with women PTs in the military.
**1956** Knott and Voss collaborate on PNF text.
**1956** Salk Vaccine is introduced in massive vaccination program.
**1956** Public Health (Community Home Health) Section is formed.
**1956** Elson resigns and is succeeded by Mary Haskell.
**1957** The Physical Therapy Fund is established to further research.
**1958** The Bobaths first tour of the U.S.
**1958** National membership dues are raised to $25.
**1959** McMillan dies at 79.
**1959** "The Return" is produced and distributed.
**1959** Lucy Blair succeeds Anetta Cornell Wood as Executive Director.
**1960** Case Western Reserve University launches 2-year graduate program in physical therapy which will be phased out 11 years later.
**1961** Voss resigns as editor of the *Review* and Helen Hislop takes over. In observance of the Association's 40th anniversary, the *Review* publishes special issue including Gertrude Beard's engaging history entitled "Foundations For Growth."
**1962** *Review* changes name to the *Journal of Physical Therapy.*
**1962** National Foundation for Infantile Paralysis ends financial support of APTA and Catherine Worthingham leaves NFIP to commence an exhaustive "Study of Physical Therapy Education" with an Office of Vocational Rehabilitation grant.
**1963** McMillan Scholarship Fund is established.
**1963** Unionism issue surfaces, starting with New York Chapter.
**1964** Committee on Research formed.
**1964** First Mary McMillan Lecture delivered by Mildred Elson.
**1965** Section on Research organized.
**1965** Medicare legislation enacted.
**1966** First physical therapists go to Vietnam.
**1967** Foundations of PTA program laid.
**1967** First Lucy Blair Service Award winners named.
**1969** Blair resigns as Executive Director.
**1970** Temporary affiliate membership offered to physical therapy (later therapist) assistants and made permanent three years later.
**1970** Sections for State Licensure and Regulation (later Health Policy, Legislation, and Regulation) and for Administration formed.
**1970** Royce Noland becomes Executive Director of APTA. National office moves to Washington, D.C.
**1970** Signe Brunnström's techniques are described in *Movement Therapy in Hemiplegia.*
**1971** American Registry dissolved by AMA.
**1972** Joint Commission on Accreditation of Hospitals attempts to interpose physiatrists between PTs and primary care physicians.
**1973** Sports Physical Therapy Section formed.
**1973** NYU inaugurates first PhD program in physical therapy.
**1974** Pediatrics, Clinical Electrophysiology, and Orthopaedic Sections formed.
**1974** Howard University, Washington, D.C., establishes the first physical therapy department at a historically black college or university and graduates eight students.
**1975** Cardiopulmonary Section formed.
**1975** At the Annual Conference in Anaheim, CA, Helen Hislop delivers McMillan lecture entitled, "The Not So Impossible Dream."

**1976** First combined Sections Meeting held in Washington D.C.
**1976** American Registry disbanded.
**1976** House of Delegates revises "Essentials of an Acceptable School of Physical Therapy."
**1977** Council on Post-Secondary Accreditation (COPA) grants recognition to APTA as a second independent accrediting agency.
**1977** Obstetrics and Gynecology (later Women's Health) Section formed; Electrophysiology, Section formed.
**1978** Geriatrics Section formed.
**1978** "Plan to Foster Clinical Research" adopted. Mechanism on "Certification of Advanced Clinical Competency" established.
**1978** Marilyn Lister begins 10-year stint as Journal editor.
**1979** Foundation for Physical Therapy set up as successor to PT Fund.
**1980** Catherine Worthingham Fellows (FAPTA) established as a new category of membership, with Catherine Worthingham as its first recipient.
**1980** House of Delegates sets 1991 as target year for raising minimum entry level of education to postbaccalaureate degree. Bylaws amended to limit size of House to 400 delegates (revised upward in 1992 to 432).
**1980** Veterans Affairs Section established.
**1981** APTA establishes formal Archives for its own history.
**1981** First Foundation for Physical Therapy research grants awarded.
**1982** Hand Rehabilitation Physical Therapy Section established.
**1983** Oncology Section established.
**1983** APTA national office moves to new building in Alexandria, Virginia.
**1983** APTA becomes sole accrediting agency for physical therapy education programs.
**1985** First examinations for Specialist Certification held. Linda Crane, Scot Erwin, and Meryl Cohen receive Advanced Certification Cardiopulmonary Physical Therapy.
**1986** *P.T. Bulletin* is launched.
**1986** First Specialist Certification in Clinical Electrophysiology and Pediatrics are awarded.
**1987** First Specialist Certifications in Neurology and Sports Physical Therapy are awarded.
**1987** Prime Timers group is created.
**1987** William D. Coughlin named Chief Executive Officer of APTA.
**1988** Steven Rose takes over as *Journal* editor.
**1988** Setting of "Goals and Objectives" becomes part of APTA's annual self-review process.
**1988** APTA Office of Minority affairs created.
**1989** First Foundation undergraduate scholarships awarded.
**1988** TriAlliance of Health and Rehabilitation Professions established
**1989** First Specialist Certifications in Orthopedics awarded.
**1989** Upon Rose's death, Jules Rothstein succeeds to Journal editorship.
**1989** Bylaws are amended to establish Affiliate Assembly for PTAs.
**1990** Two major federal initiatives affect physical therapy profession: the Americans with Disabilities Act is passed and the National Center for Medical Rehabilitation Research is created.
**1991** Student Assembly formed.
**1992** First Specialist Certification in Geriatrics awarded.
**1992** APTA expands offices, purchasing second building in TransPotomac complex.
**1992** APTA administration reorganized into seven distinct operations.
**1992** Resource Center for Research and Learning established by House action.
**1993** *PT Magazine* launched, combining quarterly *Clinical Management* and monthly *Progress Report.*
**1993** First "Impact" Conference on Postbaccalaureate Entry-level curricula held. Creighton University, Omaha, Nebraska, inaugurates pioneer "professional" D.P.T. program.
**1993** First Foundation consensus conference held.
**1994** APTA creates Office of Women's Issues. Francis J. Mallon, Esq, succeeds Coughlan as Chief Executive Officer.
**1995** American Board of Physical Therapy Specialties inaugurates nationwide electronic testing.
**1995** World Confederation for Physical Therapy convenes in Washington, D.C.
**1995** APTA celebrates 75th anniversary of Association and profession.

APPENDIX II

# The Model Practice Act for Physical Therapy

**A Tool for Public Protection and Legislative Change**

Revised 1999 (Original Printing 1997)

Federation of State Boards of Physical Therapy
509 Wythe Street • Alexandria, VA 22314
Telephone: 800.200.3031 • 703.299.3100
Fax: 800.981.3031 • 703.299.3110
www.fsbpt.org

# Preface

This second edition of *The Model Practice Act for Physical Therapy: A Tool for Public Protection and Legislative Change* (MPA) follows 2 years after the original edition was published in 1997. Although only 2 years, this edition contains numerous and significant modifications and improvements to the original edition. The development of this second edition benefitted in part from the considerable experience of several states that used the original version of the MPA to make everything from minor to major revisions of existing practice acts.

Indeed, the MPA is a living document. This edition embodies the experience of physical therapist regulators and clinicians, public members of state boards, legislators, and legal counsel of state legislatures, professional associations and the Federation of State Boards of Physical Therapy. It continues to be a necessary, timely and useful document for the benefit of jurisdictions desiring to ensure that their statutes and rules are effectively meeting the goal of public protection. It is intended to provoke ongoing and lively discussion of the best means to protect the public and provide legal standards that will ensure a competent profession.

This edition contains editorial improvements throughout its model statute language to clarify and lend a user-friendly theme to professional regulatory language. It also contains numerous substantive changes and additions, especially regarding patient care management, supervision and use of assistive personnel.

Licensing boards and local APTA chapters are encouraged to work together in full cooperation to review and, when appropriate, change current statutes and rules in the light of this model language. The Federation is available through the Vice President of Professional Standards and its Legislative Committee to assist in the use of this tool. We will work closely at the jurisdictional level with all parties involved in effectuating statutory and regulatory change.

We welcome continuing feedback regarding this document. Although we believe that the MPA language provides solid guidance in the area of regulation, we realize that there may be additional valid considerations not included here. Further recommendations relative to any aspect of *The Model Practice Act for Physical Therapy: A Tool for Public Protection and Legislative Change* may be sent to Federation Headquarters for consideration in further analysis and later revision by the Legislative Committee.

# Acknowledgments

The Model Practice Act Task Force of the Federation of State Boards of Physical Therapy served from November 1994 until the completion of their task in March 1997. Acknowledgment and appreciation is also extended to Federation staff and many others who reviewed and contributed comments of early drafts and the field review.

Acknowledgment and appreciation is also extended to the many states, through the work of licensing boards and APTA chapters, that have already used this tool to effectively modernize state practice acts.

## Task Force Members/State

J. Kent Culley, Esq., *Federation Counsel*, Pennsylvania
Ann Giffin, PT, Tennessee
Anne H. Harrison, PT, Alabama
Ron J. Hruska, PT, Nebraska
Mark Lane, PT, Washington
Christine A. Larson, PT, *FSBPT Board*, Washington
Mary Hass Sheid, PT, OCS, Missouri
Deborah B. Tharp, PT, Kentucky
Blair J. Packard, PT, *Task Force Chair*, Arizona

# Introduction

The Federation of State Boards of Physical Therapy had its beginning in 1986. Shortly thereafter, discussion began about the feasibility of developing model language for an entire physical therapy practice act. Later, tools were developed that allowed for easier electronic gathering and analysis of all current state practice acts. The feasibility of successfully completing such a task then came within reach. In late 1994 the FSBPT Board appointed a nine-member task force and gave them their charge to develop a model practice act in a timely manner.

At the outset of the project, the task force envisioned a final document that could be used cafeteria style. If a particular state wanted to change a specific section of their practice act, it was thought that they could use the model act as a reference for their particular needs, selecting what was of worth to them at the time. Certainly, statute language in state practice acts is often amended this way. The Model Practice Act can indeed be used for such piecemeal amending of practice acts.

However, the longer the task force worked to complete their task, the more apparent something became. Nearly all practice acts contain quite functional and useful regulatory language as well as problematic regulatory language and concepts. Most practice acts had their origins in the 1950s and early 1960s. Over the years, several amendments have left some practice acts as cobbled together collections of regulatory models that are very diverse in their approach to the basic functions of protecting the public and regulating the profession. What evolved in *The Model Practice Act for Physical Therapy: A Tool for Public Protection and Legislative Change* is perhaps different from what was initially envisioned. While it can be used cafeteria style, this document is also a tightly constructed and integrated model for the regulation of physical therapy. The component parts of this model fit together and complement each other well. And certain parts of this model act are indispensable from other parts, with changes in one area requiring additional modification of a state's practice act in other areas.

This document has three sections. The first, *Key Areas,* contains model language for statutes only, not rules. It also contains extensive discussion and commentary, as well as additional legal considerations. The second section, *Guidelines for Rules,* contains guidance and suggestions for rule development. It will be each state's responsibility, as always, to develop the procedural aspects of state regulation, the administrative rules. The last section is *Appendices* and contains, first, the entire model statutes again, but without the commentary and in a format identical to how a state physical therapy law is structured. It also contains other valuable resources helpful in planning and making legislative changes.

As regulatory changes are made in state practice acts, efforts should be made to use the terms and statute clauses in this model act as they are recommended. The model language has been carefully researched, developed, professionally and legally reviewed, and adopted. Variances from the model language should be very carefully considered. This will help preserve the concept of a model act and avoid further confusion of terminology and weakening of regulatory systems. The Legislative Committee of the Federation welcomes your inquiries about any aspect of this document and remains a continuing resource for any jurisdiction considering or making practice act changes.

When making substantial changes to an existing practice act, it is advisable to assemble a panel of experts with extensive history of involvement in both regulatory and professional issues, and then carefully compare this model act with current regulatory language.

The Federation invites your examination and use of *The Model Practice Act for Physical Therapy: A Tool for Public Protection and Legislative Change* and pledges its resources for your ongoing support.

# Contents

## KEY AREAS

### Key Area #1 • Legislative Intent



### Key Area #2 • Definitions

## Key Area #2 • continued



## Key Area #3 • Board of Physical Therapy

### Key Area #4 • Licensure and Examination



### Key Area #5 • Lawful Practice



### Key Area #6 • Use of Titles



### Key Area #7 • Patient Care Management

### Key Area #7 • continued



### Key Area #8 • Grounds for Disciplinary Action

### Key Area #9 • Disciplinary Actions/Procedures



### Key Area #10 • Unlawful Practice



### Key Area #11 • Consumer Advocacy



## GUIDELINES FOR RULES

**APPENDICES**

# Key Areas

# Key Area #1
# Legislative Intent

## MODEL LANGUAGE

### Legislative Intent

This [chapter, act, section, law] is enacted for the purpose of protecting the public health, safety, and welfare, and of providing for state administrative control, supervision, licensure and regulation of the practice of physical therapy. It is the legislature's intent that only individuals who meet and maintain prescribed standards of competence and conduct may engage in the practice of physical therapy as authorized by this [chapter, etc.]. This [chapter, etc.] shall be liberally construed to promote the public interest and to accomplish the purpose stated herein.

***Bracketed areas in the model language throughout the Model Practice Act indicate optional language each state should adapt to its own needs.***

## DISCUSSION

### Legislative Intent

This statement of legislative intent focuses on the necessity of placing public interest foremost. There is an inherent benefit to society and individuals when public health, safety and welfare are protected through licensing. However, boards often narrowly interpret the concept of "protection," which has led to a perception that boards function only as "gatekeepers" and "hand-slappers." Licensing boards can and must function in more than a defensive mode and assume a more active role in effecting positive benefit for the public.

Licensure is also inherently restrictive and exclusive. Only those who "meet" and "maintain" standards established by the board will, for the protection and benefit of the public, be allowed to profess their qualifications and provide their services to the public—which has relied on the state to affirm the qualifications of physical therapists. The addition of "maintain" in the statute language introduces many possibilities, the least of which is an ongoing commitment to maintaining standards of practice—the concept of continuing competence. What is "prescribed" as minimum standards of competence at entry level may be expected to rise to a higher level of competence with experience.

The last sentence mandates that all interpretation of the practice act and associated rules refer back to this purpose statement when the intent and meaning are being considered. Many state practice acts contain a purpose clause or statement of legislative intent. Other states may not use purpose clauses as a matter of statutory precedent. However, after review of the model language, the benefit that such a purpose statement can have in giving focus and direction to the process of licensure and regulation should be apparent.

From the beginning to the end of a practice act, an important principle of statutory construction is that no paragraph of a practice act can be taken out of context of the entire practice act. The entire practice act, including accompanying rules, constitutes the law that governs the practice of physical therapy in a state.

## ADDITIONAL LEGAL CONSIDERATIONS

In the area of statutory construction, it is most often the intent of those drafting the statute to do so free of ambiguities. Even the most tightly drafted statute, however, is subject to the interpretation (and misinterpretation) of the reader, as well as the inherent risk of perceived ambiguities, whether or not any exist. When an ambiguity does arise, the courts and the legislatures may agree that it is the intent of the body creating the statute that dictates the interpretation of the statute. For this reason, a legislative history is sometimes maintained throughout the drafting process, recording the comments and deliberations of the task force creating the statute. This history, if maintained, is then available to assist in the interpretation and resolution of any ambiguities in the final product.

Another interpretive aid is the "purpose clause" set forth at the beginning of a statute. It serves as a concise summation of the intent of those creating the statute and of the legislature enacting the statute. The careful drafting and inclusion of this clause are particularly important in the creation of a model act, especially if a legislative history is unavailable. Additionally, model acts are sometimes adopted verbatim by a state's legislature and, in the absence of a legislative history, the purpose clause often serves as the sole declaration of the intent of the legislature in adopting the act. The purpose clause establishes the tone of the legislative intent behind the statute, also decreasing the risk of ambiguities for those reviewing the statute for the first time.

# Key Area #2
# Definitions

## MODEL LANGUAGE

### Definitions

A. "Board" means the [specify the state] board of physical therapy.

B. "Physical therapy" means the care and services provided by or under the direction and supervision of a physical therapist who is licensed pursuant to this [chapter, act, section, law].

C. "Physical therapist" means a person who is licensed pursuant to this [chapter, etc.] to practice physical therapy.

D. "Practice of physical therapy" means:

1. Examining, evaluating and testing individuals with mechanical, physiological and developmental impairments, functional limitations, and disability or other health and movement-related conditions in order to determine a diagnosis, prognosis, plan of therapeutic intervention, and to assess the ongoing effects of intervention.
2. Alleviating impairments and functional limitations by designing, implementing, and modifying therapeutic interventions that include, but are not limited to therapeutic exercise; functional training in self care and in home, community or work reintegration; manual therapy including soft tissue and joint mobilization and manipulation; therapeutic massage; assistive and adaptive orthotic, prosthetic, protective and supportive devices and equipment; airway clearance techniques; debridement and wound care; physical agents or modalities; mechanical and electrotherapeutic modalities; and patient-related instruction.
3. Reducing the risk of injury, impairment, functional limitation and disability, including the promotion and maintenance of fitness, health and quality of life in all age populations.

4. Engaging in administration, consultation, education and research.

E. Assistive Personnel

1. "Physical therapist assistant" means a person who meets the requirements of this act for certification and who assists the physical therapist in selected components of physical therapy intervention.
2. "Physical therapy aide" means a person trained under the direction of a physical therapist who performs designated and supervised routine tasks related to physical therapy.

F. "Restricted license" means a license on which the board places restrictions or conditions, or both, as to scope of practice, place of practice, supervision of practice, duration of licensed status, or type or condition of patient or client to whom the licensee may provide services.

G. "Restricted certificate" means a certificate on which the board has placed any restrictions due to action imposed by the board.

H. "On-site supervision" means the supervising physical therapist is continuously on-site and present in the department or facility where services are provided, is immediately available to the person being supervised and maintains continued involvement in appropriate aspects of each treatment session in which assistive personnel are involved in components of care.

I. "Testing" means standardized methods and techniques used to gather data about the patient, including electro-diagnostic and electrophysiologic tests and measures.

J. "Consultation by means of telecommunication" means that a physical therapist renders professional or expert opinion or advice to another physical therapist or health care provider via telecommunications or computer technology from a distant location. It includes the transfer of data or exchange of educational or related information by means of audio, video or data communications. The physical therapist may use telehealth technology as a vehicle for providing only services that are legally or professionally authorized. The patient's written or verbal consent will be obtained and documented prior to such consultation. All records used or resulting from a consultation by means of telecommunications are part of a patient's records and are subject to applicable confidentiality requirements.

K. "Jurisdiction of the United States" means any state, territory or the District of Columbia that licenses physical therapists.

[Optional Statute or Rule Language] if using only the term "manual therapy" and not using the additional descriptor of manual therapy, i.e., the phrase "including soft tissue and joint mobilization and manipulation" in the "practice of physical therapy" definition.

[L. "Manual therapy" means a broad group of skilled hand movements used by physical therapists to mobilize soft tissues and joints for the purpose of modulating pain, increasing range of motion, reducing or eliminating soft tissue inflammation, inducing relaxation, improving contractile and noncontractile tissue extensibility, or improving pulmonary function.]

## DISCUSSION

A practice act conveys the basis and extent of legal authority, permission, restrictions, penalties, etc., of a given health care practitioner. The intent is to provide sufficient regulation to protect the public. The clearer and more precise a law is, the more consistent (and less variable) will be the understanding of the law by those practitioners who are regulated, and the interpretation and administration of the law by those appointed to be the regulators—the licensing boards. Such a law will also require less additional legislative modification and less legal interpretation or clarification by state attorney general offices or by the courts.

The writers of practice acts endeavor to achieve their clarity of intent by including definitions of the terms and phrases used within the act. Some of these are operational definitions that have more significance in one specific state's practice act because of the choice of language used in that law. However, other terms have overall significance in all practice acts, giving meaning to whom and what is being regulated. These are the terms recommended for inclusion in the *Definitions* section of the law. The terms defined in this section include *Board, Physical Therapy, Physical Therapist, Practice of Physical Therapy, Physical Therapist Assistant, Physical Therapy Aide, Restricted License, Restricted Certificate, On-Site Supervision, Testing, Consultation by Means of Telecommunications, Jurisdiction of the United States,* and an optional definition for *Manual Therapy.*

### Definitions

**A. "Board" means the [specify the state] board of physical therapy.**
Including this model language of "Board" in the definitions area of the model language indicates the preference for an autonomous licensing board for physical therapy. Most states have such boards. For various reasons other states have physical therapy boards as part of state medical boards or may have combined boards with other disciplines. For example, some are combined with occupational therapy, athletic trainers or others. There are also a few "super boards" where all regulatory activities are subordinate to one board, with various committees, commission or subcommittee structures for the various disciplines. There is no evidence of greater effective-

ness, efficiency or better public protection from multidisciplinary boards. (See additional discussion and rationale for an autonomous board in key area *Board of Physical Therapy.)*

**B. "Physical therapy" means the care and services provided by or under the direction and supervision of a physical therapist who is licensed pursuant to this [chapter, act, section, law].**

A weakness of several practice acts is their vulnerability to the false notion that physical therapy is a generic term. The combined language of the three definitions: "physical therapy," "physical therapist" and the "practice of physical therapy" is crucial to curtail this false idea and strengthen physical therapy practice acts in this country. Therefore, it is important that when changes in practice acts are made in this area, these definitions should be examined and changed in concert with each other. It is equally important that the exclusive use of titles and terms is included whenever such changes in definitions are made. (See *Lawful Practice, Licensure and Examination, Use of Titles*, and *Unlawful Practice* key areas.)

The very foundation of practice acts centers on the concept that the public recognizes the specific training and qualifications of a given health care profession and enacts laws governing its practice, including restrictions on how licensees represent themselves to the public. One of these restrictions is that each discipline practices within its scope of practice and uses titles and/or letters and representations that do not mislead the public. For example, a medical or osteopathic physician practices and represents to the public that he or she practices medicine, but not dentistry. A dentist practices and represents his or her practice as dentistry but not podiatry, a nurse—nursing, a podiatrist—podiatry, a chiropractor—chiropractic, a physical therapist—physical therapy, and so on. So when practitioners other than physical therapists represent that they are providing "physical therapy" or "physiotherapy" they are violating, if not always the letter of the law, at least the very spirit and core of licensure laws by misrepresentation to the public.

One reason for the vulnerability of many physical therapy practice acts and the perpetuation of the false concept that physical therapy is a generic term is our previous reliance on a definition of "physical therapy" based on physical agents and modalities. However, these same physical agents or modalities have not been the exclusive domain of physical therapy, which has resulted in conflict at times.

There is a better solution, however, than fighting turf battles. The primary solution is to define very clearly that "physical therapy is the care and services provided by (and only by) or under the direction and supervision of a physical therapist." This is also strengthened by a modernized definition of "Practice of Physical Therapy" reflective of current scope of practice, plus language in the *Use of Titles* key area restricting the use of appropriate terms to protect the public from misrepresentation.

This model language also explicitly allows that, while it is necessary for a physical therapist to always be part of the services defined and represented as physical therapy, appropriate use of assistive personnel in the delivery of physical therapy is authorized.

**C. "Physical therapist" means a person who is licensed pursuant to this [chapter, etc.] to practice physical therapy.**

This language, with minor variation, is consistent with language already used in many practice acts. This particular language reinforces the tie to licensure as a necessary prerequisite for the professional designation as a physical therapist. The requirements for licensure, as well as the regulation of practice, are appropriately determined by state law and may vary from state to state.

Several states use the definition of "physical therapist" to introduce other concepts that are better dealt with in other areas of a practice act. These include the topic of supervision, which the Model Practice Act addresses first in the definition of physical therapy, then more fully in the *Patient Care Management* key area. Also, issues of equivalency of terms (such as physiotherapy and physiotherapist), education (degree from an accredited program), the exclusive use of terms (PT, RPT), and restrictions of practice (no X-rays, surgery, etc.) are sometimes addressed in this definition. These aspects are more appropriately addressed in other areas of the Model Practice Act. (See suggested use of the definition for physiotherapy and physiotherapist under *Guidelines for Rules Key Area #2.*)

**D. "Practice of physical therapy" means:**

1. **Examining, evaluating and testing individuals with mechanical, physiological and developmental impairments, functional limitations, and disability or other health and movement-related conditions in order to determine a diagnosis, prognosis, plan of therapeutic intervention, and to assess the ongoing effects of intervention.**
2. **Alleviating impairments and functional limitations by designing, implementing, and modifying therapeutic interventions that include, but are not limited to therapeutic exercise; functional training in self care and in home, community or work reintegration; manual therapy including soft tissue and joint mobilization and manipulation; therapeutic massage; assistive and adaptive orthotic, prosthetic, protective and supportive devices and equipment; airway clearance techniques; debridement and wound care; physical agents or modalities; mechanical and electrotherapeutic modalities; and patient-related instruction.**

3. **Reducing the risk of injury, impairment, functional limitation and disability, including the promotion and maintenance of fitness, health and quality of life in all age populations.**
4. **Engaging in administration, consultation, education and research.**

Why should this language be placed in a definition titled "Practice of Physical Therapy," as opposed to a definition of "Physical Therapy?" One reason, previously stated, is to give isolated focus and added strength to the concept that physical therapy is that which is practiced solely by licensed physical therapists. However, another reason that is more important is that this represents the "statutory definition of the scope of practice of physical therapy."

The component elements of the "scope of practice" of any discipline include three determinants: 1) established history of inclusion in educational training, 2) established history of inclusion in clinical practice, and 3) specific statutory authority. When the first two are well established, specific statutory authority may also be appropriately substituted by "lack of statutory prohibition." For example, where a practice act is silent on the issue of needle insertion EMG, the fact that there is a long history of educational inclusion and an established history of clinical practice in physical therapy substantiates this procedure as within the scope of practice of physical therapy. Legal opinions in the form of affirmative court decisions will also play a role in defining scope of practice and apparently have in this specific example.

However, if there is any fear that the model definition for the "Practice of Physical Therapy" is not specific enough in regard to certain clinical procedures such as NCV and needle insertion EMG, wound management, iontophoresis or any other clinical procedure, then the model practice act offers additional definition language under paragraph (I) that follows for electrodiagnostic procedures, and also under the *Lawful Practice* key area where optional language for wound management and use of medications is suggested.

To further illustrate why a "Practice of Physical Therapy" definition will be helpful, equate scope of practice to a three-legged stool. The three legs providing the stability are 1) history of education, 2) history of clinical practice, and 3) statutory authority. Generally, progressive change in statutory authority and construction, perhaps in all the regulated professions, often lags behind change in education and practice. Since we sit, or perhaps stand, on only three legs, they all need to be strong. In some states statutory construction may be a weak leg and a significant reason to consider revisions and updates to physical therapy practice acts. The inclusion of a "Practice of Physical Therapy" clause provides a statutory definition of the scope of practice of physical therapy—the "third leg" of establishing scope of practice.

The model language above is an abbreviated version of the current "model definition" of the APTA's Board of Directors, last modified by the Board in March 1997. (See *Appendix B* for full APTA *Board's Model Definition of "Physical Therapy."*) The abbreviation presented here as model language still captures the essence of the APTA Board's language but does not try to be as all-inclusive—something probably not feasible in a statute, nor always desirable. It certainly gives a much clearer description of current practice than most definitions of physical therapy now in practice acts. Physical therapists do in fact: 1) examine and evaluate to come to conclusions (a diagnosis) regarding a patient's condition for which they will provide services, 2) plan and implement treatment intervention, 3) consider long-term implications and provide preventive care to reduce risks of injury and impairment, and 4) consult with peers from the same and other health disciplines as well as engage in education and research. This forms a well-organized and structured outline for the scope of modern physical therapy practice.

A few additional points regarding this model definition will be important to highlight:

- The language used of "patients with mechanical, physiological and developmental impairments, functional limitations and disability or other health and movement-related conditions" is sufficiently broad to allow for inclusion of any type of patient condition that physical therapists encounter.
- Physical therapists must examine and evaluate each patient prior to determining and initiating treatment interventions.
- Determining "a diagnosis" rather than "diagnosis" or "the diagnosis" is a subtle but very important point. Direct patient access to physical therapy services is now a reality in the majority of states. By education, and now by practical and legal necessity, physical therapists, prior to making patient management decisions, must come to a conclusion (a diagnosis) regarding the patient's specific condition for which they will be providing treatment intervention. Previously established diagnoses from other health practitioners are helpful and should always be considered but cannot provide the sole basis for decisions regarding physical therapy management. A diagnosis from another referral source, even the definitive diagnosis, does not rule out a physical therapist's responsibility to arrive at a diagnosis specific to the condition for which the therapist's treatment plan and intervention will be directed. Another way of appropriately stating this would be "a diagnosis for physical therapy." By contrast, an inappropriate expression, and one strongly advised against ever using, is "a physical therapy diagnosis." Although diagnostic labels, tests or tools

may vary from provider to provider, the process of diagnosis is consistent and should not be compartmentalized by provider.

- The evaluative and diagnostic process should also include a prognosis or an expectation of outcome associated with treatment intervention. This may also have certain time parameters and/or goal expectations associated with it. And, of course, the end result of the evaluative process is the design of the therapeutic intervention itself. The effects of the therapeutic intervention are regularly assessed in order to make further modifications in the intervention.
- It is not necessary or advisable to list the evaluative processes or tests and measures used by physical therapists within the definition of the "Practice of Physical Therapy." This model language is sufficiently broad as to be enabling and not restrictive. When this is combined with a licensing board comprising professional peers in physical therapy and knowledgeable public members, there should be no unreasonable restrictions on established or developing evaluative procedures or tests.
- In paragraph (2) of this definition, it is more appropriate to list some of the typical therapeutic interventions used in physical therapy. This helps exemplify the breadth and scope of practice. It will be noted, however, that it is not recommended to have a stand-alone list of physical agents or modalities as is contained in many practice acts today.
- A potential topic of political conflict arises when using the term "manipulation." An alternative in paragraph (D. 2) is to use only the term "manual therapy" or "manual therapy techniques," and further define this term. See further discussion with the optional definition language under paragraph (L).

**E. Assistive Personnel**

"Assistive Personnel" serves only as the *categorical heading* of two more specifically defined persons who may assist the physical therapist either in selected components of intervention or some other aspect of the overall care of a patient. They include "physical therapist assistants" and "physical therapy aides."

The term "assistive personnel" is preferable to "support" or "supportive personnel" because of their involvement in patient care. Support personnel, by contrast, are not involved directly in patient care, and the term would more appropriately apply to management, clerical or maintenance workers. There is no need to regulate "support" personnel or activities that are not directly involved with patient care.

Practice acts should not use the *Definitions* section of the statute to elaborate on the specifics of what assistive personnel may or may not do. For example, a state might chooses to restrict physical therapists from using physical therapy aides to directly provide any physical therapy intervention, or components of intervention. Any such supervision requirements or restrictions should be reserved for the *Patient Care Management* section and rules.

1. **"Physical therapist assistant" means a person who meets the requirements of this act for certification and who assists the physical therapist in selected components of physical therapy intervention.**

A few state practice acts continue to use the incorrect designation of physical therapy assistant. Careful attention should be used to include proper terminology. Language that equates physical therapy assistant with physical therapist assistant in order to prohibit and protect against inappropriate usage of this term is best handled in the *Use of Titles* key area.

Debate should be avoided on whether to title the physical therapist assistant a paraprofessional, a worker, an educated or a technical level provider, or other titles used in a few practice acts. Simply "a person" is preferable.

The requirement that a physical therapist assistant "has met the conditions of this act" refers to application requirements addressed in the *Licensure and Examination* key area for certification of physical therapist assistants. Educational requirements, such as being a graduate of an accredited physical therapist assistant education program, are best addressed in other areas of the practice act, not in definitions.

The role of the physical therapist assistant is to assist the physical therapist in selected components of physical therapy intervention. Although measurement and data collection activities may be part of the responsibilities of the physical therapist assistant, their role is in assisting the physical therapist with treatment interventions rather than evaluative, therapeutic intervention design and modification, or consultative activities. Other role delineation or restrictions a board may wish to include should be specified in rules.

The Model Practice Act contains further recommendations regarding supervision for physical therapist assistants and physical therapy aides under *Guidelines for Rules.* The Model Practice Act recommends uniform *certification* rather than licensure for physical therapist assistants. (See further discussion on certification in the *Licensure and Examination* key area and in *Appendix C.*)

2. **"Physical therapy aide" means a person trained under the direction of a physical therapist who performs designated and supervised routine tasks related to physical therapy.**

This definition of a physical therapy aide is similar to the definition contained in the APTA's *Guide to Physical Therapist Practice.*

A physical therapy aide is neither licensed nor certified. Others who may be licensed in another discipline and who are employees in a physical therapy service working under the supervision of a physical therapist would not fit in this category but would be included in "other assistive personnel."

Physical therapy aides are generally trained on the job. This does not preclude vocational or technical training that may exist for physical therapy aides or "techs." However, such training does not relieve the supervising physical therapist of responsibility for further on-the-job training. What this training is, and the documentation of the training, should be specifically addressed in rules.

Massage therapists, exercise physiologists, athletic trainers or other persons who may have technical or professional education or training, and who are used within a physical therapy service as assistive personnel, shall be considered and represented as physical therapy aides. The only exception to this should be if such persons are providing consultative services and their particular service is not represented or billed as physical therapy, but as the service of another specific discipline.

**F. "Restricted license" means a license on which the board places restrictions or conditions, or both, as to scope of practice, place of practice, supervision of practice, duration of licensed status, or type or condition of patient or client to whom the licensee may provide services.**

**G. "Restricted certificate" means a certificate on which the board has placed any restrictions due to action imposed by the board.**

Boards need full authority to impose restrictions on a licensee's practice or a certificate holder's employment primarily as a part of the disciplinary process. This could also be used as part of relicensure where continuing competence is in question and temporary restrictions are imposed while remedial measures are required of the licensee. These statutory definitions of the terms "restricted license" and "restricted certificate" are sufficiently broad to grant the board power to impose restrictions on a licensee or certificate holder in all situations necessary. This will be further addressed under the *Discipline: Actions/Procedures* key area and should also be addressed in rules under continuing competence as it relates to relicensure, if and when such requirements are implemented.

**H. "On-site supervision" means the supervising physical therapist is continuously on-site and present in the department or facility where services are provided, is immediately available to the person being supervised and maintains continued involvement in appropriate aspects of each treatment session in which assistive personnel are involved in components of care.**

"On-site supervision" is also an important inclusion in the definitions section. Although the term "assistive personnel" refers to physical therapist assistants and physical therapy aides, the *Patient Care Management* key area will specify that on-site supervision generally applies only to physical therapy aides.

On-site supervision could also apply to foreign-educated physical therapists under interim permits. It could also include those under a restricted license or certificate, if so specified under the conditions imposed by the restricted license or certificate.

This is an area in practice acts where there often exist multiple definitions of "supervision." Some are very specific acts where, for example, further defining "on-site" as meaning direct visual contact, or defining "immediately available" within a time parameter of so many seconds or minutes. Such definitions are overly restrictive. The supervising physical therapist remains professionally and legally responsible for care rendered under their license.

The language gives guidance that the recommended supervision should be within a close proximity—the department or facility—*and* immediately available. It also gives latitude that a building could mean the other side of a hospital. But in this instance, if injury to a patient occurred and the supervising physical therapist was on the other side of the hospital and not "immediately available," would a jury of peers on a licensing board find that this was "professionally responsible" conduct? "Immediately available" is a term of art and is frequently used in health care statutes, including Medicare. It denotes a sense of urgency in delivery of care, not a sense, necessarily, of standing next to assistive personnel at all times.

The last of this statute clause highlights an important concept needing greater attention. This also represents a subtle shift from generally used statute language using the phrase "delegation of selected tasks and procedures." That phrase will not appear in this or other statute clauses in the Model Practice Act. Instead the phrase or concept of "assisting in components of physical therapy intervention" will be emphasized for the physical therapist assistant and "assisting in components of care" for physical therapy aides. Physical therapists should be maintaining closer contact with each patient on each treatment date than is now occurring in some practice settings. Generally, it is not appropriate to delegate the entire physical therapy intervention to assistive personnel. Physical therapists should remain actively involved on a daily basis with their patient's care. Therefore, "components" infers that assistive personnel might be appropriately involved in certain aspects of care, but not all.

Within patient management, direction and supervision are functions that belong solely to the licensed physical therapist. The physical therapist directs and supervises all patient care activities of any assistive personnel. When certain tasks or procedures are performed by a physical therapist assistant, the assistant may need the help of a physical therapy aide. Nevertheless, the physical therapist assistant does not assume the responsibility to "direct and supervise" the provision of care. That responsibility remains with the supervising physical therapist and, by law, cannot be relinquished to another.

There are many situations where physical therapists in extended care, home health or school settings train others to carry out certain exercises or activities for the benefit of patients or clients. Such training in exercise or activities is appropriate as an extension of the educational and consultative responsibilities a physical therapist has, as set forth in the definition of the "Practice of Physical Therapy." (See *Definitions* key area.) But unless a physical therapist is on-site and directing and supervising such activities as an integral part of a physical therapy plan of care and intervention, this is no different than giving instruction to a family member who assists the patient with their home exercise program. Activities carried out under such circumstances and without proper on-site supervision from a physical therapist should not be represented or billed as physical therapy services.

I. **"Testing" means standardized methods and techniques used to gather data about the patient, including electrodiagnostic and electrophysiologic tests and measures.**

The definition of "Practice of Physical Therapy" in paragraph (D.1) includes a reference to "testing." The statutory definition is purposely and necessarily broad and does not specify any particular tests. (See previous *Discussion* under paragraph (D) and following under *Additional Legal Considerations* in this section.) This statutory paragraph, however, does two things: it incorporates the profession's standard definition of "tests and measures" as found in the *Guide to Physical Therapist Practice* which acts to further clarify the meaning of "tests" or "testing," and it also includes a reference to particular diagnostic testing procedures that are within the scope of physical therapy practice but have often been challenged legally or legislatively.

Some states already have, and others may wish to include, rules specifying additional training and certification procedures. This language also reflects direct access and decision-making relating to electrodiagnostic and electrophysiologic procedures.

J. **"Consultation by means of telecommunication" means that a physical therapist renders professional or expert opinion or advice to another physical therapist or health care provider via telecommunications or computer technology from a distant location. It includes the transfer of data or exchange of educational or related information by means of audio, video or data communications. The physical therapist may use telehealth technology as a vehicle for providing only services that are legally or professionally authorized. The patient's written or verbal consent will be obtained and documented prior to such consultation. All records used or resulting from a consultation by means of telecom-**

**munications are part of a patient's records and are subject to applicable confidentiality requirements.**

This definition is tied to a specific exemption (see *Licensure and Examination, Exemptions from Licensure* key area) that relates to the emergence of telehealth as a means of delivering professional services. This allows only for consultation, not treatment intervention, by means of telecommunication. The nature of physical therapy practice requires the *evaluative components* of practice (i.e. examination, evaluation, reevaluation and testing in order to determine a diagnosis, prognosis and plan of care) to occur with a physical therapist in the physical presence of the patient. Further restrictions on consultations are not necessary to protect the patient so long as the physical therapist in the state where the patient is being provided evaluation or intervention retains ultimate responsibility for the care of the patient.

Most states already have provisions for off-site supervision of physical therapist assistants. How components of intervention are rendered by physical therapist assistants under off-site supervision, or even rendered directly to a patient by a physical therapist through some means of telecommunication, may be areas of statute or rules needing further clarification.

**K. "Jurisdiction of the United States" means any state, territory or District of Columbia that licenses physical therapists.**

This necessary clarifying definition specifies the range of possible licensing jurisdictions within the United States.

**[Optional Statute or Rule Language] if using only the term "manual therapy" and not using the additional descriptor of manual therapy, i.e. the phrase "including soft tissue and joint mobilization and manipulation" in the "practice of physical therapy" definition.**

**[L. "Manual therapy" means a broad group of skilled hand movements used by physical therapists to mobilize soft tissues and joints for the purpose of modulating pain, increasing range of motion, reducing or eliminating soft tissue inflammation, inducing relaxation, improving contractile and noncontractile tissue extensibility, or improving pulmonary function.]**

Paragraph (D) is the preferred and recommended model language defining the practice of physical therapy. However, because of political sensitivities over the term "manipulation" it may occasionally be necessary to find an acceptable alternate that still authorizes, *and in no way inhibits*, the use of manipulative therapy procedures by physical therapists. If another approach is required, an acceptable alternative is to retain in the definition of Practice of Physical Therapy (paragraph D. 2.) the term "manual therapy" or "manual therapy techniques" (without using the term "manipulation") and then further define "manual therapy" by inclusion of the above optional clause within the statute definitions. This definition comes from the glossary of terms in APTA's *Guide to Physical Therapist Practice*, minus any reference to "manipulation" or "joint mobilization."

Another important point that supports either the primary or the alternate approach to this definition is that in 1998 the American Medical Association approved specific CPT coding for use by M.D. physicians and physical therapists for "manual therapy techniques." This code also contains the terms "mobilization" and "manipulation" as part of the CPT code description.

## ADDITIONAL LEGAL CONSIDERATIONS

The inclusion of a definition section in a model practice act is a necessary standard for statutory construction. From a legal point of view, definitions are very important in establishing the basis and direction of the professional practice in question. In statutory drafting, internal consistency in the use of terms is critical and the definition section serves as an anchor for this well-recognized maxim. Moreover, definitions serve as an important guide to courts when a statute is being scrutinized and interpreted. Courts are not particularly interested in labels per se. Courts look, rather, at what someone specifically does in his or her practice and at the scope of education and training. For this reason, clear, concise definitions serve the purpose of giving the courts a road map in weaving through a statutory or regulatory maze.

Definitions, however, should not be so limiting or strict that they fail to allow for change and interpretation that transcends the actual time the definition is established. Physical therapy is a dynamic profession in which education and practice evolve. Thirty-five years ago, the concept of direct access was virtually unknown; now a majority of states have a form of or protocol for direct access. Care should be given to this point, also, when drafting definitions that will effect a change in any statutory scheme. It is not always easy to run to the legislature and revise a practice act. Therefore, careful attention must be given to the content of the definitions, as they may—and probably will—be in use for a lengthy period of time following a revision to the statute.

Attention to the manner in which definitions are drafted is also important to ensure that there exists the requisite basis for the regulators to interpret the definitions in a manner that best benefits and meets the needs of the public and an ever changing profession. However, being overly specific can also create certain problems. A simple example of this might be the use of testing or the word "test." If a definition section attempted to list all the existing tests utilized by physical therapists, tests devised at a later time may well be excluded because they were not originally included. Under general statutory construction rules, such an interpretation is possible. In describing that part of practice that includes testing, the word "tests" provides the basis for the authority of the physical therapists to provide testing. The rules, based on education and experience in actual practice, should be the vehicle to describe more fully the type of testing, the scope and perhaps the limits of tests. As testing methods change and new tests are added, the rules can address these issues because the statutory basis always existed by simply stating the authority to test in the definition.

Past definitions relating to physical therapy practice have often relied too heavily on the utilization of physical modalities. In reality, the most important functions of the physical therapist's practice should focus on the evaluative, diagnostic, plan of intervention and clinical skills of the licensed physical therapist. The proposed definitions section sets forth a description of practice that is far removed from the simple application of modalities.

# Key Area #3
# Board of Physical Therapy

## MODEL LANGUAGE

### Board of Physical Therapy

A. The board of physical therapy shall consist of five members appointed by the governor. Three members shall be physical therapists who are residents of this state, possess unrestricted licenses to practice physical therapy in this state and have been practicing in this state for no less than 5 years before their appointments. The governor shall also appoint two public members who shall be residents of this state and who are not affiliated with, nor have a financial interest in, any health care profession and who have an interest in consumer rights.
B. Board members serve staggered 4-year terms. Board members shall serve no more than two successive 4-year terms nor for more than 10 consecutive years. By approval of the majority of the board, the service of a member may be extended at the completion of a 4-year term until a new member is appointed or the current member is reappointed.
C. If requested by the board the governor may remove any member of the board for misconduct, incompetence or neglect of duty.
D. Board members are eligible for reimbursement of expenses pursuant to [cite applicable statute relating to reimbursement] to cover necessary expenses for attending each board meeting or for representing the board in an official board-approved activity.
E. A board member who acts within the scope of board duties, without malice and in the reasonable belief that the member's action is warranted by law is immune from civil liability.

## Powers and Duties of the Board

The board shall:

1. Evaluate the qualifications of applicants for licensure and certification.
2. Provide for the national examinations for physical therapists and physical therapist assistants and adopt passing scores for these examinations.
3. Issue licenses, permits, or certificates to persons who meet the requirements of this [chapter, act, section, law].
4. Regulate the practice of physical therapy by interpreting and enforcing this [chapter, etc.].
5. Adopt and revise rules consistent with this [chapter, etc.]. Such rules, when lawfully adopted, shall have the effect of law.
6. Meet at least once each quarter in compliance with the open meeting requirements of [cite applicable statute].

   A majority of board members shall constitute a quorum for the transaction of business. The board shall keep an official record of its meetings.
7. Establish mechanisms for assessing continuing competence of licensees.
8. Establish and collect fees for sustaining the necessary operation and expenses of the board.
9. Elect officers from its members necessary for the operations and obligations of the board. Terms of office shall be 1 year.
10. Provide for the timely orientation and training of new professional and public appointees to the board regarding board licensing and disciplinary procedures, this [chapter, etc.] and board rules, policies and procedures.
11. Maintain a current list of all persons regulated under this chapter, including the person's name, current business and residential address, telephone numbers and license or certificate number.
12. Provide information to the public regarding the complaint process.
13. Employ necessary personnel to carry out the administrative work of the board. Board personnel are eligible to receive compensation pursuant to [cite specific statute].
14. Enter into contracts for services necessary for adequate enforcement of this chapter.
15. Report final disciplinary action taken against a licensee or certificate holder to a national disciplinary database recognized by the board or as required by law.
16. Publish, at least annually, final disciplinary action taken against a licensee or certificate holder.

17. Publish, at least annually, board rulings, opinions, and interpretations of statutes or rules in order to guide persons regulated pursuant to this [chapter, etc.].
18. Participate in or conduct performance audits of the board.

### Disposition of Funds

[No model language is offered under this section heading. See *Discussion* for further information.]

## DISCUSSION

The language in this section is constructed to create an autonomous licensing board. Combined boards may have inherent conflicting and competing interests where overlapping scope of practice issues influence decisions. This could detract from the work of public protection, whereas an autonomous board may have a less-distracted and more-enhanced focus on public protection.

This section title could also be modified, if necessary, to apply to other models of board structure. For example, if a state board is actually a panel within a larger *Board of Healing Arts,* the title might be *The Physical Therapy Panel of the State Board of Healing Arts.*

### Board of Physical Therapy

**A. The board of physical therapy shall consist of five members appointed by the governor. Three members shall be physical therapists who are residents of this state, possess unrestricted licenses to practice physical therapy in this state and have been practicing in this state for no less than 5 years before their appointments. The governor shall also appoint two public members who shall be residents of this state and who are not affiliated with, nor have a financial interest in, any health care profession and who have an interest in consumer rights.**

Most states have licensing boards appointed by an elected official, usually the governor. This process, although often political in nature, assures a public focus to licensing boards. Public members are commonly members of the board, but often there may be only one public member. Some boards currently have fewer than five total members, and larger states have greater numbers serving on their boards. The recommendation in the Model Practice Act of not having less than five members is based on the assumption and recommendation of a minimum of two public members. With that minimum, there should also be at least three professional members.

The recommended language supports several views. First, greater public participation is recommended. The following ratios of professional to public members are the recommended ratios for various board sizes.

| BOARD SIZE | PROFESSIONAL | PUBLIC MEMBERS |
|---|---|---|
| 5 | 3 | 2 |
| 6 | 4 | 2 |
| 7 | 5 | 2 |
| 8 | 5 | 3 |
| 9 | 6 | 3 |
| 10 | 7 | 3 |

It is recommended that a majority of the board members be physical therapists. The concept of peer review, with public involvement as well, is valid. Professional peers who are respected by others in the state should be sought to fill these positions. Generally, physical therapists are in a more knowledgeable position to render judgment upon the actions of other physical therapists and physical therapist assistants. Public members heighten the sensitivity of the board to public concerns. A board made up of a majority of professionals with a well represented component of public members will be better able to deal with the many complex and technical issues related to educational preparation and practice procedures.

Better training needs to be incorporated into public and professional member orientation. It often takes an extended period of time for public members to become knowledgeable and comfortable in their decision making, rather than deferring to other professional members on the board. (See further discussion under paragraph 10 of *Powers and Duties of the Board.)*

Physical therapist members of the board must reside in the state, have practiced for a period of 5 years preceding their appointments, and have no restrictions on their licenses. There are no other restrictions, and the Model Practice Act has no reference to a nomination process or guarantee of a position on the board from a professional association. This does not preclude a professional association or any other organization from making such a nomination. But ties to such a process in the statute are an inappropriate link between a public board and a private professional association, a practice based more on tradition than need. There is an inherent understanding that professional appointees should have the respect of their peers since they will sit in seats of judgement. Public appointees likewise should be competent to serve and effectively advocate for the public.

If licensing boards are to be seen as more responsive to public concerns, the public members should not be members of any other health care discipline or be close enough to one that they may have a financial or professional interest in the decisions made. This model language precludes, in addition to those actually working as health care providers, spouses or immediate family members and those employed by any health care provider or organization, for example, a lobbyist for a health care professional association. The intent is to obtain representation in public members who can be uncompromised in their interests and advocacy on behalf of the public.

A state may also want to consider in rules a process of appointment that includes recommending that those making nominations consider geographical, practice setting and gender distribution in the nomination process. Considering geographical distribution helps ensure the board's knowledge of individuals and practice circumstances throughout a state; practice setting variety ensures an equitable distribution of practice types or settings, as well as avoiding multiple appointments from the same practice setting or company; and gender distribution helps avoid situations where sensitive issues of sexual misconduct or accusations of abuse could be heard by a board made up of the same or opposite sex to the complainant or the accused. (See *Guidelines for Rules, Key Area #3.*)

**B. Board members serve staggered 4-year terms. Board members shall serve no more than two successive 4-year terms nor for more than ten consecutive years. By approval of the majority of the board, the service of a member may be extended at the completion of a 4-year term until a new member is appointed or the current member is reappointed.**

There is considerable inconsistency from state to state on the length and limitation of terms. A 4-year term provides sufficient time to become thoroughly familiar with board functions and processes. Serving consecutive 4-year terms for a total of 8 years may not be as imposing an obstacle if considering consecutive terms than when a single term is 5 or more years in length. Limiting service to two full terms or a maximum of no more than ten consecutive years also avoids the issue of "ownership" of a board position and fosters periodic turnover. The ten consecutive year provision addresses the circumstances in which someone is appointed to fill a partial term and, in addition, fills two consecutive terms. States certainly have the prerogative to select a different number of years than proposed in this model.

**C. If requested by the board the governor may remove any member of the board for misconduct, incompetence or neglect of duty.**

Many statutes specify that a member can be removed for cause and list several causes, but they may not list a mechanism. The governor appoints those who serve on licensing boards. Therefore, the governor should also be the one with power to remove any members, within certain restrictions.

The causes for removal, the process for board consideration and action, and the recommendation to the governor for removal should all be specified in rules.

**D. Board members are eligible for reimbursement of expenses pursuant to [cite applicable statute relating to reimbursement] to cover necessary expenses for attending each board meeting or for representing the board in an official board-approved activity.**

Most states provide per diem and reimbursement for members, but the method varies. Reimbursement procedures should be specified by reference to applicable statutes or in rules.

**E. A board member who acts within the scope of board duties, without malice and in the reasonable belief that the member's action is warranted by law is immune from civil liability.**

Immunity from liability or suit while serving on a licensing board is standard. However, this statute paragraph points out that even this protection has its limits if a board member's conduct is determined to be unwarranted or with malice.

### Powers and Duties of the Board

**The board shall:**

In the subsequent paragraphs the various powers and duties of the board are delineated.

**1. Evaluate the qualifications of applicants for licensure and certification.**

Establishing application requirements and review of credentials and other application material is often the first interaction a board has with a prospective licensee. This is the first duty and power listed.

**2. Provide for the national examinations for physical therapists and physical therapist assistants and adopt passing scores for these examinations.**

This language construction authorizes testing of both physical therapists and physical therapist assistants by their respective standardized national examinations. The name of the examinations can be specified in rules. Although national examinations may contain a determined passing score the board should retain in statute the authority to set passing scores for the physical therapist and physical therapist assistant examinations. The passing scores for the examinations and the mechanism of scoring, e.g. criterion-referenced scoring, may be specified in rules.

**3. Issue licenses, permits, or certificates to persons who meet the requirements of this [chapter, act, section, law].**

Boards are authorized, by this paragraph, to issue the appropriate license, interim permit or certificate after all requirements have been met as stated in the statutes and rules.

4. **Regulate the practice of physical therapy by interpreting and enforcing this [chapter, etc.].**

Interpretation of the statutes and rules, enforcement of the same and disciplinary activity are major duties of licensing boards. This clause empowers boards to fulfill these duties. Interpretation of the statutes and rules always falls first to members of the licensing board. These interpretations often take the form of substantive board policy, actions and opinions of the board. Board decisions form a consistent pattern over time that further guides actions consistent with the statutes and rules of that state. Rules may also be considered that would create a more formal process in recording and compiling such substantive board policy, decisions and opinions. States may also have administrative statutes relating to substantive board policies or opinions.

5. **Adopt and revise rules consistent with this [chapter, etc.]. Such rules, when lawfully adopted, shall have the effect of law.**

This rule-making authority is essential to the entire regulatory process. The construction of this Model Practice Act is such that only necessary, empowering or authorizing language is included in statutes, with the remainder of administrative process and procedure being left to the rules. But, as the second sentence points out, rules are integral to—and have equal weight in regulating—the practice of physical therapy. States vary considerably in the process used to adopt rules. Some licensing boards have wide latitude and discretion; others are under governor or state legislative oversight nearly as restrictive as that required to change the statutes. There are generally other administrative codes or laws that address the rule-making procedure. (See additional discussion in *Guidelines for Rules, Key Areas #1* and *#3.)*

6. **Meet at least once each quarter in compliance with the open meeting requirements of [cite applicable statute]. A majority of board members shall constitute a quorum for the transaction of business. The board shall keep an official record of its meetings.**

This language sets a minimum meeting frequency to comply with the law. Board meetings are subject to open meeting laws, but provisions in rules should specify when executive sessions are permissible or advisable. Of necessity, boards require that a majority of members be present to conduct business. Record keeping is always legally required.

7. **Establish mechanisms for assessing continuing competence of licensees.**

This paragraph empowers the board to set the requirements for assessing continuing competence to practice physical therapy.

*Note:* As valid mechanisms are developed for assessing continuing competence and states consider implementing continuing competence requirements for relicensure, the following language might be considered for addition to the *Licensure and Examination: Licensure or Certificate Renewal* section:

The board shall establish, by rule, activities to periodically assess continuing competence to practice physical therapy. The board shall also have authority to implement remedial actions if necessary to require continuing competence as a condition of relicensure.

Accountability to the public of ongoing competency to practice is an area of increasing concern. All health care disciplines are searching for appropriate models to provide valid and measurable assessments of continuing competence. Both the Federation and the APTA will be working in the future to refine valid assessment models. But it is appropriate to provide this model statute language now for the time when states feel ready to implement continuing competency requirements. Mandatory continuing education as the sole model for meeting requirements for relicensure *is not* recommended. Requirements for demonstrating continued competence to practice physical therapy apply only to the relicensing of physical therapists who have a defined scope of practice. Physical therapist assistants should also maintain and improve their knowledge and skills to be effective providers. As they function under the direction and supervision of the licensee, the licensee accepts some responsibility for the physical therapist assistant's ongoing skill development. However, continuing competence requirements should not be applied to recertification of physical therapist assistants, as this would be an inappropriate and overburdensome form of regulation.

Models that could be considered in the future for assessing continuing competence of physical therapists include the following:

a. Development of an examination for the purpose of relicensure. Obviously, the Federation would need to develop this testing option. If such a test is developed, consideration may need to be given for those involved in specialty practice. Evolving testing technology may use multimedia or other technologies allowing visual case presentations. Future testing, however innovative in its design, should have the intent of increasing knowledge and competency, even through the testing process itself.
b. Use of specialty board certification in physical therapy. Achievement of a board-certified clinical specialty may, with periodic re-certification in that specialty, serve as demonstration of continuing competence and be sufficient to waive further requirements of any other type of reassessment.
c. The use of an in-office audit or on-site peer review. In addition, submitted case presentations to the board that would follow a set form approved by the board. These models may also be considered if triggered by actions such as a threshold of a certain number of complaints against a licensee within a given period of time. For example, if a licensee had more than

three complaints within a five-year time period, an in-office audit or a standardized case evaluation may be required to demonstrate ongoing competency, even before the scheduled time for relicensure. These options may be used in addition to other models.

d. Standardized simulated case evaluation, which could also be integrated with the testing described in (1.) above.
e. Continuing professional education, but only where measurable outcome assessment can be achieved. This would require the use of valid pre- and post-course test instruments. Continuing education, if used as an assessment tool, must examine individuals on a wide range of information that includes the full scope of clinical practice. It is emphasized again that currently neither the Federation nor the APTA supports mandatory continuing education in state regulation. The various models to be considered should *not include* the exclusive use of mandatory continuing education.
f. Use of an outcome measurement tool that would demonstrate the physical therapist's competence.

As states have used the Model Practice Act language and subsequently developed supporting rules, in some instances these states are also adopting continuing competence requirements. It may be helpful to consult recently adopted rules from these states. The Federation office will serve as a resource for those seeking this information.

8. **Establish and collect fees for sustaining the necessary operation and expenses of the board.**

In rules there should exist a breakout of all the fees, including application fees for licensure and certification, testing fees, renewal fees, reinstatement fees and late penalties, etc. This clause empowers boards to establish and collect such fees. Placing this listing of the fees in the rules may give greater latitude to changes that may occur from time to time in fee structure.

Legislators generally expect licensing boards to be self-funding through the licensing and renewal fees of those being regulated. Other enabling legislation that addresses the funding of state regulatory boards should be reviewed. As in any enterprise, several expenses are not always apparent. Staffing, space, supplies, equipment costs and maintenance, investigative services or staff, consultants, legal counsel through a state attorney general's office, etc., add to the cost of running a licensing board. The majority of fees usually go to fund these direct expenses. Some boards are 90/10 boards, where 90% of fees pay direct board expenses, and 10% goes to the state's general fund to defray the general state overhead costs that are not as easily allocated. (See additional discussion under the *Licensure and Examination* key area regarding fees.)

**9. Elect officers from its members necessary for the operations and obligations of the board. Terms of office shall be 1 year.**

Rules can specify the offices created, when elections occur, any eligibility requirements and any particular duties related to the various offices. All board members, public and professional, should be eligible for each office.

**10. Provide for the timely orientation and training of new professional and public appointees to the board regarding board licensing and disciplinary procedures, this [chapter, etc.] and board rules, policies and procedures.**

A significant omission of several jurisdictions is in orientation and training of new appointees. This is especially true of public member appointees. The public member's experience with all aspects of the profession may be minimal. For the benefit and protection of the public, timely and adequate training of new appointees needs to be a statutory requirement of boards. In addition, just because a physical therapist has a long record of practice or of professional leadership involvement, it does not always indicate a thorough knowledge of the statutes and rules governing the practice of physical therapy. So professional appointees are in no less need of timely and thorough orientation. Responsibility for the training should be that of the board officers and they should utilize board staff to help in this tasks. Appropriate materials provided to a new appointee may include the statutes and rules, substantive board policies, other board operational policies, procedures and historical documents.

**11. Maintain a current list of all persons regulated under this chapter, including the person's name, current business and residential address, telephone numbers and license or certificate number.**

Boards may exercise some discretion on how they distribute or share such information. For example, board policy may need to include whether information is shared or sold to individuals or organizations for commercial purposes. The public should have access to information regarding those licensed or certified by the state. This is public information and should be made available to any interested party. A state board directory of licensees and certificate holders may be one mechanism for sharing this information appropriately. Technological advances may make other avenues of electronic access to this information easier in the future. Home addresses and telephone numbers are not public records unless they are the only address and telephone numbers of record, as stated in *Consumer Advocacy: Rights of Consumers* section.

**12. Provide information to the public regarding the complaint process.**

Boards should provide assistance wherever needed to facilitate the complaint process by the public. If a person needs information on how to file a complaint, the board should have easy- to-follow information available to aid them in the process. Another action that some states have implemented is to require that a notice be posted within a physical therapy department identifying those regulated by the state who work in that office or department and listing the name, address and phone number of the state licensing board. Such a requirement with the actual language to be used could be specified in rules.

**13. Employ necessary personnel to carry out the administrative work of the board. Board personnel are eligible to receive compensation pursuant to [cite specific statute].**

The board should have statutory authority, as granted in this paragraph, to employ necessary personnel to carry out duties of the board. The board must comply with state administrative employment guidelines including relevant compensation guidelines. However, the final decisions to hire, release, give direction relative to duties, review for pay increases, etc., should ideally reside with the board.

**14. Enter into contracts for services necessary for adequate enforcement of this chapter.**

This provides for additional latitude needed to carry out the work of the board. This could include contracts for investigators, administrative law judges or hearing officers and board consultants.

**15. Report final disciplinary action taken against a licensee or certificate holder to a national disciplinary database recognized by the board or as required by law.**

This paragraph refers to informing the Federation of State Boards of Physical Therapy of disciplinary action for their national database of disciplinary action. Any state licensing board may, and should, access this information when an application is received from an applicant previously licensed or certified in another state. The effect of this program will be to prevent someone from moving from one state to another to escape disciplinary consequences. The *Grounds for Disciplinary Action* key area contains the statute clause allowing previous disciplinary action to be sufficient grounds to continue a disciplinary action in the new state or to deny the applicant a license or certificate.

The ending phrase, ". . . or as required by law," is in reference to the federally mandated reporting system known as the Healthcare Integrity and Protection Data Bank (HIP-DB). After mid-1999 state boards are required to report adverse action against anyone regulated by the board to the HIP-DB. This requirement is a result of the Health Insurance Portability and Accountability Act (HIPAA) which was signed into law in 1996.

**16. Publish, at least annually, final disciplinary action taken against a licensee or certificate holder.**

The public, which also includes other physical therapists and actual or potential employers of physical therapists and physical therapist assistants, has the right to know of disciplinary actions taken against any regulated health care provider. The purpose of discipline is to correct deficiencies in conduct and address violations of the law. Some of these violations or deficiencies may create situations of potential public harm or may have actually resulted in harm. Discipline is first corrective in nature but may become punitive if violations are repeated or are serious enough to constitute a threat of harm or actual harm to the public. Whether it is potential or actual harm and whether the discipline is corrective or punitive, the public still has the right to access public records pertaining to disciplinary measures against those regulated by the practice act.

Paragraphs 15 and 16 specify making "final disciplinary action" known to others. But boards may be required to release only general information about pending complaints, for example, that "the licensee has two pending complaints being processed or under investigation," but not to release further information about the exact nature of the complaint until it is final. The open meeting laws of a particular state will also affect what a board must do in this situation. The board may also need to address in rules, in consultation with legal counsel, the extent to which complaint information appears in the minutes of their proceedings. There are various confidentiality laws that may influence such decisions.

Information being released or published could also be in other forms. The above statute language speaks of at least two. First, boards must publish at least annually a notice of final disciplinary action against any licensed physical therapist or certified physical therapist assistant. This could occur through the board's own newsletter, through a professional association newsletter, or through normal local print media. Second, boards should develop a method to easily accommodate consumer requests for status on any given licensee or certificate holder. If a consumer has a question about any provider, he or she should be able to call the board office and receive information on how to access the public records relating to the board and its actions.

17. **Publish, at least annually, board rulings, opinions, and interpretations of statutes or rules in order to guide persons regulated pursuant to this [chapter, etc.].**

Boards are frequently asked by licensees or other public members to offer advisory opinions clarifying definitions or practice issues. This statute clause gives boards authority to issue such advisory opinions and to publish them periodically as a guide to those regulated under the practice act.

18. **Participate in or conduct performance audits.**

Many states are conducting regular performance audits of their boards or state agencies. There may be a specific agency that performs such audits, such as an Office of the Auditor General. It is important that board activity and overall function be analyzed and a record maintained of the audit. This is important from a self-assessment standpoint so improvements can be made in board performance. It may also be important if policy makers ever question the need for a board to exist. Substantiation of actions taken in the role of public protection will be an important focus in demonstrating continued public benefit from the board's existence. This or an additional clause may also specify an annual reporting process to the governor.

### Disposition of Funds

No model language is offered under this section, but the heading is noted in the Model Practice Act because this section is necessary and this is the proper location to include such a section within a practice act. Each state handles their financial structure and disposition of funds so differently that it is difficult to suggest an actual model.

This section would not include fees or the setting of various fees. But it would cover such topics, for example, as specifying 1) which state fund monies are deposited into, 2) how funds are used to cover board expenses, including compensation for appointee's expenses, and 3) if there is a division of fees between a state's general fund and that used specifically by the physical therapy board. There may also be references or a deferring to other state statutes that guide or direct state agency funding issues.

### Additional Legal Considerations

Of paramount importance in establishing and maintaining a state licensing board is the provision of the legal authority and tools needed to properly administer the law. With such authority and tools, the board can deal effectively with its licensees and others who may be regulated or impacted by the law. The board, as noted in the previous Discussion, is the first line in interpreting and enforcing a practice act. Having adequate personnel including board members, having the ability to be self-sustaining and having the ability to be wholly independent are all important provisions that enable the board to operate in accordance with the legislative purpose of the practice act. However, the board's broad rule making power is one of its most important tools. While states differ on final enactment of rules, it is almost universal that rules emanate initially from an administrative body such as a licensing board.

Rules give the board the guidance to judiciously administer the law affecting its licensees. Also, rules, as well as board rulings and opinions provide the courts guidelines in determining the meaning and application of the law. Finally, rules, once legally promulgated, almost universally have the effect of statutory law. It is important to clearly define the effect of the final rule, especially where there is any chance that rule making may only be given the weight of "policy." "Policy" decisions, most likely, are not legally enforceable.

Another legal consideration is the need for autonomy in official board actions even where a board may be operating under an administrative umbrella board. In order to maintain this autonomy, it is important that the board avoid possible conflicts of interest with professional associations, and that board members themselves also be free of pecuniary or other types of conflicts. Such autonomy will preserve and strengthen the integrity and effectiveness of the licensing board in the view of the state, the peers within the board's jurisdiction and, more importantly, the public.

Additionally, great care should be taken in drafting and implementing board provisions on reporting disciplinary action. Because of due process concerns, such information regarding pending disciplinary actions, short of court subpoena, should be dealt with on a confidential basis. Reporting final action after due process has been met is not only appropriate but is a responsibility of the board.

Although many states have separate statutes dealing with licensure board member immunity from liability, each state's law should be carefully analyzed to ensure that no further mention need be made in the practice act. In light of the increased threat of litigation against state administrative bodies, care should be taken to ensure, by way of the statute, the immunity of board members when they are acting without malice and within the scope of their duties.

Under this key area, the board is given authority to establish mechanisms to assess continuing competence. As pointed out in the *Discussion,* mandatory continued education by itself is not an adequate measure of continuing competence. Continuing competence is an entirely different standard from a legal standpoint and legally will require a great deal of attention if such a standard is adopted by a state. The *Discussion* also affords a good "road map" of what additional standards may be considered in this area. It will become extremely important in rule making to adequately and clearly set forth criteria and standards as guidelines in determining where competency is lacking. Licensure to practice, once achieved, is a property right (see *Additional Legal Considerations* under the *Licensure and Examination* key area) and can only be burdened or removed with appropriate due process of law. Standards that are vague or unreasonable may be deemed unenforceable in a court of law.

# Key Area #4 Licensure and Examination

## MODEL LANGUAGE

### Qualifications for Licensure and Certification

A. An applicant for a license as a physical therapist shall:
   1. Be of good moral character.
   2. Have completed the application process.
   3. Be a graduate of a professional physical therapy education program accredited by a national accreditation agency approved by the board.
   4. Have successfully passed the national examination approved by the board.

B. An applicant for a license as a physical therapist who has been educated outside of the United States shall:
   1. Be of good moral character.
   2. Have completed the application process.
   3. Provide satisfactory evidence that the applicant's education is substantially equivalent to the requirements of physical therapists educated in accredited educational programs as determined by the board. If it is determined that a foreign-educated applicant's education is not substantially equivalent the board may require the person to complete additional course work before it proceeds with the application process.
   4. Provide written proof that the applicant's school of physical therapy education is recognized by its own ministry of education.
   5. Provide written proof of authorization to practice as a physical therapist without limitations in the country where the professional education occurred.
   6. Provide proof of legal authorization to reside and seek employment in a jurisdiction of the United States.

7. Have the applicant's educational credentials evaluated by a board-approved credential evaluation agency.
8. Have passed the board-approved English proficiency examinations if the applicant's native language is not English.
9. Have participated in an interim supervised clinical practice period prior to being approved to take the national examination.
10. Have successfully passed the national examination approved by the board.

C. Notwithstanding the provisions of subsection (B), if the foreign-educated physical therapist applicant is a graduate of an accredited educational program as approved by the board, the board may waive the requirements in subsection (B), paragraphs 3, 4, 7 and 9.

D. An applicant for certification as a physical therapist assistant shall:
1. Be of good moral character.
2. Have completed the application process.
3. Be a graduate of a physical therapist assistant education program accredited by an agency approved by the board.
4. Have successfully passed the national examination approved by the board.

## Application, Statement of Deficiencies, Hearing

A. An applicant for licensure or certification shall file a complete application as required by the board. The applicant shall include application and examination fees as prescribed in [reference the specific statute and/or rules specifying the fees].

B. The board shall notify an applicant of any deficiencies in the application. An applicant who disagrees with the identified deficiencies may request in writing and, upon request, shall be granted a hearing pursuant to [reference the section of the state administrative procedures act where an appeals process is addressed].

## Examination

A. The board shall conduct examinations within the state at least quarterly at a time and place prescribed by the board. The passing score shall be determined by the board.

B. An applicant may take the examination for licensure after the application process has been completed. The national examination shall test entry-level competency related to physical therapy theory, examination and evaluation, diagnosis, prognosis, treatment intervention, prevention, and consultation.

C. An applicant may take the examination for certification after the application process has been completed. The national examination shall test for requisite knowledge and skills in the technical application of physical therapy services.

D. An applicant for licensure or certification who does not pass the examination after the first attempt may retake the examination one additional time without reapplication for licensure or certification within 6 months the first failure. Before the board may approve an applicant for subsequent testing beyond two attempts, an applicant shall re-apply for licensure or certification and shall demonstrate evidence satisfactory to the board of having successfully completed additional clinical training or course work, or both, as determined by the board.

### Interim Permit

A. If a foreign-educated applicant satisfies the requirements of section [specify the *Qualifications for Licensure and Certification* section], subsection B, the board shall issue an interim permit to the applicant for the purpose of participating in a supervised clinical practice period prior to the applicant being approved to take the national examination. An applicant who has previously failed the national examination is not eligible for an interim permit until the applicant passes the examination.
B. The board may issue an interim permit for at least 90 days but not more than 6 months.
C. An interim permit holder shall complete, to the satisfaction of the board, a period of clinical practice in a facility approved by the board and under the on-site supervision of a physical therapist who holds an unrestricted license issued pursuant to this [chapter, act, section, law].
D. An interim permit is immediately revoked when the board notifies an interim permit holder that the permit holder has failed the licensing examination.

### Licensure by Endorsement

The board shall issue a license to a physical therapist who has a valid unrestricted license from another jurisdiction of the United States if that person, when granted the license, met all requirements prescribed in section [specify the *Qualifications for Licensure and Certification* section], subsections (A) and (B) and any applicable board rules. [See *Guidelines for Rules, Key Area #4.*]

### Exemptions from Licensure

A. This [chapter, act, section, law] does not restrict a person licensed under any other law of this state from engaging in the profession or practice for which that person is licensed if that person does not represent, imply or claim that he/she is a physical therapist or a provider of physical therapy.

B. The following persons are exempt from the licensure requirements of this [chapter, etc.] when engaged in the following activities:
   1. A person in a professional education program approved by the board who is pursuing a course of study leading to a degree as a physical therapist and that person is satisfying supervised clinical education requirements related to the person's physical therapy education while under on-site supervision of a licensed physical therapist.
   2. A physical therapist who is practicing in the United States Armed Services, United States Public Health Service or Veterans Administration pursuant to federal regulations for state licensure of health care providers.
   3. A physical therapist who is licensed in another jurisdiction of the United States or a foreign-educated physical therapist credentialed in another country if that person is performing physical therapy in connection with teaching or participating in an educational seminar of no more than sixty days in a calendar year.
   4. A physical therapist who is licensed in another jurisdiction of the United States if that person is providing consultation by means of telecommunication to a physical therapist licensed under this [chapter, etc.].

### License or Certificate Renewal, Changes of Name or Address

A. A licensee or certificate holder shall renew the license or certificate pursuant to board rules. A licensee or certificate holder who fails to renew the license or certificate on or before the expiration date shall not practice as a physical therapist or work as a physical therapist assistant in this state.

B. Each licensee and certificate holder is responsible for reporting to the board a name change and changes in business and home address within 30 days after the date of change.

### Reinstatement of License or Certificate

A. The board may reinstate a lapsed license or certificate upon payment of a renewal fee and reinstatement fee.

B. If a person's license has lapsed for more than 3 consecutive years that person shall reapply for a license and pay all applicable fees. The person shall also demonstrate to the board's satisfaction competence to practice physical therapy, or shall serve an internship under a restricted license or take remedial courses as determined by the board, or both, at the board's discretion. The board may also require the applicant to take an examination.

[Optional statute language] For states requiring maximum fee ceilings within the statutes.

### [Fees

The board shall establish and collect fees not to exceed:

1. __________dollars for an application for an original license or certificate. This fee is nonrefundable.
2. __________dollars for an examination for licensure or certification.
3. __________dollars for a certificate of renewal of a license or certificate.
4. __________dollars for an application for reinstatement of a license or certificate.
5. __________dollars for each duplicate license or certificate.]

## DISCUSSION

### Qualifications for Licensure and Certification

**A. An applicant for a license as a physical therapist shall:**

1. **Be of good moral character.**
2. **Have completed the application process.**
3. **Be a graduate of a professional physical therapy education program accredited by a national accreditation agency approved by the board.**
4. **Have successfully passed the national examination approved by the board.**

Every licensing board has written procedures for applying for licensure. Those detailed procedures should be outlined in rules rather than statutes. Within those rules would be the place to more specifically define terms used in this statute paragraph. For example, states may wish to define the term "good moral character." Sometimes the application form itself will define what this means through the requirements listed or questions asked. For instance, does the applicant have a criminal record? Questions regarding a criminal record sometimes appear on applications for licensure. Character references are also sometimes required. These requirements will further define what good moral character means.

Being a graduate of an accredited educational program also is an important inclusion in practice acts. Because accrediting bodies occasionally change, it is not recommended that the actual accrediting agency be specified in statutes. That agency is now the Commission on Accreditation of Physical Therapy Education (CAPTE) and this can be indicated either by rule or by board policy. The model language specifies that it is the accrediting agency, rather than each educational program, that needs the approval of the board.

It is also important to understand that it is a constitutionally protected right of states for a licensing board to require the accreditation process. The U.S. Supreme Court (*Dent v. West*, 1889) upheld the constitutional right of state licensing boards to require a specific educational credential. Accreditation is the means of assuring standardized professional education, thereby giving licensing boards a degree of comfort in licensing a new graduate from any accredited educational program outside their state, or granting licensure by endorsement to an applicant previously licensed in another state who graduated from an accredited educational program.

**B. An applicant for a license as a physical therapist who has been educated outside of the United States shall:**

1. **Be of good moral character.**
2. **Have completed the application process.**
3. **Provide satisfactory evidence that the applicant's education is substantially equivalent to the requirements of physical therapists educated in accredited educational programs as determined by the board. If it is determined that a foreign-educated applicant's education is not substantially equivalent the board may require the person to complete additional course work before it proceeds with the application process.**
4. **Provide written proof that the applicant's school of physical therapy education is recognized by its own ministry of education.**
5. **Provide written proof of authorization to practice as a physical therapist without limitations in the country where the professional education occurred.**
6. **Provide proof of legal authorization to reside and seek employment in a jurisdiction of the United States.**
7. **Have the applicant's educational credentials evaluated by a board-approved credential evaluation agency.**
8. **Have passed the board-approved English proficiency examinations if the applicant's native language is not English.**
9. **Have participated in an interim supervised clinical practice period prior to being approved to take the national examination.**
10. **Have successfully passed the national examination approved by the board.**

**C. Notwithstanding the provisions of subsection (B), if the foreign-educated physical therapist applicant is a graduate of an accredited educational program as approved by the board, the board may waive the requirements in subsection (B), paragraphs 3, 4, 7 and 9.**

Another factor that may extensively influence this entire process is the "Illegal Immigration Reform and Immigrant Responsibilities Act of 1996." It requires prescreening of foreign-educated applicants for physical therapist licensure before granting work visas or a change in immigrant status. Screening includes credentials review, English proficiency examinations and determination of prior license or authority to practice in the country where the professional education was completed. There may be consideration in the future for administering the actual licensing examination as part of this prescreening process. If this occurs, the clinical internship, if still required, could be offered *after* the licensing examination is successfully passed. In this instance it would be more appropriate to eliminate the "interim permit" altogether and grant a restricted license in order to require a period of supervised clinical practice in the U.S. prior to final granting of an unrestricted license. The Federation will share further recommendations relative to this as the prescreening program develops. In the meantime, the regulatory model proposed in this Model Practice Act is recommended.

Physical therapy licensing boards and their staffs spend considerable time processing applications for licensure by foreign-educated applicants. It is crucial in this regard that a) greater consistency occur in the licensing standards from state to state, and b) that the entire application process be detailed, both in statute and in rules.

If consistency from state to state can be achieved, states can then be comfortable in the endorsement process when a currently licensed foreign-educated physical therapist chooses to relocate to another state. There is not a current level of comfort by state boards due to the lack of uniform licensing standards. Because some states have licensing standards that are not deemed equivalent to those applied to U.S. graduates, state boards are simply not defaulting to the weaker standards when considering foreign-educated applicants. Therefore, many states require all foreign-educated applicants to complete the entire application process, including additional education and clinical supervision, even though they may have been licensed and practicing in another state for several years. When uniform licensing standards are achieved, the endorsement process can be applied when considering applications from foreign-educated physical therapists previously licensed in another state. (See *Licensure and Examination: Licensure Endorsement* key area.)

The more detailed the application process is addressed in rules, the easier it will be for licensing boards to deal with the oftentimes complicated process of foreign-educated applications for licensure. The following items, which conform to the statute language above, should be specified in rules:

1. It is appropriate to define what a "foreign-educated applicant" means. For example:

"A 'foreign-educated applicant' means a physical therapist who graduated from any physical therapy educational program outside the fifty states, Puerto Rico, District of Columbia, or U.S. territories."

2. Educational equivalency should be defined. Requiring a certain number of credit hours in specific areas of both general and professional education curricula may accomplish this. However, this may not guarantee equivalency of course content. Again, the more specific a practice act is, the more consistent a board can be with foreign-educated applications. It would be appropriate to also specify a grade standard, for example, the foreign-educated applicant must have obtained a grade of C or better in professional education courses. Three resources to consult for additional guidance are (1) the Federation's *Course Work Evaluation Tool for Persons Who Received Their Physical Therapy Education Outside the United States,* (2) CAPTE's criteria for accrediting foreign educational programs, and (3) APTA's *A Normative Model of Physical Therapist Professional Education, Version 97.*
3. In board policy or rules, specify the process by which credential review agencies become board approved. Indicate what information must be submitted to a credential review agency.
4. Rules or board policy should specify the exact English proficiency examinations required and under what circumstances they are required. The Federation recommends the following three tests be taken and passed: *Test of English as a Foreign Language* (TOEFL), *Test of Spoken English* (TSE), and *Test of Written English* (TWE). In addition, states may wish to include the passing scores required for each test. The Federation's passing score recommendations for each test are:
   TOEFL: 560 TSE: 50 TWE: 4.5 (See *Appendix F.*)

**D. An applicant for certification as a physical therapist assistant shall:**
1. **Be of good moral character.**
2. **Have completed the application process.**
3. **Be a graduate of a physical therapist assistant education program accredited by an agency approved by the board.**
4. **Have successfully passed the national examination approved by the board.**

As with the licensure application process for a physical therapist, the application process for certification as a physical therapist assistant should be detailed, in writing and included in rules.

The position of the Federation of State Boards of Physical Therapy regarding the appropriate regulation of physical therapist assistants is addressed in detail in the "FSBPT Position Paper: Physical Therapist Assistant Regulation, Oct 1998, Federation of State Boards of Physical Therapy," attached as *Appendix C.* The summation of that position is as follows:

It is the position of the Federation of State Boards of Physical Therapy that the least restrictive form of regulation available within a state should be used for physical therapist assistants that allows for 1) minimal educational requirements,

2) entry competency examination, 3) title protection, and 4) the board's power to discipline. This can usually be accomplished by statutory certification. When this is the case, regulation by licensure should be reserved for the physical therapist.

The full position paper in *Appendix C* outlines 1) the importance of regulating physical therapist assistants, 2) defines regulatory terms such as "registration," "certification" and "licensure," and 3) discusses the appropriate form of regulation for the physical therapist assistant based on the various forms of state regulation available. The reader is encouraged to review this position carefully.

*Note:* States adopting the Model Practice Act language extensively but electing to retain or adopt licensure for physical therapist assistants need to be careful in modifying Model Practice Act language in several areas. *Appendix D* provides alternate model statute language where licensure rather than certification is used for regulation of the physical therapist assistant.

There is no provision in the Model Practice Act for regulating foreign-educated physical therapist assistants. The physical therapist assistant does not have professional level health care provider standing with the U.S. Immigration and Naturalization Service that is required for entry to the United States, and it is not anticipated that this will change. It is also not appropriate to certify as a physical therapist assistant a foreign-educated physical therapist who has not met the requirements for licensure as a physical therapist in the United States.

## Application, Statement of Deficiencies, Hearing

**A. An applicant for licensure or certification shall file a complete application as required by the board. The applicant shall include application and examination fees as prescribed in [reference the specific statute and/or rules specifying the fees].**

Each state should clearly list the information required of each applicant for licensure or certification and the forms or format in which the information is to be submitted. Generally, this information is placed in rules.

The Model Practice Act recommends that the amount of all fees be placed in rules. However, some states place in statute either a range of fees or a ceiling on fees, and then set the actual fees in rules. Where most states require at least a notification and public hearing process for rule changes, the above language is adequate. However, the use of fee ranges or ceilings in statute language would also be appropriate. Where a state chooses to include such language in statute, optional model language is included within this key area.

**B. The board shall notify an applicant of any deficiencies in the application. An applicant who disagrees with the identified deficiencies**

**may request in writing and, upon request, shall be granted a hearing pursuant to [reference the section of the state administrative procedures act where an appeals process is addressed].**

Mechanisms should exist that allow an applicant to appeal to the board if they feel there is a discrepancy with a determination of deficiencies in their application for licensure or certification. A "hearing" normally would be accomplished through a scheduled appearance at a regular board meeting, where the deficiencies would be discussed with the board. This process is usually already specified in the Administrative Procedures statutes of each state.

## Examination

**A. The board shall conduct examinations within the state at least quarterly at a time and place prescribed by the board. The passing score shall be determined by the board.**

**B. An applicant may take the examination for licensure after the application process has been completed. The national examination shall test entry-level competency related to physical therapy theory, examination and evaluation, diagnosis, prognosis, treatment intervention, prevention, and consultation.**

**C. An applicant may take the examination for certification after the application process has been completed. The national examination shall test for requisite knowledge and skills in the technical application of physical therapy services.**

**D. An applicant for licensure or certification who does not pass the examination after the first attempt may retake the examination one additional time without reapplication for licensure or certification within 6 months the first failure. Before the board may approve an applicant for subsequent testing beyond two attempts, an applicant shall reapply for licensure or certification and shall demonstrate evidence satisfactory to the board of having successfully completed additional clinical training or course work, or both, as determined by the board.**

Taking the examination for licensure as a physical therapist or the examination for certification as a physical therapist assistant should not occur until all application processes are complete. Requirements are outlined under *Qualifications for Licensure and Certification* and may be further specified in rules.

Examination for licensure as a physical therapist should be "competency specific" and appropriately cover the entire scope of practice, including theory, examination and evaluation, diagnosis, prognosis, treatment intervention, prevention and consultation, which parallels the definition of the "Practice of Physical Therapy." (See *Definitions* key area.)

The minimum frequency of testing by statute is established in the model language as quarterly. However, computerized testing will allow for the availability of candidate testing almost daily.

Paragraph (D) specifies that an applicant who fails the examination once does not have to go through an entire application process in order to take the examination a second time, provided the examination is taken within 6 months after the initial failure. The computerized testing now requires at least a 30 day wait before a subsequent test. The rationale for requiring a complete application after the 6 months is to recheck for such factors as verification of continued good moral conduct. Two failures may indicate a need for remedial didactic and/or clinical work before being qualified to take the exam again.

## Interim Permit

**A. If a foreign-educated applicant satisfies the requirements of section [specify the *Qualifications for Licensure and Certification* section], subsection B, the board shall issue an interim permit to the applicant for the purpose of participating in a supervised clinical practice period prior to the applicant being approved to take the national examination. An applicant who has previously failed the national examination is not eligible for an interim permit until the applicant passes the examination.**

There may be more than one way to approach the credentialing of foreign-educated physical therapists during a supervised interim period. For example, in the past some states have used "probationary" permits, while others have exempted the applicants as they do student physical therapists. Other possibilities include temporary or even restricted licenses. One prominent goal of the Model Practice Act is to promote greater uniformity as well as decrease unusual regulatory barriers where the public can benefit and still be protected. The Model Practice Act recommends unifying the regulation and terminology under an "interim permit." The very term "probationary" has a connotation of discipline, which is not the intent. Temporary licenses are not being recommended in the Model Practice Act due to the availability of computerized testing that enable scores to be reported back within several days to a few weeks.

**B. The board may issue an interim permit for at least 90 days but not more than 6 months.**

**C. An interim permit holder shall complete, to the satisfaction of the board, a period of clinical practice in a facility approved by the board and under the on-site supervision of a physical therapist who holds an unrestricted license issued pursuant to this [chapter, act, section, law].**

**D. An interim permit is immediately revoked when the board notifies an interim permit holder that the permit holder has failed the licensing examination.**

The time period of supervised clinical practice is an interim period between application and final licensure to allow for direct observation of clinical orientation and competence by another licensed physical therapist, prior to the foreign-educated physical therapist being granted final clearance to take the examination. The parallel exists here with CAPTE accredited program graduates, where they *always* participate in supervised clinical internships, whereas there is no assurance that a clinical internship is part of the educational training of foreign-educated physical therapists.

While there are many similarities between the foreign-educated applicant for licensure and the U.S.-educated physical therapy student intern, there are enough differences to warrant a separate form of regulation. The "interim permit" offers the best option.

Additional rule requirements must be adopted to conform to these statute paragraphs. These additional rule requirements should address at least the following:

1. Specify the parameters of supervised clinical experience prior to eligibility for licensure examination. This should include the length of time (both the minimum and maximum number of weeks or months the supervised clinical experience can occur), the minimum and maximum number of hours worked per week, the options for types of facilities or clinical settings that will be approved (for example, a facility providing broader exposure to general physical therapy, as opposed to narrow specialty care), the nature of supervision (direct on-site, for example), the qualifications of a clinical supervisor (for example, the length of time they have been licensed), the reporting requirements and forms used by the clinical supervisor for reporting back to the board, provisions for extension of time or for transfer to another clinical setting if the first supervised clinical experience is not deemed successful, and options for a second supervised clinical experience.
2. Rules should specify that once an examination is taken and failed by a foreign-educated applicant, continued clinical work, even under supervision, is not permitted. This same standard applies to U.S.-educated graduates as well. U.S.-educated physical therapists participate in clinical training as part of their educational curriculum prior to graduation. They then are eligible to take the licensing examination. The reason a supervised clinical training period is required of foreign-educated applicants is the variance in educational inclusion of clinical experience in foreign educational programs, and the importance of exposure to clinical practice in the United States. When the application for licensure

is completed by a foreign-educated physical therapist and he or she is approved for an interim supervised clinical education period, there exists an assumption of competence. If an examination is subsequently failed, that assumption of competence is deemed void and approval for continued clinical practice should not be extended. The U.S. Immigration and Naturalization Service should then be notified of the applicant's status. The language in the second sentence of the statute clause states: "An applicant who has failed the national examination is not eligible for an interim permit until after he or she has passed the examination." This clause prevents a foreign-educated applicant who has failed the examination in one state from moving to another state and working under an interim permit in that state.

No temporary licenses are proposed under the Model Practice Act. In case of revocation of an interim permit due to failure of the examination, reexamination should be subject to the same provisions as specified in the *Examination* section, paragraph (D).

### Licensure by Endorsement

**The board shall issue a license to a physical therapist who has a valid unrestricted license from another jurisdiction of the United States if that person, when granted the license, met all requirements prescribed in section [specify the *Qualifications for Licensure and Certification* section], subsections (A) and (B) and any applicable board rules. [See *Guidelines for Rules, Key Area #4.*]**

When greater regulatory consistency is achieved from state to state, states will confidently grant licensure by endorsement to physical therapists currently licensed in other states. A phrase now common in many practice acts in their endorsement or reciprocity sections is: ". . . having licensing requirements substantially similar to those prescribed in this [chapter, act, etc.] at the time the license was originally granted." That language is probably closer to reciprocity than endorsement. But when combined with a process of having most states enact over time the Model Practice Act requirements for licensure of foreign-educated physical therapists, this model language will eventually lead to true endorsement. Standardized prescreening, mentioned earlier as being under consideration and development, will also have an effect on greater standardization for entry to practice in the United States.

Any other requirements for endorsement should be specified. These may include submission of verification of a current license in the state of previous residency, affidavit of previous practice within 3 years, freedom from pending or current disciplinary action or restricted license, continuing education history if mandatory for licensing requirements, specific continuing education required such as HIV continuing education, or the requirement to take a jurisprudence test.

### Exemptions from Licensure

A. **This [chapter, act, section, law] does not restrict a person licensed under any other law of this state from engaging in the profession or practice for which that person is licensed if that person does not represent, imply or claim that he/she is a physical therapist or a provider of physical therapy.**

This is a crucial area of language construction. Some states have seemingly granted blanket exemption status, e.g., "Other licensed health care providers are exempt from the provisions of this act." Other professional disciplines have challenged such weak language, interpreting it to mean that they are completely exempt from all provisions of the physical therapy practice acts, including title protection. Although such existing statute language may be weak, it was never intended to grant blanket exemption status, which is contrary to the very purpose of licensure laws. Some have made the claim that physical therapy is not only a generic term, but a term they are not prevented from using because of statute language like the example above that seems to grant blanket immunity.

Legal challenges have tested this line of reasoning. Such reasoning is completely counter to the purpose of practice acts and the power of a state to enact scope of practice and title protection statutes. Scope of practice does overlap, but that does not justify misleading or inappropriate use of titles and terms.

This model language, when combined with other language in this Model Practice Act under the *Definitions, Licensure and Examination, Lawful Practice*, and *Use of Titles* key areas, will significantly help in public protection and clarification of the services being provided. It will also provide greater strength against legal challenges.

In practice acts there is a tendency to exempt other practitioners such as massage therapists, athletic trainers, etc., who may be providing services similar to physical therapy. The Model Practice Act does not include such exemptions, and caution should be used in the drafting of any type of exemption.

This statute clause will be sufficient for all those who are licensed to practice another discipline. For those not licensed, there never should be a blanket exemption granted. If language is required because of the political necessities of adopting a practice act, then the statute language should be very narrowly and tightly worded so that it does not allow the illegal practice of physical therapy. Following are examples of such language that could apply to massage therapists and athletic trainers:

*Massage Therapy:* This [chapter, act, section, law] shall not prohibit a masseur, a masseuse or massage therapist from giving a massage as long as such service is not represented in any way as being physical therapy or as being provided by a physical therapist.

*Athletic Training:* This [chapter, act, section, law] shall not prohibit an athletic trainer certified by a national athletic trainers' association approved by the board from providing athletic training services to participating athletes of an educational institution or a professional or bona fide amateur sports organization at the institution or the organization's athletic training facility or at the site of athletic practice or competition.

**B. The following persons are exempt from the licensure requirements of this [chapter, etc.] when engaged in the following activities:**

1. **A person in a professional education program approved by the board who is pursuing a course of study leading to a degree as a physical therapist and who is satisfying supervised clinical education requirements related to the person's physical therapy education while under on-site supervision of a licensed physical therapist.**
2. **A physical therapist who is practicing in the United States Armed Services, United States Public Health Service or Veterans Administration pursuant to federal regulations for state licensure of health care providers.**
3. **A physical therapist who is licensed in another jurisdiction of the United States or a foreign-educated physical therapist credentialed in another country if that person is performing physical therapy in connection with teaching or participating in an educational seminar of no more than 60 days in a calendar year.**
4. **A physical therapist who is licensed in another jurisdiction of the United States if that person is providing consultation by means of telecommunication to a physical therapist licensed under this [chapter, etc.].**

The purpose of exemption from licensure is that a person so exempted is generally engaged in providing or practicing physical therapy, but there is a compelling reason not to require state licensure for that person when performing specific activities. The categories of those exempted should therefore be limited. The above three categories represent physical therapists or soon-to-be licensed physical therapists (in the case of physical therapist students).

Physical therapy students in clinical internships prior to graduation will obviously not yet have met the requirements for licensure but will need to perform at almost the same level as an entry-level physical therapist while under the direct, on-site supervision of a licensee. Although they will work under the on-site supervision of a licensee, they will need the authority to examine, evaluate, diagnose, and initiate treatment intervention, consult, etc.—which essentially is practicing physical therapy. Physical therapist assistant students do not require an exemption because they do not have an independent scope of practice and they function as assistive personnel under the authority of a licensed physical therapist.

In continuing education courses involving physical therapist assistants, where patient treatment is involved, the supervision statutes and rules of a given state would apply. For example, if a physical therapist assistant were involved in a long-term course (more than 60 days) that involved patient care, the physical therapist assistant would still need to be providing care under the supervision of a licensed physical therapist. A physical therapist assistant would not be providing physical therapy intervention independent of a physical therapist, even in a continuing education setting. Therefore, no exemption from certification is necessary.

Physical therapists in federal employment such as in the Veterans Administration, U.S. Public Health Services, or the military services have historically been exempt from licensure while practicing specifically in those governmental environments. The statute language above reflects changing federal regulations that now require federally employed health care professionals to be licensed in at least one state, though not necessarily the state where they are based or practicing.

Paragraph (B.3) addresses the need for those physical therapists participating either as instructors or as students in continuing professional education. Frequently these individuals are participating in offerings outside the state where they are licensed, and occasionally patient contact and treatment may be part of this educational offering. As long as this is a short-term course, or multiple courses, of no more than 60 days in a calendar year, this exemption allows the latitude needed. A longer period of time would constitute something more like a fellowship or an advanced clinical residency and should definitely require licensure in that state.

Paragraph (B.4) provides statutory exemption for telehealth or consultation by means of telecommunications. This paragraph is also linked to the *Definitions* paragraph (J) that defines "Consultation by Means of Telecommunications." Exemption from licensure is provided specifically for consultation with a physical therapist who is licensed in the state where the patient is located. This exemption extends only to consultation and does not extend to any other aspect of patient management including treatment intervention. It allows for consultation across state lines. Any aspect of patient care other than this exempted consultation must occur with a physical therapist who possesses a full and unrestricted license from the state where the patient is located.

### License or Certificate Renewal, Change of Name or Address

**A. A licensee or certificate holder shall renew the license or certificate pursuant to board rules. A licensee or certificate holder who fails to renew the license or certificate on or before the expiration date shall not practice as a physical therapist or work as a physical therapist assistant in this state.**

States should specify in rules the terms of license and certification renewal along with the exact renewal date. It should also be stated in rules that all licensees and certificate holders are responsible for keeping the board advised of their current mailing address, practice or employment location. Failure to receive a renewal in the mail should not constitute a sufficient excuse for not renewing in a timely manner. It should be specifically detailed in rules the date that renewal notices are mailed, and the time period allowed for a response. It should be further specified that failure to meet the time limit will constitute a lapsed license or certificate and will be treated as such under authority of the following paragraph, *Reinstatement of License or Certificate*. License and certificate holders also should not rely on an employer to renew the license or certificate. Timely renewal is the responsibility of the licensee or certificate holder even where an employer may be funding the expense of such renewal.

**B. Each licensee and certificate holder is responsible for reporting to the board a name change and changes in business and home address within 30 days after the date of change.**

At the time of license or certificate renewal, a licensing board should not have to deal with an excuse that the board did not have the correct address. This clause places the responsibility for updating name and address changes on those regulated. In addition, beyond the issue of renewal, there are other circumstances where the board should have available to it the correct name and mailing address of those regulated under its jurisdiction.

### Reinstatement of License or Certificate

**A. The board may reinstate a lapsed license or certificate upon payment of a renewal fee and reinstatement fee.**

**B. If a person's license has lapsed for more than 3 consecutive years that person shall reapply for a license and pay all applicable fees. The person shall also demonstrate to the board's satisfaction competence to practice physical therapy, or shall serve an internship under a restricted license or take remedial courses as determined by the board, or both, at the board's discretion. The board may also require the applicant to take an examination.**

A single section of rules should address all fees, including renewal and reinstatement fees.

Having a license to practice is part of being a professional. There is a general expectation of meeting the requirements and maintaining a license throughout one's career. Where a license has been allowed to lapse for a lengthy period of time, it may evidence a break in continuity of practice and professional development, and potentially a loss of ongoing competence. It is recommended that a 3-year time period be used to determine when the further requirement of re-application for licensure should be instituted. The board should be given discretion in assessing continuing competence to practice physical therapy in the case of a 3-year or greater lapse. This may include the options of 1) a supervised internship, 2) remedial or refresher course work, and 3) retesting, or any combination of these options. Further provisions for applicant interview by the board should be specified.

Where a license lapses due to a licensee moving to another state, but the licensee returns to the original state, the requirement for successfully demonstrating competence, as stated in paragraph (B) above, may be satisfied by verification of licensure and practice in the other state.

During a period of remedial action as described in the above paragraph, the physical therapist would have a restricted license. This would be an example of an occurrence outside of a disciplinary action where the use of a restricted license is appropriate.

A lapse of a certificate disqualifies a physical therapist assistant from further employment as a physical therapist assistant until appropriate renewal and reinstatement fees are paid. As the physical therapist assistant resumes employment, the supervising licensed physical therapist who always remains professionally and legally responsible for care given under the authority of his or her license should direct what remedial measures are appropriate if a physical therapist assistant who has not worked for an extended time is found to have inadequate skills. There should not be a system of demonstrating competence as part of an application for reinstatement as there is with physical therapists. The physical therapist assistant remains subject to disciplinary procedures, including responsibility for not violating paragraph (5) of key area *Grounds for Disciplinary Action* section which reads:

5. *Engaging in the performance of substandard care by a physical therapist assistant, that includes exceeding the authority to perform tasks selected and delegated by the supervising licensee regardless of whether actual injury to the patient is established.*

**[Optional statute language] For states requiring maximum fee ceilings within the statutes.**

**[Fees**

**The board shall establish and collect fees not to exceed:**

**1. ____________ dollars for an application for an original license or certificate. This fee is nonrefundable.**
**2. ____________ dollars for an examination for licensure or certification.**
**3. ____________ dollars for a certificate of renewal of a license or certificate.**
**4. ____________ dollars for an application for reinstatement of a license or certificate.**
**5. ____________ dollars for each duplicate license or certificate.]**

This is optional statute language to use if fee ceilings or ranges are required in statute, rather than being addressed entirely in rules. Using this model, a ceiling for fees would be established in statute, and the actual fees would be set by the board in the rules. The model language here sets the same dollar amount for licenses and certificates in the different categories. However, in rules the fees for licensees and certificate holders could easily be established at different amounts for each of the categories.

## ADDITIONAL LEGAL CONSIDERATIONS

Licensure of professionals is one of the cornerstones of a state's methods to provide protection to its citizens. The state acts under its police powers to ensure the protection of the health, safety and welfare of its citizens by requiring a license for the physical therapist to practice and provide care. A license of a professional, such as a physical therapist, physician or lawyer, has been held to be a property right as contrasted to a privilege such as driver's license. The state, therefore, as noted in the *Discussion,* has wide latitude in professional licensing to exact appropriate standards and qualifications. Such qualifications should be as clear and concise as possible. Legally, for example, as suggested in the *Discussion,* such qualifications as "moral character," may be clarified in rules to help not only the licensing board in its deliberations but to avoid potential litigation by prospective licensees who may have to demonstrate this qualification.

Establishing clear standards is particularly important with foreign-educated applicants where equivalency measures are employed. With the high influx of foreign-educated applicants has come increased litigation to obtain U.S. state licensure. State licensing laws that do not have adequate legal criteria and standards relating to issues of equivalency run a serious risk of enabling unqualified persons to achieve licensure through aggressive legal advocacy.

The Model Practice Act encourages states to use *licensure* as the form of regulation for physical therapists and *certification* as the form of regulation for physical therapist assistants. Licensing laws, such as physical therapy practice acts, set forth a definitional scope of practice. A physical therapist's license allows the unrestricted right to practice that statutory scope of practice without supervision. By contrast and by definition, a physical therapist assistant is an assistant to a licensed physical therapist and factually, the physical therapist assistant has no independent scope of practice. The Model Practice Act has accordingly recommended a separate credentialing standard for the physical therapist assistant through certification. Certification for the assistant is most appropriate, as it denotes qualifications to perform an act or provide a service, but does not exclude the physical therapist from acting or providing such services. Physical therapy scope of practice does exclude the physical therapist assistant from providing physical therapy practice in the manner defined by law. Factually, the entire body of knowledge of the physical therapist and application of that knowledge in practice encompasses all aspects of the knowledge and application of the physical therapist assistant. The opposite, however, is not true, thus, the basis for separate and distinct credentialing standards. The use of credentialing standards does not in any manner compromise the protection of the public. The control and supervision of the physical therapist assistant's activities by a licensed physical therapist are otherwise well defined by the Model Practice Act.

# Key Area #5
# Lawful Practice

## MODEL LANGUAGE

### Lawful Practice

A. A physical therapist licensed under this act is fully authorized to practice physical therapy as defined herein.
B. A physical therapist shall refer a patient or client to appropriate health care practitioners if the physical therapist has reasonable cause to believe symptoms or conditions are present that require services beyond the scope of practice or when physical therapy is contraindicated.
C. A physical therapist shall adhere to the recognized standards of ethics of the physical therapy profession and as further established by rule. [Rules should specify ethical conduct or specifically reference the APTA's *Code of Ethics* and *Guide for Professional Conduct* at *Appendix E.]*

*Special Note:* The following two paragraphs are optional and each state may wish to consider whether such clauses are needed in their particular practice act. These procedures are already within the scope of physical therapy practice, and statutory authority allowing and not prohibiting them is already contained in language in the Definitions key area. (See *Discussion* under *Definitions: Practice of Physical Therapy.)*

Caution needs to be used when considering adding authorizing statutes for these or any other procedures to a practice act. From a statutory and regulatory standpoint, it is better to define physical therapy broadly so as to have these types of procedures included within that definition rather than list several procedures that seem to fall outside of the definition and need special affirmative statute clauses. This will effectively avoid challenges to the legitimacy of their inclusion in the scope of practice. If an attempt is made to legislatively add the following clauses to state statutes, and such an attempt fails, the failure may signal a legislative intent that the procedure should not be included within the scope of physical therapy practice, when it may have been part of physical therapy practice for decades. Scope of practice evolves, but sometimes it must evolve in education and practice before it evolves statutorily.

However, there may be circumstances that require, or may benefit from, specific statutory inclusion affirming these procedures as within the scope of physical therapy practice. So each state needs to examine its circumstances carefully with respect to these statute clauses. Where physical therapy practice acts in some states currently contain statutes affirmatively authorizing the following procedures, it is advisable to retain the current authorizing language or substitute the model language below.

Another approach is to place guidelines for a specific practice procedure in rules rather than statutes.

[Optional Statute Clauses]

[D. A physical therapist may perform wound management that includes, but is not limited to, sharp debridement, debridement with other agents, dry dressings, wet dressings, topical agents including enzymes, and hydrotherapy.

E. A physical therapist may purchase, store and administer topical and aerosol medications as part of the practice of physical therapy as defined herein. A physical therapist shall comply with any regulation duly adopted by the [specify the state] Board of Pharmacy (or other regulatory board) specifying protocols for storage of medications.]

## DISCUSSION

### Lawful Practice

**A. A physical therapist licensed under this act is fully authorized to practice physical therapy as defined herein.**

This language is an affirmative statement of the legal authority of a physical therapist to practice physical therapy within its full scope. It eliminates language that poses "thou shalt not" restrictions. Many states have simply eliminated the word or phrase that addressed "referral" to allow direct access to physical therapy services by consumers. This model language leaves no room for doubt regarding the basis of this authority.

If a legislature insists on some limitations to paragraph (A), this positive statement should still be maintained. For example, if the legislature wishes to maintain restrictions on X-rays, or electrocauterization, etc., paragraphs (A) could still remain intact and be included in the statutes, but with the added item of another paragraph such as: "B. Physical therapy does not include . . . ." Such restrictive clauses are common in current practice acts but are not recommended, nor included, in this Model Practice Act.

**B. A physical therapist shall refer a patient or client to appropriate health care practitioners if the physical therapist has reasonable cause to believe symptoms or conditions are present that require services beyond the scope of practice or when physical therapy is contraindicated.**

This language is similar to language in the APTA's *Guide for Professional Conduct.* Similar language has been used in several practice acts as a safety net when direct access legislation has been adopted. It stands on its own merit, however, and should be included.

**C. A physical therapist shall adhere to the recognized standards of ethics of the physical therapy profession and as further established by rule. [Rules should specify ethical conduct or specifically reference the APTA's *Code of Ethics* and *Guide for Professional Conduct at Appendix E.*]**

A foundational tenet of a profession is that it has a code of ethics—a codified standard that encourages a higher standard of conduct among its members. Professional associations are recognized as the rightful authors of these codes of conduct. Individual states, however, retain the right to adopt practice acts or laws relating to the health professions. These state laws establish minimum levels of acceptable conduct for a profession. One is a higher, but voluntary, standard; the other is a lower, but mandatory, standard—voluntary and mandatory in the sense of the law. However, both would be mandatory in the sense of ethics. For example, it would be unethical to violate one's professional code of ethics or to break the law. On the other hand, one may be able to violate a tenet of an ethical code without necessarily violating the law.

Ethics and law are certainly related, and in this section of model language, that relationship becomes closer. In the discussion under the Legislative Intent key area, it was mentioned that licensing boards should have a sense of duty beyond the "gatekeeper" and "hand-slapper" level. To do this, licensure laws must give the boards who administer them some latitude to foster a higher level of conduct. The importance of including this clause is for this purpose, and many states have this type of clause. A similar clause is also included in the model language of the *Grounds for Disciplinary Action* key area. The inclusion of the clause in both areas is encouraged.

The model language is "generic" language, in that it does not specifically reference the American Physical Therapy Association, or the APTA's *Code of Ethics* with its accompanying *Guide for Professional Conduct* at *Appendix E.* But the inference is clear. These documents are the only recognized standards of ethics of the entire profession.

Another reason for using the generic version of this language is the recommendation of many state legislatures' legal counsel *not* to have specific reference to national associations in their statutes. This language avoids such a conflict while preserving a clear tie to recognized national standards. The link can be specifically made in rules by referencing the APTA *Code of Ethics* and *Guide for Professional Conduct*. (See *Guidelines for Rules, Key Area #5*.)

In the past, a few state practice acts have referred specifically to the APTA *Code of Ethics*. Other states did not use the name of the APTA but simply adopted the *Code* verbatim as their own ethical code. Still other states adopted their own written code of ethics with their own variations of the APTA *Code* as a model.

In addition, it is *not recommended* that statutes include references to the *Standards of Ethical Conduct for the Physical Therapist Assistant* and the *Guide for Conduct of the Affiliate Member*. Ultimately, the responsibility for ethical practice rests with the licensed professional physical therapist. If necessary, a state may add a sentence such as, "Physical therapist assistants shall conduct themselves in an ethical manner."

**[Optional Statute]**

**[D. A physical therapist may perform wound management that includes, but is not limited to, sharp debridement, debridement with other agents, dry dressings, wet dressings, topical agents including enzymes, and hydrotherapy.]**

Wound management in burn care, ulcer care and other conditions is well established as within the scope of practice of physical therapy. Debridement and wound management are specifically included in the model definition of the practice of physical therapy. Yet occasionally this may be challenged, especially when physical therapists use sharp debridement. It may be helpful to have specific enabling statute language in practice acts.

**[Optional Statute]**

**[E. A physical therapist may purchase, store and administer topical and aerosol medications as part of the practice of physical therapy as defined herein. A physical therapist shall comply with any regulation duly adopted by the [specify the state] Board of Pharmacy (or other regulatory board) specifying protocols for storage of medications.]**

Similar to wound management, the use of topical and aerosol medications for such purposes as iontophoresis, phonophoresis, pulmonary physical therapy, or in aiding wound debridement have long been established as within the scope of practice of physical therapy. The model language is enabling language that codifies in statute what has been well established in education and practice.

The reference to pharmacy statutes is an appropriate tie to storage safeguards. If this issue is not addressed in the physical therapy law, it may also be appropriate, as some states have done, to amend only the pharmacy statute to allow the permissive use of certain medications and/or their storage by physical therapists.

This may also be an area where restrictive language may be necessary for political reasons. An example would be:

Nothing in this paragraph shall be construed to authorize a physical therapist to prescribe or dispense medications.

However, such a clause is unnecessary and inadvisable since there is no educational or practice history of physical therapists prescribing medication. This is an argument that could be used against adopting any similar restrictive clauses.

## Additional Legal Considerations

Paragraph (A), affirmatively stated, gives physical therapists in jurisdictions which adopt this language the legal authority, without limitation, to practice all aspects of the scope of physical therapy within the meaning of the act. Paragraph (B) modifies this unlimited authority to so act based only on the exercise of the professional judgment of the attending physical therapist that a referral of the patient to another practitioner may be necessary.

Regarding the use of ethical standards in a practice act, adherence to the profession's ethical code and standards of practice further strengthens the legal argument that the profession and practice are unique and separate from other professions. One of the legal determinants of a profession is that it has a code of ethics. The statutory adoption of, or clear reference to, the profession's code of ethics, in whole or in part, also provides an enhanced basis for utilizing unethical behavior as grounds for discipline. However, the drafters of specific statutory or regulatory disciplinary measures involving ethical behavior should understand the need for clear standards and guidelines regarding such provisions. These provisions, particularly in the rules, should spell out the unethical conduct specifically. Unethical behavior is not necessarily illegal unless it is legally prohibited by law or rule. In the realm of quasi-penal statutes, such as a practice act with penalty provisions, standards are important to provide the basis for prosecution. If the described behavior is too vague, the provision may be unenforceable.

# Key Area #6
# Use of Titles

## MODEL LANGUAGE

### Use of Titles, Restrictions, Classification of Violation

A. A physical therapist shall use the letters "PT" in connection with the physical therapist's name or place of business to denote licensure under this [chapter, act, section, law].

B. A person or business entity, its employees, agents or representatives shall not use in connection with that person's name or the name or activity of the business, the words "physical therapy," "physical therapist," "physiotherapy," "physiotherapist" or "registered physical therapist," the letters "PT," "LPT," "RPT," or any other words, abbreviations or insignia indicating or implying directly or indirectly that physical therapy is provided or supplied, including the billing of services labeled as physical therapy, unless such services are provided by or under the direction of a physical therapist licensed pursuant to this [chapter, etc.]. A person or entity that violates this subsection is guilty of a [cite specific legal sanction].

C. A physical therapist assistant shall use the letters "PTA" in connection with that person's name to denote certification hereunder.

D. A person shall not use the title "physical therapist assistant," the letters "PTA," or any other words, abbreviations or insignia in connection with that person's name to indicate or imply, directly or indirectly, that the person is a physical therapist assistant unless that person is certified as a physical therapist assistant pursuant to this [chapter, etc.]. A person who violates this subsection is guilty of a [cite specific legal sanction].

## DISCUSSION

Two of the most significant sections of a practice act are 1) the granting of a scope of practice and 2) title protection. The state legislature, acting on behalf of the public and their protection, grants scope of practice privileges and imposes certain restrictions on that practice. Because of the licensee's unique education and skill and his or her potential to provide beneficial service when such knowledge and skill is used properly, as well as his or her potential to harm the public, the public is afforded some assurance that licensed health care providers are who they say they are and can do what they say they can do. So a scope of practice is granted along with the protected and exclusive use of titles and letter designations that identify a given practitioner to the public. The language used in this area of statute is, therefore, very important.

Title protection encompasses names and titles, as well as the letters and abbreviations that are associated with professional degrees. Titles such as medical doctor, nurse, podiatrist, physical therapist, chiropractor, dentist, etc., are examples of titles protected under title protection clauses of practice acts. Corresponding names of professions such as medicine, nursing, podiatry, physical therapy, chiropractic, dentistry, etc., should also be protected professional names. Examples of letter abbreviations include MD, DO, RN, DPM, PT, DC, DDS, etc., and are appropriately protected designations. Paragraph (B) above addresses all such titles, designations and abbreviations applicable to physical therapy.

The reason for including such terms as "physiotherapy," which is the international title of the profession, is to preclude misleading use of terms by other individuals or professions. Some claim that "physical therapy" and "physiotherapy" are generic terms and that they are entitled to their use. This claim that physical therapy is a generic term is misleading, and legislatures should be made aware of the importance of protecting any such related terms that imply physical therapy is being provided. The argument is not against members of other professions using various physical agents, modalities or procedures. The argument is against the inappropriate labeling of those modalities and procedures as, or equating them to, physical therapy. "Physiotherapy" is already a restricted term in about one-half of the state physical therapy practice acts, but, should be included as a restricted term in all acts. (See additional discussion under key area *Unlawful Practice:* paragraph (A), and *Guidelines for Rules, Key Area #2: Physiotherapy/ Physiotherapist Definition.*)

The various combinations of letter designations encompass those generally used, or expected to be used, in physical therapy. But the use of the phrase " . . . or any other words, abbreviations or insignia indicating or implying directly or indirectly that physical therapy is provided or supplied . . .," will provide latitude to address other violations that may occur.

Paragraph (A) indicates the legally required use of a professional letter designation in association with one's name. "PT" is the most common designation, but not the only designation currently used by physical therapists. It is desirable to have a consistent standard throughout the profession and from state to state. This statute clause emphasizes that "PT" is the consistent standard, just as MD, DO, RN, DPM, etc., are consistent designations used by other professions. There is no prohibition against adding—but not substituting—other letter designations indicating academic degree (e.g., MS, PhD), professional degree (e.g., DPT), certification (e.g., ATC), or honorary status (e.g., FAPTA), but all such additional designations should follow the standard "PT" designation. For example, a board-certified orthopedic specialist would be appropriately designated as Jane Doe, PT, OCS. Archaic designations such as RPT or LPT, while they may be protected designations, should not be used. Rules may be considered that even prohibit the use of such archaic designations. (See *Guidelines for Rules, Key Area #6.*)

Licensing boards should print original licenses and certificates and renewal cards with the letters "PT" and "PTA" respectively following the names of those licensed or certified. Often these licenses and certificates are printed without any letter designations. If licenses are to be displayed for public view, the proper designations should be included.

Paragraphs (C) and (D) add much stronger title protection to physical therapist assistants. In view of other disciplines that may claim they are providing "physical therapy" and delegate the provision of modalities to office staff or aides under their supervision, this clause becomes more important. It should be noted that this is one area where title protection is granted without a corresponding granting of a scope of practice. This is a regulatory concept proposed by the Pew Commission and is appropriately applied in this situation. Physical therapist assistants, while being granted title protection, do not practice physical therapy. They assist physical therapists in the provision of physical therapy services. (See *Definitions, Lawful Practice, Patient Care Management, Licensure and Examination* key areas, and *Appendix C, FSBPT Position Paper: Physical Therapist Assistant Regulation,* October 1998.)

An inappropriate use of letter terminology is where students use, or are required to use, the letters SPT or SPTA on nametags, in signing notes or with other means of identification. This portrays a false representation of achieved professional credentials, when, in fact, the professional credentials are yet to be obtained. The proper approach is simply to use the term "physical therapy student," "physical therapist assistant student" or the name or letters of the academic institution followed by "student" following their name (e.g., Jane Doe, Duke Student). Statutes or rules should not be adopted that allow for the use of the SPT or SPTA letter designations, and rules may be adopted prescribing appropriate terminology for students. (See *Guidelines for Rules.*)

## Additional Legal Considerations

Legally, it is important not only to statutorily establish a title but also give it protection. This area accomplishes this task and also integrates with the *Definitions, Licensure and Examination,* and *Unlawful Practice* key areas. Such use of the title legally denotes education, degree and position and demonstrates, for the benefit of the public, a legal basis for providing qualified physical therapy practice and the support of that practice. This, together with the legislative enactment of the scope of practice, is the legal foundation for title protection. Based on such demonstration of legislative intent, the term "physical therapy" and the title "physical therapist" and the designation "PT" are not generic and are not to be used in the public domain without a legal basis.

Title protection should not necessarily be seen as protecting the provider but as that which protects the public from misrepresentation, confusion and harm. If the public believes they are receiving "physical therapy" because a non-physical therapist provider, licensed or otherwise, is administering physical agents and calling it "physical therapy," then the public is being defrauded and may be at risk. Great efforts should be made to ensure that the focus and content of this area should not be diluted in the legislature to change its full import of consumer protection and professional integrity.

# Key Area #7
# Patient Care Management

## MODEL LANGUAGE

### Patient Care Management

A. A physical therapist is responsible for managing all aspects of the physical therapy care of each patient. The physical therapist shall provide:
   1. The initial written evaluation for each patient;
   2. Periodic written re-evaluation of each patient;
   3. A written discharge plan for the patient and the patient's response to treatment at discharge.

B. A physical therapist shall assure the qualifications of all assistive personnel to perform specific designated tasks through written documentation of the assistive personnel's education or training.

C. For each date of service, a physical therapist shall provide all therapeutic interventions that require the expertise of a physical therapist and shall determine the use of assistive personnel that provides delivery of service that is safe, effective, and efficient for each patient.
   1. A physical therapist assistant shall work under a physical therapist's supervision. A physical therapist assistant may document care provided without the co-signature of the supervising physical therapist. [Any further limitations on supervision of the physical therapist assistant should be specified here and/or clarified in rules.]
   2. A physical therapist may use physical therapy aides for designated routine tasks. A physical therapy aide shall work under the on-site supervision of a physical therapist who is continuously on-site and present in the facility. This may extend to an off-site setting only when the physical therapy aide is accompanying and working directly with a physical therapist assistant with a specific patient. [Any further

limitations on the use of physical therapy aides should be specified here and/or clarified in rules.]

D. A physical therapist may concurrently utilize no more than any combination of [specify the number] assistive personnel. In addition to [specify the number] assistive personnel, a physical therapist may supervise any combination of [specify the number] additional persons who are physical therapist students, physical therapist assistant students or physical therapists under restricted license or interim permit.

E. A physical therapist's responsibility for patient care management shall include oversight of all documentation for services rendered to each patient, including awareness of fees charged or reimbursement methodology used. A physical therapist shall also be aware of what constitutes unreasonable or fraudulent fees.

## DISCUSSION

### Patient Care Management

**A. A physical therapist is responsible for managing all aspects of the physical therapy care of each patient. The physical therapist shall provide:**

**1. The initial written evaluation for each patient;**

**2. Periodic written re-evaluation of each patient;**

**3. A written discharge plan for the patient and the patient's response to treatment at discharge.**

Central to practice and patient care management is the fact that licensed physical therapists always remain professionally and legally responsible for the therapeutic interventions they personally render plus those components of intervention rendered by assistive personnel under their supervision. This responsibility is not diminished even when assistive personnel are licensed or otherwise regulated. The practice of physical therapy includes examination, evaluation and testing for purposes of determining a diagnosis (for physical therapy), a prognosis, a plan of therapeutic intervention, and assessing the ongoing effects of intervention. These responsibilities of a physical therapist are evaluative in nature and are non-delegable. They comprise the subject matter of what should be documented in consequence of subparagraphs 1–3 of the model statute paragraph above.

**B. A physical therapist shall assure the qualifications of all assistive personnel to perform specific designated tasks through written documentation of the assistive personnel's education or training.**

The use of assistive personnel is a patient care management decision made by each physical therapist with each patient and on each date of service. The first decision that the physical therapist must make is whether assistive personnel are qualified to assist in a particular component of patient care. Such qualifications should be written and documented. For the physical therapist assistant, this should at least include documentation of educational training and regulatory credentialing. For physical therapy aides, this should at least include written evidence of on-the-job training by the physical therapist.

C. **For each date of service, a physical therapist shall provide all therapeutic interventions that require the expertise of a physical therapist and shall determine the use of assistive personnel that provides for delivery of service that is safe, effective, and efficient for each patient.**

Physical therapy practice includes various therapeutic interventions, and after the evaluative components of care, the next responsibility that a physical therapist has is to determine and provide those portions of any physical therapy intervention requiring their expertise and direct involvement.

Determining when to use assistive personnel on each date of service and for each patient also includes the knowledge that the use of assistive personnel will be safe or will enhance the safety of the patient, that interventions will continue to be effective, and that the use of assistive personnel is an efficient use of resources.

1. **A physical therapist assistant shall work under a physical therapist's supervision. A physical therapist assistant may document care provided without the co-signature of the supervising physical therapist. [Any further limitations on supervision of the physical therapist assistant should be specified here and/or clarified in rules.]**

The default language of this model paragraph assumes that the physical therapist assistant is authorized under the practice act to work in an off-site setting and under the general supervision of a physical therapist. If a state chooses any variation from this it should be specified in this paragraph. For example, any state requiring on-site supervision of physical therapist assistants would insert the single word "on-site" prior to the word "supervision" in the first sentence so that it would read " . . . shall work under a physical therapist's on-site supervision." There may be other supervisory requirements and procedures related to communication and documentation that are more appropriately addressed in rules.

2. **A physical therapist may use physical therapy aides for designated routine tasks. A physical therapy aide shall work under the on-site supervision of a physical therapist who is continuously on-site and present in the facility. This may extend to an off-site setting only when the physical therapy aide is accompanying and working directly with a physical therapist assistant with a specific patient. [Any further limita-**

**tions on the use of physical therapy aides should be specified here and/or clarified in rules.]**

The definition of "on-site supervision" is an important definition included in the *Definitions* key area, paragraph (H). Part of that definition is reiterated here but the entire definition applies.

In 1999 the American Physical Therapy Association's House of Delegates addressed issues related to using physical therapy aides to assist in physical therapy interventions. The intent of adopted APTA positions is to restrict or limit use of physical therapy aides in direct physical therapy interventions, although the extent of such limitations were not fully defined.

To guide states in practice act construction, the Model Practice Act suggests the following for consideration:

a. States should at least adopt the basic language in this subparagraph 2. This language limits use of aides to onsite (previously defined), allows use of an aide in a off-site setting only when working directly with a physical therapist assistant, and allows the physical therapist to determine what "designated routine tasks" mean for the particular department or practice. The phrase "designated routine tasks" is distinctly different from "selected components of intervention" as used in model definition for physical therapist assistants.
b. Where a state chooses to enact more explicit restrictions, a functional definition may be included within this statute paragraph. For example, "For purposes of this subparagraph, 'designated routine tasks' means [or includes, or does not include, etc.] . . ." The Model Practice Act does not specify what such restrictions should be, but instead leaves any such additional restrictions to the jurisdictions for their consideration.

There are situations where physical therapists in extended care, home health or school settings train others to carry out certain exercises or activities for the benefit of patients or clients. Such training in exercise or activities is appropriate as an extension of the educational and consultative responsibilities of a physical therapist, as set forth in the definition of the "Practice of Physical Therapy." (See the *Definitions* key area.) However, unless a physical therapist is on-site and personally involved with such activities as an integral part of a physical therapy plan of care and intervention it is no different than giving instruction to a family member to assist a patient with their home exercise program. Activities carried out under such circumstances should not be represented as, or billed as, physical therapy services.

**D. A physical therapist may concurrently utilize no more than any combination of [specify the number] assistive personnel. In addition to [specify the number] assistive personnel, a physical therapist may supervise any combination of [specify the number] additional persons**

**who are physical therapist students, physical therapist assistant students or physical therapists under restricted license or interim permit.**

It is a reasonable assumption that there are limits to the capacity of a physical therapist to perform their responsibilities in patient care and management and also fulfill a supervisory role with others. For purposes of patient protection and in the interest of assuring quality care, the Model Practice Act recommends that states adopt this statute paragraph with appropriate limitations on the number of assistive personnel and others that a physical therapist may personally supervise. It would also be appropriate to move such a paragraph to rules rather than place it in statutes, especially if this is a number that might be expected to change over time.

E. **A physical therapist's responsibility for patient care management shall include oversight of all documentation for services rendered to each patient, including awareness of fees charged or reimbursement methodology used. A physical therapist shall also be aware of what constitutes unreasonable or fraudulent fees.**

Professional services include all documentation associated with such services and the professional fees for the services. These responsibilities are inherent and are non-delegable in professional practice. Awareness of fees charged or the reimbursement methodology used relates directly to the physical therapist's legal and ethical responsibility to ensure that fees are reasonable and that fraudulent billing practices are not employed.

## ADDITIONAL LEGAL CONSIDERATIONS

It is axiomatic that within the professional scope and practice of physical therapy, the physical therapist is ultimately and comprehensively responsible for patient care management. The physical therapist's position, from a practice and legal perspective, is not unlike the head surgeon during an operation, which has developed into the legal doctrine of "Captain of the Ship." While the physical therapist may utilize assistive personnel in caring for the patients' needs, it is the skill, education and expertise of the physical therapist that makes the critical patient care management decisions from the initial evaluation to the final patient discharge under the Model Practice Act. In exercising responsibility for care management decisions, the patients' health, safety and welfare must be at the forefront of the physical therapist's decisions. To assist the proper management of the patients' care, the following legal points may be instructional and useful:

- In the area of patient care management, standards and guidelines are very important, particularly with assistive personnel such as physical therapist assistants who may have more off-site supervised work opportunities in certain jurisdictions. It is important to know and document the physical therapist assistant's experience, training and education, his or her skill level as well as the status and complexity of the condition of the patient. The supervising physical therapist's management decisions regarding the use of assistive personnel for components of the treatment intervention will differ based on these details.

- Another reason to develop management standards is the potential for liability for the licensed physical therapist. Management of acts, procedures, etc. to such personnel assisting the licensed physical therapist brings to the foreground the legal principle of "vicarious liability." Plainly stated, the old common-law principle means the employer is responsible for the acts of his or her employees who work within the scope of the employer's business. This legal principle operated in the physical therapist's favor in the past when physical therapy was more of a prescriptive practice and the therapist basically carried out the physician's orders. In that era, strictly following the physician's prescription gave the physical therapist great protection from liability based on the above legal principle. Now it is essentially the physical therapist who effectively determines and manages the plan of physical therapy care for the patient and supervises how it is carried out. Further, the establishment of such management standards is even more important considering the physical therapist often manages multiple assistive personnel in providing patient care.

For the above reasons, the statutes and the profession's *Code of Ethics* made the licensed physical therapist responsible for managing physical therapy care. Employing adequate management standards, guidelines and procedures with the assistive personnel is not only necessary, but is a safeguard to limit the potential liability of each physical therapist who is involved in the management of patient care through physical therapy intervention.

# Key Area #8 Grounds for Disciplinary Action

## MODEL LANGUAGE

### Grounds for Disciplinary Action

The following are grounds for disciplinary action:

1. Violating any provision of this [chapter, act, section, law], board rules or a written order of the board.
2. Practicing or offering to practice beyond the scope of the practice of physical therapy.
3. Obtaining or attempting to obtain a license or certificate by fraud or misrepresentation.
4. Engaging in the performance of substandard care by a physical therapist due to a deliberate or negligent act or failure to act regardless of whether actual injury to the patient is established.
5. Engaging in the performance of substandard care by a physical therapist assistant, including exceeding the authority to perform components of intervention selected by the supervising licensee regardless of whether actual injury to the patient is established.
6. Failing to supervise assistive personnel in accordance with this [chapter, etc.] and board rules.
7. Having been convicted of a felony in the courts of this state or any other state, territory or country. Conviction, as used in this paragraph, shall include a finding or verdict of guilt, an admission of guilt, or a plea of nolo contendere.
8. Practicing as a physical therapist or working as a physical therapist assistant when physical or mental abilities are impaired by the use of controlled substances or other habit-forming drugs, chemicals or alcohol.

9. Having had a license or certificate revoked or suspended, other disciplinary action taken, or an application for licensure or certification refused, revoked or suspended by the proper authorities of another state, territory or country.
10. Engaging in sexual misconduct. For the purpose of this paragraph sexual misconduct includes:
    a. Engaging in or soliciting sexual relationships, whether consensual or non-consensual, while a physical therapist or physical therapist assistant/patient relationship exists.
    b. Making sexual advances, requesting sexual favors or engaging in other verbal conduct or physical contact of a sexual nature with patients or clients.
    c. Intentionally viewing a completely or partially disrobed patient in the course of treatment if the viewing is not related to patient diagnosis or treatment under current practice standards.
11. Directly or indirectly requesting, receiving or participating in the dividing, transferring, assigning, rebating or refunding of an unearned fee, or profiting by means of a credit or other valuable consideration such as an unearned commission, discount, or gratuity in connection with the furnishing of physical therapy services. This does not prohibit the members of any regularly and properly organized business entity recognized by law and comprising physical therapists from dividing fees received for professional services among themselves as they determine necessary to defray their joint operating expense.
12. Failing to adhere to the recognized standards of ethics of the physical therapy profession.
13. Charging unreasonable or fraudulent fees for services performed or not performed.
14. Making misleading, deceptive, untrue or fraudulent representations in violation of this [chapter, etc.] or in the practice of the profession.
15. Having been adjudged mentally incompetent by a court of competent jurisdiction.
16. Aiding or abetting a person who is not licensed or certified in this state and who directly or indirectly performs activities requiring a license or certificate.
17. Failing to report to the board any act or omission of a licensee, certificate holder, applicant or any other person who violates the provisions of this [chapter, etc.].
18. Interfering with an investigation or disciplinary proceeding by willful misrepresentation of facts or by the use of threats or harassment against any patient or witness to prevent them from providing evidence in a disciplinary proceeding or any legal action.

19. Failing to maintain patient confidentiality without prior written consent of the patient or unless otherwise required by law.
20. Failing to maintain adequate patient records. For the purposes of this paragraph, "adequate patient records" means legible records that contain at a minimum sufficient information to identify the patient, an evaluation of objective findings, a diagnosis, the plan of care, the treatment record and a discharge plan.
21. Promoting an unnecessary device, treatment intervention or service for the financial gain of the practitioner or of a third party.
22. Providing treatment intervention unwarranted by the condition of the patient, or continuing treatment beyond the point of reasonable benefit.
23. Participating in underutilization or overutilization of physical therapy services for personal or institutional financial gain, or participation in services that are in any way linked to the financial gain of a referral source.

## DISCUSSION

### Grounds for Disciplinary Action

**The following are grounds for disciplinary action:**

The following list itemizes the various causes or grounds for which a licensed physical therapist, and in many cases a certified physical therapist assistant, may be disciplined under the provisions of the law. These two persons are the only ones falling under this disciplinary authority. Others who may be attempting to practice physical therapy unlawfully come under the powers granted a licensing board in the *Unlawful Practice* key area. In many practice acts this list is referred to as "Unprofessional Conduct." The term "Grounds for Disciplinary Action" is more precise and descriptive and is the recommended title for this section. This statute section needs to be comprehensive and broad enough to cover all areas of potential violation. The clarity and intent of this language is important as it empowers licensure boards to act in areas pertaining to discipline of licensees and certificate holders.

Ignorance of the law should not be considered a defense for acting or not acting. This is where use of a jurisprudence exam, even an open book exam, at the time of initial licensure or certification helps to underscore this legal responsibility and develops greater familiarity with the following potential violations of conduct.

1. **Violating any provision of this [chapter, act, section, law] board rules or a written order of the board.**

This clause provides the broadest enabling foundation for disciplinary action. It encompasses statutes, rules and written disciplinary orders.

2. **Practicing or offering to practice beyond the scope of the practice of physical therapy.**

   The determination and interpretation of what constitutes practice beyond the scope of practice of physical therapy will largely rest with the members of licensure boards. They will be guided by the three determinants of scope of practice: history of educational inclusion, history of practice inclusion, and enabling statute authority or lack of statutory prohibition when educational and practice inclusion are established. (See discussion in *Definitions: Practice of Physical Therapy.*) Scope of practice may be somewhat dynamic, and boards will need the latitude to determine the appropriateness of certain procedures as they relate to established scope of practice.
3. **Obtaining or attempting to obtain a license or certificate by fraud or misrepresentation.**

   Unfortunately, this potential violation is more common than might be imagined. It has been especially true in recent years with increased demand for physical therapists and the pressure to license more foreign-educated physical therapists, many of whom may not meet licensure requirements and may resort to fraudulent applications. Another potential use of this clause is where a licensee or certificate holder who has previously been disciplined in another state makes application and withholds information regarding previous disciplinary action.
4. **Engaging in the performance of substandard care by a physical therapist due to a deliberate or negligent act or failure to act regardless of whether actual injury to the patient is established.**

   This clause makes it clear that substandard care, deliberate or negligent acts, or failure to act by the licensee—whether or not actual injury is established—all constitute grounds for disciplinary action. This includes a deliberate act, a negligent act, a deliberate failure to act, or a negligent failure to act. Injury does not need to be established when those acts become substandard or potentially injurious to a patient. Refer to discussion in *Guidelines for Rules, Key Area #8*, for a definition of "substandard care."
5. **Engaging in the performance of substandard care by a physical therapist assistant, including exceeding the authority to perform components of intervention selected by the supervising licensee regardless of whether actual injury to the patient is established.**

   Where the previous clause focuses on the acts of licensees, this clause deals similarly with the acts of certified physical therapist assistants. "Substandard care" may need further clarification and even definition within rules. (See *Guidelines for Rules, Key Area #8: Substandard Care.*) At the very least, it is defined here to include "exceeding the authority to perform components of intervention that have been selected by the supervising licensee."

6. **Failing to supervise assistive personnel in accordance with this [chapter, etc.] and board rules.**

A physical therapist remains responsible for the entire scope of patient management (examination, evaluation, diagnosis, prognosis, and intervention), and is responsible as well for the use of assistive personnel in delivering selected components of intervention on each date of service. It is a practice act and the adopted rules that govern supervisory requirements. The practice act always takes precedence over such things as Medicare policy, APTA policy, or hospital standards. Adequate supervision is further clarified and discussed under key areas *Definitions, Patient Care Management,* and *Guidelines for Rules, Key Area #7: Patient Care Management.*

7. **Having been convicted of a felony in the courts of this state or any other state, territory or country. Conviction, as used in this paragraph, shall include a finding or verdict of guilt, an admission of guilt, or a plea of nolo contendere.**

This paragraph gives the board broad authority to deal with either a licensee or certificate holder who has been convicted of a felony. However, conviction per se may not necessarily be grounds for any of the potential disciplinary actions a board may take as listed under *Disciplinary Actions/ Procedures.* Legal counsel to state licensure boards may advise boards that before any discipline or restriction of practice may be imposed, there must be a relationship between the felony the licensee or certificate holder is convicted of and a risk to the public due to impaired judgement or other factors. This should always be an area for legal counsel review before board action.

8. **Practicing as a physical therapist or working as a physical therapist assistant when physical or mental abilities are impaired by the use of controlled substances or other habit-forming drugs, chemicals or alcohol.**

The *Consumer Advocacy* key area has a section on the impaired professional. It provides for the option of allowing for a first-time voluntary participation in a substance abuse program rather than disciplinary proceedings. Here, this paragraph grants the board authority to initiate and carry out disciplinary action where appropriate. This would generally be where convictions have already occurred or occurred with repeated impairment. Any restrictions on a licensee or certificate holder related to substance abuse will require this enabling statute. The safety and welfare of patients is of highest priority and is the focus of this statute language. The treatment of the impaired professional recognizes the need to pursue active rehabilitation with anyone so impaired.

9. **Having had a license or certificate revoked or suspended, other disciplinary action taken, or an application for licensure or certification**

**refused, revoked or suspended by the proper authorities of another state, territory or country.**

Disciplinary action invoked under the authority of this paragraph would obviously require further discovery and collaboration of other issues that suggest the need for restrictions of a license or certificate, more severe ongoing discipline, or the actual loss of—or refusal to issue—a license or certificate. Again, as stated in the discussion of paragraph (7) above, action of previous revocation, suspension or other disciplinary action may not be a per se reason for further disciplinary action. But this statute gives boards full latitude to address this circumstance.

10. **Engaging in sexual misconduct. For the purpose of this paragraph sexual misconduct includes:**
    (a) **Engaging in or soliciting sexual relationships, whether consensual or non-consensual, while a physical therapist or physical therapist assistant/patient relationship exists.**
    (b) **Making sexual advances, requesting sexual favors or engaging in other verbal conduct or physical contact of a sexual nature with patients or clients.**
    (c) **Intentionally viewing a completely or partially disrobed patient in the course of treatment if the viewing is not related to patient diagnosis or treatment under current practice standards.**

The first sentence is the focus of the law: Do not engage in sexual misconduct. The remainder of the clause is the operational definition of what constitutes sexual misconduct. A significant number of the disciplinary actions against physical therapists involve sexual misconduct. To violate the provisions of this law, physical therapists or physical therapist assistants do not need to actually engage in sexual relations—even the solicitation of such is a violation. The violation is not excused, even in the case of a consensual sexual relationship with a patient. California statutes, for example, go as far as to say that "a patient, client, or customer of a licentiate under this chapter is conclusively presumed to be incapable of giving free, full, and informed consent to any sexual activity . . ." Any sexual relationship or sexual contact with a patient, consensual or nonconsensual, is prohibited under law. Sexual misconduct also includes activities specified in subparagraph (b) above, which essentially defines sexual harassment. Subparagraph (c) above is language that is beginning to appear in some practice acts and expands sexual misconduct to inappropriate examination or treatment that exposes a patient unnecessarily and for improper motives. The practice of physical therapy at times may truly involve the examination and treatment of nearly the entire human body. Yet there are principles of decency and modesty that are basic to proper professional conduct and, when violated for improper motives, will constitute grounds for disciplinary action.

11. **Directly or indirectly requesting, receiving or participating in the dividing, transferring, assigning, rebating or refunding of an unearned fee, or profiting by means of a credit or other valuable consideration such as an unearned commission, discount, or gratuity in connection with the furnishing of physical therapy services. This does not prohibit the members of any regularly and properly organized business entity recognized by law and comprising physical therapists from dividing fees received for professional services among themselves as they determine necessary to defray their joint operating expense.**

Ethical standards encourage physical therapists to always base clinical and business decisions on the needs of the patient, and never on financial remuneration. Ideally, this particular ethical standard should also be the legal standard, or that which is required rather than simply encouraged. The complexity of business and practice environments, however, requires a fairly specific and identifiable standard like this paragraph.

The Model Practice Act does not directly address employment relationships with referral sources. While this issue has been debated for two decades in professional circles, it is impossible and impractical to legislatively address every practice or employment situation. There will always be some decisions in which the licensee must use his or her own ethical and moral compass as a guide. Beyond this section, the Model Practice Act does, however, give some guidance regarding this issue in several places. In paragraphs (21) and (22) of this section, model language deals with patient exploitation. Paragraph (22) clearly states, "providing treatment intervention unwarranted by the condition of the patient, or continuing treatment beyond the point of reasonable benefit," would constitute grounds for disciplinary action. Disclosure is also a topic under *Consumer Advocacy: Rights of Consumers* key area.

12. **Failing to adhere to the recognized standards of ethics of the physical therapy profession.**

This important clause empowers a licensing board to raise the level of conduct of those regulated by the practice act. It allows the recognized ethical standards of the profession to be used in disciplinary actions. (See full discussion under *Lawful Practice,* paragraph C.) As previously mentioned, states approach this differently. Some may simply adopt the clause under *Lawful Practice,* paragraph (C) in combination with this statute paragraph, and not include further specific detail about what the ethical standards are. In such a case, the history and consistency of a licensing board's actions in referring to and using the profession's established ethical code and guide would be important. In other states the legislature or rules process may require the professional code to either be specifically referenced or even the code's language being included in statutes or rules, preferably rules if this is the case. Nevertheless, either way, there is clear legal precedence for state regulatory boards utilizing the established ethical standards of the profession in disciplinary matters. (See *Additional Legal Considerations* following, and *Guidelines for Rules, Key Areas* #5 and #8.)

13. **Charging unreasonable or fraudulent fees for services performed or not performed.**

The charging of unreasonable fees and fraudulent billing of services performed or not performed occurs and must be addressed by licensing boards. Even with the advent of managed care and mandated fee schedules, there are still opportunities for fee-for-service arrangements where fees that might be considered unreasonable could be charged. For the protection of the public, boards need the authority to address public complaints focusing on unreasonable fees. The two issues of "unreasonable" and "fraudulent" fees are combined here with the implication that a clearly unreasonable fee may reach the proportion of being considered fraudulent. (See *Guidelines for Rules, Key Area #8, Unreasonable Fees.*)

The possibility also exists that a case rate or capitated contract rate could be so unreasonably *low* that adequate quality of care could not be expected. A case might be made under such a scenario for a public protection concern by a licensing board.

14. **Making misleading, deceptive, untrue or fraudulent representations in violation of this [chapter, etc.] or in the practice of the profession.**

Part of the basis of professional practice is the legal right to "profess" to others certain qualifications, knowledge, skills and abilities in a particular healing art and science. Potential violations of this clause may include private or public statements or representations of one's ability to diagnose or provide treatment for conditions outside the scope of physical therapy practice, or to make false or misleading advertisement or promotion regarding one's services. This clause is not intended in any way to restrict or limit advertisement or promotion.

The statute language is broad enough that it could also be applied to business operations, employment-related issues, billing practices or any other activity related to the operation of physical therapy services that may be misleading, deceptive, untrue or fraudulent.

15. **Having been adjudged mentally incompetent by a court of competent jurisdiction.**

Mental incompetence is a judgment made outside the scope of a physical therapy licensing board's responsibility. There may be situations where disease or injury, e.g., an auto injury, renders a physical therapist only marginally able to perform the duties of a practicing physical therapist. Concern for patient safety and concern that a patient receives appropriate care may merit board action restricting or denying licensure in a situation where a court of law has made the determination of mental incompetence. The *Disciplinary Actions/Procedures: Investigative Powers* section, paragraph (6) authorizes and empowers the board to require a licensee to be examined for mental, physical or professional competence.

16. **Aiding or abetting a person who is not licensed or certified in this state and who directly or indirectly performs activities requiring a license or certificate.**

The most frequent use of this paragraph will generally be with a licensee who is very loosely supervising and lending his or her license to the illegal practice of physical therapy. This occurs where someone not licensed or certified is providing services represented to be physical therapy without the legal and proper supervision of a physical therapist. There have been occurrences of other health care providers utilizing an aide to provide services represented and billed as physical therapy, and the physical therapist has only done an evaluation or records review, thereby illegally lending his or her license to the billing of services that are not, in fact, physical therapy.

17. **Failing to report to the board any act or omission of a licensee, certificate holder, applicant or any other person who violates the provisions of this [chapter, etc.].**

Regulated health care professionals have an obligation to be knowledgeable about what constitutes legal and ethical conduct. This not only applies to personal conduct, but also the conduct of those supervised. For the protection of the public, this responsibility extends even further. If a licensee or certificate holder has knowledge of *anyone* violating the provisions of this act, he or she has a legal obligation to protect the public and report such acts or omissions to the board.

18. **Interfering with an investigation or disciplinary proceeding by willful misrepresentation of facts or by the use of threats or harassment against any patient or witness to prevent them from providing evidence in a disciplinary proceeding or any legal action.**

This provision is specific enough that it needs little in the way of further explanation. Any attempt to interfere with or cover up the facts of an investigation or disciplinary proceeding would be a violation of the statute and subject a licensee or certificate holder to further disciplinary action.

19. **Failing to maintain patient confidentiality without prior written consent of the patient or unless otherwise required by law.**

Patient/provider confidentiality is an inherent aspect of professional services. Initial patient registration information generally contains provisions for the proper and legal release of medical information upon written approval by the patient. This may include releases for transmittal of information to the patient's referring physician, insurance company, legal counsel, or others as appropriate. Violation of this patient/provider trust will, therefore, be more than just the violation of a trust, but also a violation of law. There may be other disclosure laws in a state that will govern or modify the provisions of this paragraph.

The Model Practice Act includes another, perhaps more definitive, statement on provider/patient confidentiality. This is located under *Consumer Advocacy: Rights of Consumers* section, paragraph (F).

**20. Failing to maintain adequate patient records. For the purposes of this paragraph, "adequate patient records" means legible records that contain at a minimum sufficient information to identify the patient, an evaluation of objective findings, a diagnosis, the plan of care, the treatment record and a discharge plan.**

Documentation is the means of recording the elements of physical therapy patient management. It is essential that those providing physical therapy maintain adequate records, from the initial history and examination to the discharge summary. Records are important not only for the reference of the one doing the documenting, but also for co-workers and colleagues, payors, patients and, in some cases, licensing boards. Numerous judgments and determinations are made based on these records. The model statute here also specifically defines the minimum standards for "adequate patient records."

**21. Promoting an unnecessary device, treatment intervention, or service for the financial gain of the practitioner or of a third party.**

**22. Providing treatment intervention unwarranted by the condition of the patient, or continuing treatment beyond the point of reasonable benefit.**

These ethical *principles* of conduct in paragraphs (21) and (22) are hereby made legal *requirements* of conduct for the benefit of the consumer of physical therapy services. Unnecessary devices, unnecessary treatment intervention, or overutilization are all prohibited under these paragraphs and would subject the provider to potential disciplinary action.

The focus of paragraph (21) involves a motive of financial gain. Paragraph (22), however, focuses on the effectiveness or lack of effectiveness of intervention, and whether the intervention is warranted at all or is extended beyond a reasonable period of time when no further benefit is apparent.

**23. Participating in underutilization or overutilization of physical therapy services for personal or institutional financial gain, or participation in services that are in any way linked to the financial gain of a referral source.**

An ethical issue that all health care professionals face relates to fees and patient management decisions. Under a fee-for-service payment methodology, an increase of intervention may result in realization of greater financial gain to the provider or employer. On the other hand, in a managed care system the denial or limitation of intervention may result in greater financial gain to a provider or employer. These types of conflicts are inherent in either system of payment. The problem comes when, in either system, the financial gain or loss becomes a greater driving force than the welfare of any single patient. When overutilization or underutilization are occurring in a pattern that clearly highlights that a patient's welfare is in the position of lower priority to provider or institutional financial gain, then there is a public protection interest that a board can and should act upon. This statute paragraph would authorize board intervention.

## ADDITIONAL LEGAL CONSIDERATIONS

Although most categories listed above as grounds for disciplinary action are self-explanatory, several legal points should be addressed. First, the grounds listed are only grounds, not legal violations per se. Each ground charged is still subject to the right of notice, hearing, adjudication and appeal under general due process requirements. (See *Disciplinary Actions/Procedures* key area.)

Additionally, some enumerated grounds, such as (2), (4), (11), (12), (13) and (23), as stated, are somewhat difficult to measure from a legal perspective. The previous *Discussion* of (2) illustrates the type of criteria the board should consider in such areas. However, matching the grounds with legally adequate evidence may be difficult in some instances. To the extent possible, therefore, standards and guidelines should be established in rules to assist the board or its prosecution arm in clarifying the more subjective grounds for discipline.

Paragraph (12), for example, is a good illustration of what could normally be a difficult ground to handle legally. A breach of ethics is not, *per se,* a violation of any law unless a particular code of ethics, in whole or in part, is adopted under such provision as law or in rules, or at least clearly cited or referenced as the accepted standard within the profession. There is precedent for states to adopt provisions of the American Physical Therapy Association's *Code of Ethics* into law or rules as well as relevant provisions of the *Guide for Professional Conduct.* In either instance, once specific *Code* or *Guide* provisions are adopted in law or rules, the proven violation of such ethical prohibition would be a violation of law.

Legal considerations relating to this section must be considered in concurrence with the *Disciplinary Actions/Procedures* key area.

# Key Area #9 Disciplinary Actions/Procedures

## MODEL LANGUAGE

### Investigative Powers, Emergency Action, Hearing Officers

A. To enforce this [chapter, act section, law] the board is authorized to:
   1. Receive complaints filed against licensees or certificate holders and conduct a timely investigation.
   2. Conduct an investigation at any time and on its own initiative without receipt of a written complaint if the board has reason to believe that there may be a violation of this [chapter, etc.].
   3. Issue subpoenas to compel the attendance of any witness or the production of any documentation relative to a case.
   4. Take emergency action ordering the summary suspension of a license or certificate or the restriction of the licensee's practice or certificate holder's employment pending proceedings by the board.
   5. Appoint hearing officers authorized to conduct hearings. Hearing officers shall prepare and submit to the board findings of fact, conclusions of law and an order that shall be reviewed and voted on by the board.
   6. Require a licensee to be examined in order to determine the licensee's mental, physical or professional competence.

B. If the board finds that the information received in a complaint or an investigation is not of sufficient seriousness to merit disciplinary action against a licensee or certificate holder it may take the following actions:
   1. Dismiss the complaint if the board believes the information or complaint is without merit.
   2. Issue a confidential advisory letter to the licensee or certificate holder. An advisory letter is non-disciplinary and notifies a licensee or

certificate holder that, while there is insufficient evidence to support disciplinary action, the board believes that the licensee or certificate holder should modify or eliminate certain conduct or practices.

### Hearings

[No model statute language is offered under this section heading. See *Discussion* for additional information.]

### Disciplinary Actions/Penalties

Upon proof that any grounds prescribed in section [cite section on *Grounds for Disciplinary Action*] have been violated, the board may take the following disciplinary actions singly or in combination:

1. Issue a censure.
2. Restrict a license or certificate. The board may require a licensee or certificate holder to report regularly to the board on matters related to the grounds for the restricted license or certificate.
3. Suspend a license or certificate for a period prescribed by the board.
4. Revoke a license or certificate.
5. Refuse to issue or renew a license or certificate.
6. Impose a civil penalty of at least ______________ but not more than ______________. [Include minimum and maximum dollar amounts of civil penalties.] In addition the board may assess and collect the reasonable costs incurred in a disciplinary hearing when action is taken against a person's license or certificate.
7. Accept a voluntary surrendering of a license or certificate.

### Procedural Due Process

Actions of the Board shall be taken subject to the right of notice, hearing and adjudication and the right of appeal in accordance with [specify the state] law relating to administrative law and procedure. [Or specify the state statute that addresses appeals or review of board decisions.]

## DISCUSSION

Most states have entire sections of administrative law, referred to as an Administrative Procedures Act, which may direct the disciplinary process, especially when dealing with the potential for a loss of one's license or certificate. At the very least, all procedural aspects of discipline need to be carefully delineated in rules. This process should outline the disciplinary procedures which, at the minimum, should include:

- Initiation and handling of complaints
- Investigation
- Informal disposition of complaints
- Summons and complaint issued by the board
- Pre-hearing discovery
- Subpoena and injunctive authority
- Informal interviews or hearings
- Formal hearings
- Settlement, consent orders, disciplinary actions

### Investigative Powers, Emergency Action, Hearing Officers

**A. To enforce this [chapter, act section, law] the board is authorized to:**

This section of the statutes is procedural in nature, but comprises the authorizing statutes allowing for receiving and investigating complaints, issuing subpoenas, emergency summary suspending of a license, and appointing hearing officers. All of these actions will have additional associated procedures in rules or in the uniform Administrative Procedures Acts of some states.

**1. Receive complaints filed against licensees or certificate holders and conduct a timely investigation.**

Rules written to conform to this statute should be very straightforward. Access to the complaint process by the public should be as simple as possible. There should be a standard complaint form, but provision should be made for complaints in any form from the public including written complaints, telephone complaints, or verbal complaints. The complainant must provide their name and address for follow-up contact. However, it should be specified that confidentiality will be maintained if the complainant so requests and within the limits of law. State confidentiality laws may be a factor in drafting conforming rules. (See *Guidelines for Rules, Key Area #9, Receiving Complaints.*)

**2. Conduct an investigation at any time and on its own initiative without receipt of a written complaint if the board has reason to believe that there may be a violation of this [chapter, etc.].**

Board members often become aware of possible infractions of the laws and rules. This may occur through inquiries to board members from physical therapists, staff, or from other sources about the legal appropriateness of certain occurrences. Boards need greater latitude to investigate such concerns without being required to wait for a formal complaint to be submitted.

**3. Issue subpoenas to compel the attendance of any witness or the production of any documentation relative to a case.**

Subpoenas may be used not only to compel witnesses to attend hearings but also to review and obtain records. A request for records often is the first step in initiating an investigation. An investigator may also need to do an on-site investigation of a practice or department that will include all pertinent records. The use of subpoenas in unannounced site investigations is occasionally a necessary part of the investigation of complaints.

Patient records that are subpoenaed under this authority should be accorded proper confidentiality. Therefore, specific model statute language is further recommended under *Key Area #11, Consumer Advocacy: Rights of Consumers*, paragraph (H), to specifically protect confidential patient information.

4. **Take emergency action ordering the summary suspension of a license or certificate or the restriction of the licensee's practice or certificate holder's employment pending proceedings by the board.**

   This statutory authority to take emergency action ordering summary suspension of a license or certificate has been lacking in many state practice acts. However, such authority is important to include in updating and modifying practice acts to improve responsiveness to the public. State boards have sometimes been required to wait weeks or months before a hearing can be conducted. The board needs authority to act on a complaint having serious implications for public protection. Conforming rules may specify parameters for the use of this authority and be responsive to other legal precedents in such summary suspension proceedings.

5. **Appoint hearing officers authorized to conduct hearings. Hearing officers shall prepare and submit to the board findings of fact, conclusions of law and an order that shall be reviewed and voted on by the board.**

   This is another area of board procedure that varies considerably from state to state. When the hearing process reaches the formal level, the preferred procedure is to use an independent hearing officer to conduct the hearing. Assistant attorneys general sometimes represent state boards in conducting such hearings, but they have a conflict of interest in conducting a hearing impartially while still representing the board. Sometimes boards themselves conduct such hearings. Administrative procedures acts may specify that hearing officers shall be administrative law judges. If that is the case, the reference to "administrative law judges" may be more appropriate than "hearing officers."

   The recommended model is to use independent hearing officers who will conduct hearings, accept pleas, preside over opening statements and closing arguments, preside over the direct, cross, re-direct and re-cross examination of the accused and witnesses, and propose an order for final decision by the board. These procedures should be specified in rules or referenced in a uniform Administrative Procedures Act.

6. **Require a licensee to be examined in order to determine the licensee's mental, physical or professional competence.**

There may be times when a person's mental, physical or professional competence as a licensee or applicant may be questioned. This paragraph empowers a board to direct appropriate evaluations for such competence if the circumstances warrant it. This is also an area of law that needs to be navigated very carefully. The Americans with Disabilities Act may pose some legal questions, perhaps valid questions, of what is appropriate or inappropriate to evaluate. However broad this model statute language is, and it is broad, it will need to be tempered with the legal counsel that state boards have at their disposal.

**B. If the board finds that the information received in a complaint or an investigation is not of sufficient seriousness to merit disciplinary action against a licensee or certificate holder it may take the following actions:**

Paragraph (b), with its two subparagraphs, addresses appropriate responses a board may take where an investigation determines that no violation of law exists.

**1. Dismiss the complaint if the board believes the information or complaint is without merit.**

The obvious outcome of a complaint and subsequent investigation that comes to a conclusion that no violation of law or rules has occurred is that the complaint is dismissed. Appropriate notification of such a dismissal is important to both parties of a complaint—the complainant and the person who is the subject of the complaint.

One other concept that is worth considering is the formation of a board complaint resolution subcommittee. This is discussed further in *Guidelines for Rules* under the topic of unreasonable fees. There may be complaints that never rise to the level of a violation of law, yet responsiveness to the public might warrant an attempted effort to resolve issues that might end in a more favorable reconciliation of both parties. Some may find this beyond the role of a board but this is well within the stated purpose clause of the model practice act to "promote the public interest."

**2. Issue a confidential advisory letter to the licensee or certificate holder. An advisory letter is non-disciplinary and notifies a licensee or certificate holder that, while there is insufficient evidence to support disciplinary action, the board believes that the licensee or certificate holder should modify or eliminate certain conduct or practices.**

Historically, boards have been inclined to deal only with whether a licensee violated a law or not, and have not provided advice to those regulated that might have averted a complaint in the first place. However, the model practice act has consistently put forth a broader role for licensing boards in its language and concepts. This statute is an important inclusion granting boards authority to address issues of conduct it deems problematic, although not illegal. This paragraph will offer a board a means to give guidance, in the spirit of public protection, which may avert future violation of law and potential injury to the public.

Because such an action is clearly advisory—not disciplinary and not punitive in any way—it is recommended that such an advisory letter not be a matter of public record where it might be misconstrued.

## Hearings

**[No model statute language is provided under this section.]**

At the very minimum there should be a statute paragraph referring to the state's Administrative Procedures Act. For states that might not have or feel they have an inadequate Administrative Procedures Act, this statute section should exist at this point in the Physical Therapy Law. Topics under this section may include:

- Authority to request informal and formal hearings
- Authority to take limited disciplinary action after informal hearings
- Authority and procedure for notice of a formal hearing
- Right of anyone appearing before the board to be represented by counsel
- Authority to administer the oath to witnesses
- Right for board to waive the technical rules of evidence in hearings
- Right to file motion for rehearing or review of board decision within specified time period.

## Disciplinary Actions/Penalties

**Upon proof that any grounds prescribed in section [cite section on *Grounds for Disciplinary Action*] have been violated, the board may take the following disciplinary actions singly or in combination:**

Licensure boards must be empowered to enact disciplinary actions upon all those regulated under the provisions of the act. Discipline so imposed serves two primary functions. First, to protect the health, safety and welfare of the public from individuals and their actions that does, or might, cause harm or injury. Second, it serves as corrective action for those disciplined.

The board reserves the discretion to take appropriate disciplinary action against a licensee or certificate holder who has violated any law or rule and to decide on a case-by-case basis the type and extent of disciplinary action appropriate by applying at least the following considerations:

(a) The seriousness of the infraction,
(b) The detriment to the health, safety and welfare of the public, and
(c) Past and pending disciplinary actions relating to the licensee or certificate holder.

Based on these considerations, the following constitute the options for action that a board may have:

1. **Issue a censure.**

   A censure is the mildest form of discipline. It may be used where infractions of the law or rules do not merit a more serious disciplinary action. A censure, like a letter of concern, may include items for correction, advice or warning from the board. However, a censure remains a part of the licensee or certificate holder's file.

2. **Restrict a license or certificate. The board may require a licensee or certificate holder to report regularly to the board on matters related to the grounds for the restricted license or certificate.**

   The use of a restricted license or certificate is an essential provision of disciplinary authority of boards. Use of a restricted license or certificate can also be in combination with other disciplinary options. Boards must be free to place restrictions on scope of practice, place of practice, supervision of practice and duration of the restricted license, and the type of patients served, as established under the definition of "restricted license." For example, the licensee could only practice under on-site supervision of a board-approved licensee. Various restrictions may also be imposed on a certificate holder. There is no "probation" as one of the disciplinary options. Probation is, in a sense, a form of a restricted license so is subsumed under that category of discipline.

   A restricted license, as presented in this model, is generally not intended to be used for a purpose other than a disciplinary situation. For example, it should not be used to replace the lack of a temporary license nor should it be used at the present time to substitute for the interim permit of the foreign-educated physical therapist. There are two exceptions for use of a restricted license other than for disciplinary actions. They are 1) with a voluntary substance abuse program and 2) with a professional re-entry after a 3-year lapse of a license. A third possible use in the future may be if pre-screening of foreign-educated physical therapists is implemented and such candidates for licensure take the examination *prior* to completing their supervised interim clinical period in the United States. If this occurs then a supervised interim clinical period required after the applicant has passed the licensure examination would most appropriately be completed under a restricted license rather than an interim permit.

3. **Suspend a license or certificate for a period prescribed by the board.**

   Suspension is a temporary disciplinary action. It will always have a fixed period of time that will end either in reinstatement of a license or some other level of discipline. Combined with paragraph A.4 under *Investigative Powers; Emergency Action,* authority is granted to a board to take emergency action temporarily suspending a license or certificate. When danger to the public health, safety and welfare requires immediate action, the board may take such action. The conditions and process for when and how this action may be imposed should be further clarified in rules. This provision of the statute grants the board authority to take such an action.

**4. Revoke a license or certificate.**

The most severe penalty, and the most drastic step taken to protect the public, is the revocation of a license to practice physical therapy or of a certificate allowing employment as a physical therapist assistant. Licenses and certificates that are revoked are not reinstated, but reapplication for licensure or certification could occur in conjunction with the reconvening of a formal hearing process. (See *Guidelines for Rules, Key Area #9: Reapplication for Licensure After Revocation.*)

**5. Refuse to issue or renew a license or certificate.**

There may be conditions, such as fraudulent applications or discipline imposed in another state, where a board may refuse to issue a license or certificate. There may also be pending relicensure or recertification where the conclusion of a disciplinary proceeding is to refuse renewal of a license or certificate. This paragraph grants such authority.

**6. Impose a civil penalty of at least ________________ but not more than ________________. [Include minimum and maximum dollar amounts of civil penalties.] In addition the board may assess and collect the reasonable costs incurred in a disciplinary hearing when action is taken against a person's license or certificate.**

Most states have provisions for imposing fines or civil penalties associated with disciplinary decisions. States vary considerably on the use of such monetary penalties. Some states use fines to reimburse the board for the cost of investigating and conducting the disciplinary process. Some states use fines for punitive measures. It is recommended that the amount or possible ranges of such fines or penalties be specified in statute or in the rules. The Model Practice Act under the fees section does not address fines or penalties. Therefore, the monetary amount of such penalties should be addressed under this section or in rules. State Administration Procedures Acts may place limits on cost recovery in disciplinary action.

**7. Accept a voluntary surrendering of a license or certificate.**

There may be times when a licensee or certificate holder desires to surrender his or her license or certificate at a certain point in a disciplinary action, rather than continue with an entire disciplinary proceeding. Many states currently do not have the authority in statutes to accept a voluntary surrender of a license or certificate. One thing that should be clear by placement of this paragraph under this section is that such an act of surrendering one's license is still considered a level of discipline, subject to record-keeping information about the alleged violation of law, reporting to the Federation's nationwide disciplinary database and publication of the disciplinary action taken by the board. The language still allows a board the latitude to accept or not accept the surrender of a license or certificate. If a violation is deemed serious enough that a board wishes not to accept a voluntary surrender and proceed with an investigation and hearing process, this language allows that avenue. By contrast, someone simply not wanting to be licensed or certified any longer would accomplish this by allowing his or her license or certificate to lapse without renewal.

### Procedural Due Process

**Actions of the Board shall be taken subject to the right of notice, hearing and adjudication and the right of appeal in accordance with [specify the state] law relating to administrative law and procedure. [Or specify the state statute that addresses appeals or review of board decisions.]**

Adherence to this provision affords the licensee or certificate holder their due process of law. Most states have separate statutory provisions related to this area that should be referenced and linked under this paragraph.

## ADDITIONAL LEGAL CONSIDERATIONS

This section illustrates the procedure by which a license or certificate may be encumbered or revoked with the application of due process elements including charge, notice, hearing, final adjudication and appeal rights. Most states have clear procedures, as the Model Practice Act suggests, to facilitate the due process requirements.

Regarding the section on *Investigative Powers*, etc., while some states have similar provisions or separate administrative enabling laws, each state should carefully analyze the powers given to their board in this instance. These are the "tools" discussed in the *Board of Physical Therapy* key area which give "teeth" to the law. The board should not be hamstrung in dealing with proven violations by its licensees or legal emergencies requiring swift and decisive action. It should also be noted that the Model Practice Act suggests the board give final approval to determinations made by administrative hearing officers. It is important to note that some states permit the board to waive this responsibility, thereby establishing the hearing officer's determination as final judgment (subject to appeal). States preparing legislative action need to understand this type of provision before deciding how to respond legislatively. It may mean divesting the board of some power.

# Key Area #10
# Unlawful Practice

## MODEL LANGUAGE

### Unlawful Practice, Classification, Civil Penalties, Injunctive Relief

A. It is unlawful for any person to practice or in any manner to represent, imply or claim to practice physical therapy or use any word or designation that implies that the person is a physical therapist unless that person is licensed pursuant to this [chapter, act, section, law]. A person who engages in an activity requiring a license pursuant to this [chapter, etc.] or uses any word, title, letters, or any description of services that incorporates one or more of the terms, designations or abbreviations in violation of section [cite specific *Use of Titles* section] that implies that the person is licensed to engage in the practice of physical therapy is guilty of a [cite specific legal sanction, e.g., class 1 misdemeanor.]

B. The board may investigate any person to the extent necessary to determine if the person is engaged in the unlawful practice of physical therapy. If an investigation indicates that a person may be practicing physical therapy unlawfully, the board shall inform the person of the alleged violation. The board may refer the matter for prosecution regardless of whether the person ceases the unlawful practice of physical therapy.

C. The board, through the [Office of the Attorney General or the appropriate county attorney], may apply for injunctive relief in any court of competent jurisdiction to enjoin any person from committing any act in violation of this [chapter, etc.]. Injunction proceedings are in addition to, and not in lieu of, all penalties and other remedies prescribed in this [chapter, etc.]. [It may be the Justice Department, a county attorney, or other appropriate agency other than or in addition to the office of the Attorney General. Language should reflect those options.]

D. A person who aids or requires another person to directly or indirectly violate this [chapter, etc.] or board rules, who permits a license to be used by another person, or who acts with the intent to violate or evade this [chapter, etc.] or board rules is subject to a civil penalty of not more than [$ amount of violation] for the first violation and not more than [$ amount of violation] for each subsequent violation. [At least one thousand dollars and five thousand dollars, respectively, are suggested.]

[Optional Statute]

[E. The board shall transmit all monies it collects from civil penalties pursuant to this [chapter, etc.] to the [specify the disposition of these funds if different from other funds].]

## DISCUSSION

### Unlawful Practice, Classification, Civil Penalties, Injunctive Relief

**A. It is unlawful for any person to practice or in any manner to represent, imply or claim to practice physical therapy or use any word or designation that implies that the person is a physical therapist unless that person is licensed pursuant to this [chapter, act, section, law]. A person who engages in an activity requiring a license pursuant to this [chapter, etc.] or uses any word, title, letters, or any description of services that incorporates one or more of the terms, designations or abbreviations in violation of section [cite specific *Use of Titles* section] that implies that the person is licensed to engage in the practice of physical therapy is guilty of a [cite specific legal sanction, e.g., class 1 misdemeanor.]**

The primary focus of this entire section is to put in place legal safeguards and sanctions that extend to those who are not regulated providers of physical therapy but who may falsely claim to provide, or attempt to provide, physical therapy services contrary to provisions of the practice act. The specific civil sanctions may vary from state to state, but states generally consider a first-time violation of this statute a misdemeanor of some type. The bigger issue often is finding the legal jurisdiction to prosecute the case. The state attorney general's office, a county or a city attorney are all possibilities, but there is an occasional reluctance of law enforcement agencies to devote resources to such a violation unless injury to the public is evident. The threat of prosecution may, by itself, impose an impediment to some who would otherwise violate the provisions of this statute.

The statute paragraphs of this key area may apply equally to an ordinary citizen or to other regulated health care providers who violate the provisions of the physical therapy practice act. This would especially be applicable where claims of providing physical therapy were made by someone not licensed under the physical therapy practice act. The second sentence in the statute paragraph is very important language for inclusion because it specifically defines "representing" oneself and how a person claims or "implies" that he or she is a physical therapist by the use of the terms and letter designations protected under the *Use of Titles* section of physical therapy practice acts.

**B. The board may investigate any person to the extent necessary to determine if the person is engaged in the unlawful practice of physical therapy. If an investigation indicates that a person may be practicing physical therapy unlawfully, the board shall inform the person of the alleged violation. The board may refer the matter for prosecution regardless of whether the person ceases the unlawful practice of physical therapy.**

Under the key area *Disciplinary Actions/Procedures: Investigative Powers,* the board is authorized to investigate, issue subpoenas and compel witnesses in any case involving someone *regulated* under the practice act. This paragraph is an important additional power of the board that extends the board's authority of investigation beyond that of those regulated under the practice act. This is a necessary additional power because violations of the act, and potential violators of the act, certainly fall outside those primarily regulated by the practice act as providers.

Where an investigation reveals a violation of the act by someone not regulated under the physical therapy law, the board is empowered to inform the violator and request that he or she immediately cease the unlawful behavior—essentially a cease and desist order. The threat of the board referring the case for legal action if the violator does not cease and desist the unlawful conduct may be the main deterrent of this statute clause as well. If a violator were prosecuted under this clause, all rights of due process would apply.

**C. The board, through the [Office of the Attorney General or the appropriate county attorney], may apply for injunctive relief in any court of competent jurisdiction to enjoin any person from committing any act in violation of this [chapter, etc.]. Injunction proceedings are in addition to, and not in lieu of, all penalties and other remedies prescribed in this [chapter, etc.]. [It may be the Justice Department, a county attorney, or other appropriate agency other than or in addition to the office of the Attorney General. Language should reflect those options.]**

In addition to the threat of action that an investigation and subsequent cease and desist letter may pose, the board must also be empowered to actually bring about a cessation of illegal action when necessary. Unsuspecting and uninformed members of the public may be harmed or injured by someone engaged in illegal practice. Avenues for preventing such illegal and harmful conduct, therefore, should exist. On occasion, preventing illegal acts needs to be accomplished quickly, which is the intent of an injunction, until all the pertinent facts of the case can be fully investigated and determined and damages, if any, assessed. Usually, an injunction is initiated by the board through the state's Office of the Attorney General. An assistant attorney general is assigned to work with the board and assists the board in filing an injunction to protect the public from someone violating the law. An injunction does not preclude any additional actions, penalties or remedies that may be imposed according to law.

**D. A person who aids or requires another person to directly or indirectly violate this [chapter, etc.] or board rules, who permits a license to be used by another person, or who acts with the intent to violate or evade this [chapter, etc.] or board rules is subject to a civil penalty of not more than [$ amount of violation] for the first violation and not more than [$ amount of violation] for each subsequent violation. [At least one thousand dollars and five thousand dollars, respectively, are suggested.]**

This statute provision certainly applies to those outside the regulation of the physical therapy practice act, but could also include those regulated by the act—physical therapists and physical therapist assistants. This is often the case in the kind of violation where a physical therapist may assist, condone, or supposedly lend the authority of his or her license illegally to someone not regulated by the practice act. In such a case, in addition to the disciplinary provisions under *Key Areas #10* and *#11*, someone regulated under the act may also be exposed to the monetary penalties stated above.

This paragraph could also be applied to a non-physical therapist employer or supervisor who may exert influence on a licensee requesting or requiring conduct in violation of a practice act.

**[Optional Statute]**

**[E. The board shall transmit all monies it collects from civil penalties pursuant to this [chapter, etc.] to the [specify the disposition of these funds if different from other funds].]**

A state may make the determination that the monies received by the board from civil penalties do not go into the physical therapy fund or the operating funds of the board, but rather they would go into the general fund of the state. This is the usual procedure, and in a way, it sets up a precautionary barrier against the temptation of using civil penalties to increase the funds of the board. The board does have the authority under *Disciplinary Actions/Procedures: Disciplinary Actions/Penalties* section, paragraph (6) to assess and collect the reasonable costs incurred in a hearing. There may need to be further clarification as to whether such monies would be deposited in the physical therapy fund or a state's general fund, according to each state's disposition of funds policies.

## ADDITIONAL LEGAL CONSIDERATIONS

It is essential in developing a practice act for a profession with a limited scope of practice to not only define the scope of such practice (see *Definitions* key area) but to establish a legal basis to prevent those not legally qualified from utilizing the titles and scope of practice in any manner. This is not simply an exercise in "turf protection," as overlaps of activities appear in almost all fields of health care. Rather, this is an attempt to limit misrepresentation to the public for both the actual practice and the holding out to practice physical therapy.

When a jurisdiction passes a law with a provision such as paragraph (A) in this section, it is a recognition by that jurisdiction that this specific practice and title are protected and limited to those who meet the statutory requirements, such as education, and are licensed by that jurisdiction to so act. The *Exemptions From Licensure* section in the *Licensure and Examination* key area makes it equally clear that the protection afforded the profession in question in no way limits other licensed professions from legally conducting the practice for which they are licensed. However, this would not permit other health care practitioners from representing themselves as physical therapists or providing physical therapy.

This key area also delineates between those regulated as licensees and certificate holders under this act and persons not regulated by this act, addressing the legal options against the latter. This is an important provision in view of the numerous attempts by certain non-physical therapists to utilize the term or practice of physical therapy. Relating to paragraph (B), an example may be of a person advertising that they provide "physical therapy" when they are, in fact, not licensed in the state and are prohibited from making such a claim or using the term "physical therapy." In addition to the monetary penalties that may be assessed under (A), the board can also seek, by injunction, to stop or prevent further advertisement of the term "physical therapy," or the use of other terms protected under the title protection clause. An injunction is a court-dictated method of preventing or stopping the illegal activity before monetary damages can be subsequently assessed.

# Key Area #11 Consumer Advocacy

## MODEL LANGUAGE

### Reporting Violations, Immunity

A. Any person, including but not limited to a licensee, corporation, insurance company, health care organization or health care facility and state or local governmental agencies shall report to the board any conviction, determination or finding that a licensee has committed an act that constitutes a violation of section [cite section on *Grounds for Disciplinary Action*].
B. A person is immune from civil liability, whether direct or derivative, for providing information in good faith to the board pursuant to paragraph (A) of this section.
C. The board shall not disclose the identity of a person who provides information unless such information is essential to proceedings conducted *pursuant to sections [cite the Disciplinary Actions/Procedures: Investigative Powers and Hearings* section] or unless required by a court of law.

### Substance Abuse Recovery Program

In lieu of a disciplinary proceeding prescribed by this [chapter, act, section, law], the board may permit a licensee or certificate holder to actively participate in a board-approved substance abuse recovery program if:
A. The board has evidence that the licensee or certificate holder is impaired.
B. The licensee or certificate holder has not been convicted of a felony relating to a controlled substance in a court of law of the United States or any other territory or country.
C. The licensee or certificate holder enters into a written agreement with the board for a restricted license or certificate and complies with all the

terms of the agreement, including making satisfactory progress in the program and adhering to any limitations on the licensee's practice or certificate holder's work imposed by the board to protect the public. Failure to enter into such an agreement shall activate an immediate investigation and disciplinary proceeding by the board.

D. As part of the agreement established between the licensee or certificate holder and the board, the licensee or certificate holder signs a waiver allowing the substance abuse program to release information to the board if the licensee or certificate holder does not comply with the requirements of this section or is unable to practice or work with reasonable skill or safety.

## Rights of Consumers

A. The public shall have access to the following information:
   1. A list of licensees and interim permit holders that includes place of practice, license or interim permit number, date of license or interim permit expiration and status of license.
   2. A list of physical therapist assistants certified in the state, including place of employment, certification number, and date of certificate expiration.
   3. A list of official actions taken by the board.

B. The home address and telephone numbers of physical therapists and physical therapist assistants are not public records and shall be kept confidential by the board unless they are the only addresses and telephone numbers of record.

C. If a referring practitioner is deriving direct or indirect compensation from the referral to physical therapy the physical therapist shall disclose this information in writing to the patient prior to the initial evaluation.

D. A physical therapist shall disclose in writing to a patient any financial interest in products that the physical therapist endorses and recommends to the patient at the time of such endorsement or recommendation.

E. A physical therapist shall inform each patient that the patient has freedom of choice in services and products.

F. Information relating to the physical therapist-patient relationship is confidential and shall not be communicated to a third party who is not involved in that patient's care without the prior written consent of the patient. A physical therapist shall divulge to the board information it requires in connection with any investigation, public hearing or other proceedings. The physical therapist-patient privilege does not extend to cases in which the physical therapist has a duty to report information as required by law.

G. Any person may submit a complaint regarding any licensee, certificate holder, or any other person potentially in violation of this [chapter, act, section, law]. Confidentiality shall be maintained subject to law.
H. The board shall keep all information relating to the receiving and investigation of complaints filed against licensees or certificate holders confidential until the information becomes public record or as required by law. Patient records, including clinical records, files, any other report or oral statement relating to diagnostic findings or treatment of patients, any information from which a patient or his family might be identified, or information received and records or reports kept by the board as a result of an investigation made pursuant to this chapter shall not be available to the public and shall be kept confidential by the board.
I. Each licensee shall display a copy of the licensee's license or current renewal verification in a location accessible to public view at the licensee's place of practice.

### Temporary Provisions

[No model statute language is offered under this section heading. See *Discussion* for additional information.]

## DISCUSSION

This key area of the Model Practice Act contains a number of statutory clauses that are often found in various areas of practice acts but all have a common interest in consumer advocacy. A practice act by its very nature is focused on public protection, but this is a natural grouping of topics giving greater focus to consumer advocacy by the board.

### Reporting Violations, Immunity

A. **Any person, including but not limited to a licensee, corporation, insurance company, health care organization or health care facility and state or local governmental agencies shall report to the board any conviction, determination or finding that a licensee has committed an act that constitutes a violation of section [cite section on *Grounds for Disciplinary Action*].**

Many states have recently adopted similar reporting standards but usually in statutes separate from the physical therapy act, often in statutes dealing with insurance regulations. This paragraph gives the board authority to directly solicit and require such reporting by any individual or organization. However, it limits and places safeguards against any potential "witch-hunt" activity of "claimed" or "suspected" misconduct because it insists on formal conviction, determination or finding—administrative or otherwise. This language also requires a licensee to report his or her own legal entanglements that resulted in conviction, determination or finding consistent with those violations contained in *Grounds for Disciplinary Action.*

A question may arise regarding enforceability of this statute clause. Other agencies may not know the grounds for disciplinary action under the physical therapy practice act. For example, an insurance company is aware of a malpractice verdict but has not reported it to the board, or a federal agency, such as those administering the Medicare program, may not report a case of Medicare fraud to the physical therapy board. When states adopt these reporting standards, they should communicate the fact to all covered parties to encourage better cooperation. Such action will enhance consumer protection and constitutes good public policy. Petition to the courts can be made, if necessary, to gain this information.

**B. A person is immune from civil liability, whether direct or derivative, for providing information in good faith to the board pursuant to paragraph (A) of this section.**

This paragraph is a necessary companion to paragraph (A) above to protect the messenger as long as the message is delivered in good faith. A person reporting a bad faith claim of "suspected" conduct would not be granted immunity from civil liability.

**C. The board shall not disclose the identity of a person who provides information unless such information is essential to proceedings conducted pursuant to sections [cite the investigative Powers and Hearings sections] or unless required by a court of law.**

There is often a hesitancy to report violations based on perceived negative consequences of such reporting. This model paragraph gives the board greater authority to protect the confidentiality of someone providing information to the board that may be used in a board decision. There are various disclosure laws within a state that may govern what a board may and may not disclose. Those laws generally focus on the right of an accused to face his or her accuser if an action comes to the point of formal discipline. Board legal counsel will be able to advise boards in these matters.

### Substance Abuse Recovery Program

**In lieu of a disciplinary proceeding prescribed by this [chapter, act, section, law], the board may permit a licensee or certificate holder to actively participate in a board-approved substance abuse recovery program if:**

**A. The board has evidence that the licensee or certificate holder is impaired.**

**B. The licensee or certificate holder has not been convicted of a felony relating to a controlled substance in a court of law of the United States or any other territory or country.**

**C. The licensee or certificate holder enters into a written agreement with the board for a restricted license or certificate and complies with all the terms of the agreement, including making satisfactory progress in the program and adhering to any limitations on the licensee's practice or certificate holder's work imposed by the board to protect the public. Failure to enter into such an agreement shall activate an immediate investigation and disciplinary proceeding by the board.**

**D. As part of the agreement established between the licensee or certificate holder and the board, the licensee or certificate holder signs a waiver allowing the substance abuse program to release information to the board if the licensee or certificate holder does not comply with the requirements of this section or is unable to practice or work with reasonable skill or safety.**

This section is included here under the *Consumer Advocacy* key area, as opposed to earlier in the *Grounds for Disciplinary Action* key area, for two reasons. First, entry and participation in the substance abuse recovery program may not be through the formal disciplinary process. It certainly is linked to the disciplinary process if the impaired licensee or certificate holder elects either to not participate under the conditions stated above or if he or she breaks the conditions of the monitoring program and continues to engage in conduct constituting grounds for disciplinary conduct. The second reason for inclusion in this key area is the philosophy that successful recovery from substance abuse pays enormous benefits to society in general. Consumers of physical therapy services can indeed benefit from such a program from the standpoint of both the safety of the provided services and continued access to services. After a sufficient period of supervision and recovery, a knowledgeable and skilled physical therapist or physical therapist assistant with years of invested education and experience, who is otherwise free from actionable activities under the disciplinary provisions of a practice act may be able to return to or maintain a productive career.

The statute language allows for the licensee and certificate holder to either voluntarily acknowledge to the board his or her condition and willingness to participate, or for the board to initiate the action of requiring participation when it is in possession of evidence that a licensee or certificate holder is so impaired. This paragraph, when combined with paragraph (8) under *Grounds for Disciplinary Action,* gives the licensee and the board two options: either the licensee or certificate holder chooses to participate in the substance abuse program or face disciplinary proceedings.

The public will be further protected by paragraph (C) above that requires the licensee or certificate holder to adhere to any limitations on his or her practice or employment that may be imposed by the board as a condition of participation in a program.

This model language does not provide for a substance abuse recovery program that is confidential. A written agreement for participation in such a program would constitute an official action by the board. Therefore, the action would be subject to public inspection. States wishing to adopt a confidential program should seek local legal counsel.

## Rights of Consumers

**A. The public shall have access to the following information:**
   **1. A list of licensees and interim permit holders that includes place of practice, license or interim permit number, date of license or interim permit expiration and status of license.**
   **2. A list of physical therapist assistants certified in the state, including place of employment, certification number, and date of certificate expiration.**
   **3. A list of official actions taken by the board.**

**B. The home address and telephone numbers of physical therapists and physical therapist assistants are not public records and shall be kept confidential by the board unless they are the only addresses and telephone numbers of record.**

This is basic information that licensing boards should make available upon request to consumers of physical therapy services. The question arises about disciplinary actions and when it is appropriate to release information. Subparagraph (A.3) refers to "official actions taken by the board." This usually refers to final action taken against a license or certificate. For example, when a complaint is received by the board, prior to any investigation or even during the investigation and up until a determination of a violation of the statutes is made, the information regarding the case remains confidential. When official action is taken and the records of the board reflect such action, this becomes public information and may be shared upon request.

A home address and telephone number may become a public record if it is the only address and telephone number available for a licensee or certificate holder.

**C. If a referring practitioner is deriving direct or indirect compensation from the referral to physical therapy the physical therapist shall disclose this information in writing to the patient prior to the initial evaluation.**

**D. A physical therapist shall disclose in writing to a patient any financial interest in products that the physical therapist endorses and**

**recommends to the patient at the time of such endorsement or recommendation.**

Paragraph (C) is perhaps a new twist in disclosure statutes. Here the physical therapist is required to provide written disclosure that a referral source has a financial interest in the physical therapy services. The *referral source*, if the patient has been referred, is generally regulated under other practice acts. When disclosure statutes do exist in these other acts, there still may be varying success in informing patients of a financial interest. This statute places the burden of disclosure on the physical therapist providing the service. The physical therapist is licensed and regulated under this practice act and can be disciplined if necessary for violation of an activity that has consumer protection consequences.

Disclosure statutes admittedly represent a rather weak attempt at addressing a problem. By the very nature of disclosure, there is an admission that the action being disclosed represents something about which the consumer needs to be cautious. Often disclosure statutes have been applied to situations in which a referral source may derive direct or indirect financial benefit from the referral—for example, a physician-owned or invested physical therapy service. Paragraph (D) addresses this type of situation, but only as it applies to products. Physical therapists more often recommend products, rather than services, in which they may have a financial interest.

In addition to the need to disclose any financial interest in the distribution of a product or service, physical therapists must abide by legal restrictions affecting endorsements of products or services (e.g., truth in advertising). Paragraph (D) is not intended to restrict or prohibit sale or dispensing to patients of products or supplies provided by the physical therapist at cost or reasonable markup.

**E. A physical therapist shall inform each patient that the patient has freedom of choice in services and products.**

Patients have basic rights as consumers of health care services. Key among these is *the right to know* and *the right to choose.* In order for consumers to be able to "choose" effectively, there is an obligation on the part of providers to furnish accurate and sufficient information so consumers may first "know." Some would refer to this as informed consent. The application of this principle in the form of "written informed consent" is still very much a debatable legal concept as it applies to physical therapy services, where it may not be debatable as it applies to a surgeon performing surgery. For this reason, the Model Practice Act does not contain a "written informed consent" clause. Regardless of the outcome of the debate, this model language emphasizes a responsibility to which all physical therapists should adhere. They should be strong advocates for their patients having informed freedom of choice in all services being provided.

The practical application of this statute paragraph, as it applies to physical therapists, may be shown in several areas. For example, these principles should be applied in explaining the plan of treatment intervention to a patient, along with the explanation that at any time the patient may raise questions about procedures or even refuse treatment. These principles should apply at the time products or equipment are *recommended*, rather than required of a patient unexpectedly. They may also apply when a physical therapist recommends or refers a patient to a physician and offers the patient at least two or three options, answering questions fairly about each physician they may be recommending to patients.

There are times when a patient's own prior decision has placed subsequent limitations on other choices. For example, a decision to join a particular managed care plan may severely limit access to specialty services, including physical therapy. Part of the knowledge a physical therapist may be imparting to a patient is a better understanding of the implications of the patient's own decisions. The physical therapist may have limitations in being able to provide services—limitations created by a patient's prior decision. The patient can then be better informed in making future choices about health care needs, including insurance purchases.

This section also applies to so-called "gag rules" imposed by some managed care organizations on their providers. The model language does not require that a licensee is responsible for providing freedom of choice but for informing the patient that they have freedom of choice. Informing patients or clients that they have options should never be restricted. Such gag rules would be in conflict with this statute cause, and a licensee would be in violation of his or her own practice act if required to abide by such a demand.

In many of the model statute clauses in this key area, the certified physical therapist assistant is not specifically referenced. Physical therapist assistants always come under the restrictions of law and under the ethical guidelines of the physical therapy profession. They also remain at all times under the direction and supervision of the licensee, who has the primary responsibility in these consumer-related responsibilities and restrictions.

F. **Information relating to the physical therapist-patient relationship is confidential and shall not be communicated to a third party who is not involved in that patient's care without the prior written consent of the patient. A physical therapist shall divulge to the board information it requires in connection with any investigation, public hearing or other proceedings. The physical therapist-patient privilege does not extend to cases in which the physical therapist has a duty to report information as required by law.**

This model language represents the strongest statement in the Model Practice Act protecting physical therapist-patient confidentiality. It is similar to language used with other health care disciplines. Written consent of disclosure is important. It often occurs when a patient first begins seeing a physical therapist so that information can be communicated to a referring physician, insurance company and perhaps other family members. But the disclosure statements that physical therapists have their patients sign should be specific as to whom information can be released.

The last two sentences clarify that this privilege does not extend to withholding information that is required by law to be reported to the board concerning an investigation. Patient record confidentiality is further addressed in Paragraph (H) that follows. Boards have further obligation regarding confidentiality of patient records even when obtained by subpoena.

**G. Any person may submit a complaint regarding any licensee, certificate holder, or any other person potentially in violation of this [chapter, act, section, law]. Confidentiality shall be maintained subject to law.**

Most states do not allow an anonymous complaint to be filed. They may allow a confidential complaint, but not an anonymous complaint. What this means is that the name of the complainant will be held confidential as long as possible or as the law requires. With any complaint, due process may eventually require disclosure of the accuser under issues of the accused being allowed to know the nature of the complaint in order to fully defend against it or to face his or her accuser.

The emphasis in this paragraph is to remove barriers to the public filing complaints against those regulated by practice acts or others who may be in violation of a practice act. In the *Disciplinary Actions/Procedures* key area, under *Investigative Powers, Receiving and Investigating Complaints,* the discussion points out how rules need to be formulated that set forth the complaint process and that allow complaints to come to the board in writing, by phone or other electronic medium, or verbally. At the time of a complaint, the board and staff should be sensitive to a consumer's concerns or fears.

The Model Practice Act, under *Disciplinary Actions/Procedures: Investigative Powers,* also grants the board authority to investigate on its own initiative. A consumer of physical therapy who is simply too timid or fearful to initiate or follow through with the process of filing a complaint may at least notify the board of a potential violation. The board may then take the initiative to follow up on this information and begin a disciplinary process if it is warranted. This would be an instance where the identity of someone providing information to the board could conceivably remain anonymous.

**H. The board shall keep all information relating to the receiving and investigation of complaints filed against licensees or certificate holders confidential until the information becomes public record or as required by law. Patient records, including clinical records, files, any other report or oral statement relating to diagnostic findings or treat-**

**ment of patients, any information from which a patient or his family might be identified, or information received and records or reports kept by the board as a result of an investigation made pursuant to this chapter shall not be available to the public and shall be kept confidential by the board.**

This language protects the complainant, the licensee or certificate holder under investigation, and the board. Disclosure of any information relating to an investigated complaint prior to official action or ruling of the board disrupts the disciplinary process and may have a detrimental and possibly irreversible influence on both the complainant and the individual being investigated. The filing of charges constitutes information becoming part of a public record. If someone inquires about charges after charges are filed, the board would need to disclose that charges had indeed been filed against a licensee or certificate holder. However, the final ruling of the board or other details of the case could obviously not be disclosed as yet. Once final disciplinary action is taken, further information becomes public knowledge and can be disclosed. The board has further reporting requirements under *Board of Physical Therapy: Powers and Duties of the Board* that relate to reporting to a national database and the publication of final disciplinary actions.

Patient records are afforded a high level of legal protection. If such records are obtained in an investigation and retained in an investigative file they remain confidential and are not accessible as public records. The second sentence in this statute clause provides authority for the board to maintain such confidentiality.

**I. Each licensee shall display a copy of the licensee's license or current renewal verification in a location accessible to public view at the licensee's place of practice.**

It is important that patients know the name and qualifications of the persons providing their care. Posting licenses identifies by name the licensees within a facility whose qualifications have met state requirements for licensure.

As mentioned previously in the *Licensure and Examination* key area, a printed license or certificate, and the renewal cards, should always display not only the name, but also the proper PT or PTA letter designations after the names.

Physical therapist assistants fall under the supervision of the licensed physical therapist. It should be the discretion of the physical therapist or place of employment whether physical therapist assistant's certificates are posted.

Other identification such as nametags with titles are discretionary according to the facility standards or other requirements, but when worn should also include appropriate letter designations. Physical therapy aides or "techs" should never use letter designations after their name, such as PTT, but could be designated as a "physical therapy aide" or "physical therapy tech." As previously mentioned, it is inappropriate for students to use letter designations with their names. (See *Guidelines for Rules, Use of Titles.*)

Some states place a licensee's home address directly on the certificate of licensure itself or the renewal card to accommodate mailing. This is not advisable if this document is required by law to be displayed in public view. States are advised not to use this procedure.

### Temporary Provisions

**[No model statute language is offered under this section heading.]**

If major changes are enacted in a practice act, those responsible for drafting a bill will often attach what is described as session law. This describes the date such a law would become effective if passed. Other considerations would include the continuation of rules currently in place until the board would promulgate revised rules to conform to newly adopted statutes. A third area that might be addressed in such a section would be the continuation, renewal or transition to licensure or certification of those regulated, whichever would be appropriate under the new statutes. No model language is recommended under this heading, but such issues should be addressed.

## ADDITIONAL LEGAL CONSIDERATIONS

This area demonstrates the ever-changing standards not only for the actual practice of physical therapy but of public involvement that impacts practice, such as the public's legal right to know. The subject of a patient "Bill of Rights" or public reporting and access to information, virtually unknown 20 or 30 years ago, has become a major issue in modern times in all walks of life. The subject matter covered under this key area is the legal manifestation of these patient or public rights in the state's physical therapy law and for physical therapy practice.

Although the application of certain of these measures may have some legal hurdles such as how to report action "perceived" to be in violation of law, careful rule making affording clear standards, together with protection for those reporting by legal immunity, should make such statutory provisions completely viable from a legal standpoint.

In presenting these provisions, the issue of due process and confidentiality was carefully considered and utilized to protect both the licensee and the public. The inclusions of this *Consumer Advocacy* key area, under modern legal standards of consumers' rights, is no longer optional for states seeking global changes in their practice acts.

Regarding temporary provisions, when a state makes significant changes to an act regulating the practice of a licensed profession, there will undoubtedly be questions on the legal effect of the new re-enactment vis-a-vis the previous law and rules to that statute. This is particularly true if the effect of the new enactment works as a repealer of the previous law in part or in whole. Questions regarding continued licensing standards, licensing or other credentialing status and application of rules under the previous law are bound to surface. Although many states have statutory construction acts that may resolve some of these issues, inclusion of language addressing the transition status of regulatory credentialing, rules, and other administrative decisions may be helpful. There is precedent for such provisions in other jurisdictions and the drafters of revised practice acts should consider utilizing this drafting methodology to try to prevent bureaucratic paralysis after the enactment of a revised practice act.

# Guidelines for Rules

# Guidelines for Rules

## INTRODUCTION

This Model Practice Act for Physical Therapy, with exceptions evident here in *Guidelines for Rules,* does not include recommended model language for administrative rules. Individual jurisdictions should assume the task of crafting rules to fit their own needs and the requirements of their statutes. As states make regulatory changes to practice acts, and language from this model act is utilized, additional conforming rules will be required to complete the regulatory design.

One of the driving philosophies for creating this model practice act was to keep the statute language as concise as possible, focused on authorizing law, and largely free from procedural activity or description. However, those procedures should be addressed in rules. There will necessarily be some structure, policy and operational definitions that help make the administrative rules a functional and complementary part of a practice act. Some states have relatively large statute sections and small rule sections to their practice acts. Others are just the opposite. This Model Practice Act, in keeping statute recommendations concise, anticipates the "smaller statutes/larger rules" structure.

To provide assistance to jurisdictions as they work to revise practice acts, the *Guidelines for Rules* examines each of the *Key Areas* of the model statute language and lists several conforming rules that should be developed, given the structure of the model statute language. This is by no means an exhaustive list of potential rules. It follows the same order as the *Key Areas,* so it should be easy to coordinate. Regardless of the organizational structure of the rules adopted by each state, there should be a system to facilitate correlation of the rules with the corresponding statutes.

Use of "Board Policies" is the preferred way to organize procedural activities that are strictly internal and operational and have no effect on those regulated by the practice act or any other external group or individual. An example might be a board policy on office supply and equipment purchases and the authorization for such acquisitions. This should not be confused with board substantive policies, "positions" or "opinions" that may serve to interpret or give guidance regarding board interpretation of statutes or rules. Boards should not use policies as a means of avoiding the admittedly more difficult task of changing a statute or adopting rules. If a topic or issue of concern directly affects those licensed or regulated under a practice act and is not a matter of internal board or office procedure, it should be addressed through rules if not in the statutes.

## KEY AREA #1 • LEGISLATIVE INTENT

No suggestion for rule language is included under this key area. Philosophical intent is generally not appropriate for process-oriented rules.

## KEY AREA #2 • DEFINITIONS

### Rules Construction

States vary in rules construction requirements relating to definitions. For example, states may not allow the definitions section for rules to be used simply as an extension of the definitions in statute. In this case, any definition in rules should to relate directly to language within the rules itself.

### Physiotherapy/Physiotherapist Definition

Rules may need to provide further operational definitions of terms not appropriate for the *Definitions* section of the statutes. For example, here is an operational definition of the terms "physiotherapy" and "physiotherapist" that might relate to a rule about improper use of terms. Some states may feel strongly that such a definition should either be added to rules or be a part of the statutes. If in statutes rather than rules, the following would fit in either the *Definitions* or *Use of Titles* key areas of the statutes:

"Physiotherapy" and "physiotherapist" are the international terms for physical therapy and physical therapist, respectively. These terms are not used by physical therapists in the United States, but are protected titles and terminology under section [cite the specific Use of Titles statute for protected terms] and, therefore, are not to be used in any manner by any other person or organization to mislead consumers of health care and induce the false belief that physical therapy or physiotherapy is being provided by any person not licensed under this act.

### Other Definitions

Examples of other potential rule definitions include:
- accredited educational program
- credentials evaluation
- criterion-referenced passing point
- foreign-educated applicant
- good moral character
- national disciplinary database
- national examination
- recognized standards of ethics
- substandard care
- substantially equivalent
- unreasonable fees

## KEY AREA #3 • BOARD OF PHYSICAL THERAPY

### Board Appointments

Rules should be developed outlining the process of appointment to the board. The nomination process varies widely from state to state. Traditionally in some states, statute or rule clauses have specified that the appointment be made from a list supplied to the governor from the APTA chapter. However, rules should be specific to board functions and activities, not external organizations. In one state the board uses a nomination process with a mail-out ballot sent to all licensees to determine the top five recommended candidates to pass on to the governor.

As discussed under the *Board of Physical Therapy* key area, recommendations to the governor should consider geographic distribution, gender, and practice settings. (See rationale under the *Board of Physical Therapy* key area.) Suggested rules language is:

The board may provide a list of qualified candidates to the governor for appointment to the board of physical therapy. Recommendations shall consider current board geographic, gender and practice setting distribution.

### Terms of Board Appointment

Rules should specify dates or a sequence of appointment in order to stagger or overlap terms of office. This will facilitate smoother transitions so that only one or two members of a board are ever appointed in one year, rather than larger turnover in a single year that may disrupt continuity. The process of board approval for extending a term while awaiting a governor's appointment to fill a board position should also be addressed.

Where a board consists of five members, three professional and two public members, and the term of appointment is four years, suggested rules language is:

Terms of office for members of the board shall begin in January and extend for 4 years. One board member shall be appointed each year with the exception of every fourth year when both a public and professional member will be appointed.

### Removal of Board Members

The entire process for removal of a board member for misconduct should be outlined in rules. This should include the specific grounds for removal, the options for correction of a problem prior to removal, and the specific procedures used to request removal of a board member by the governor. Rule language might include:

Board members shall attend board meetings scheduled by the board. The board shall recommend to the governor that a board member who fails to attend three consecutive board meetings be removed from the board. Board members may be excused from attending board meetings for any of the following reasons:

1. Illness
2. Death in the immediate family
3. Military service
4. Inclement weather
5. Other reasons deemed appropriate by the president of the board.

The board may recommend to the governor the removal of a board member for misconduct or incompetence only upon a unanimous vote of the board following documented efforts to permit the board member to remedy the circumstances. A recommendation for removal for misconduct or incompetence requires a unanimous vote of other board members.

### Expense Reimbursement

Although probably more appropriate for board policies, rules may include the process for reimbursement of board members' expense, per diem, travel, etc., and reference any other general state guidelines or operational procedures addressing reimbursement.

### Rule Development

If not included under other statutes governing rule construction and processes, the process for administrative rule development should be detailed. This includes proper public notice, hearings and final approval mechanisms of changes to, or adoption of, any existing or proposed rule.

### Official Board Records

The maintenance of official records, confidentiality of certain records and of other discussion and distribution of board minutes are necessary inclusions in rules, as well as automatic distribution of minutes and a list of who should receive them. This may require several separate rule paragraphs. Provision should be made for a public file and a confidential investigative file, as needed, on each person regulated under the practice act.

There may be other information, legal opinions or documents that are part of board investigations but do not constitute the final action of the board. These also should be kept confidential. The following language is recommended for rules:

> The Board shall maintain a separate confidential investigative file for each licensee or certificate holder that may contain a record of complaints filed against a licensee or certificate holder, investigative reports, medical records, legal opinions, briefs, or other legal papers. Only the formal disciplinary actions taken by the Board against a licensee or certificate holder as a result of such complaints shall be open to public inspection.

### Election of Board Officers

The process for the election of board officers may be referred to board policies but could be detailed in rules. This includes eligibility, the dates of elections and any other restrictions, e.g., consecutive terms in the same office.

### Orientation

Rules should also be developed for the orientation of each new board member. This was discussed previously as a major weakness of licensing boards, and especially in regards to new public members of boards. Proper orientation and training should be a high priority.

### Public Notice of Meetings

If not addressed under state open meetings statutes, a rule should be included requiring public notice of meeting dates and agendas. This would include how and when notice is provided.

## KEY AREA #4 • LICENSURE AND EXAMINATION

### Professional Education Registering

When clinical education courses involve actual patient contact or when participants practice procedures upon each other, it may be desirable to enact a registration process to ensure that the exemption granted to instructors and participants in these continuing education offerings is specifically restricted to short-term courses not extending more than 60 days in a calendar year. If this time frame is surpassed, licensure would be required. The board may choose not to be overburdened in regulating continuing education by only requiring registration for those courses exceeding, for example, 30 days.

### Application Procedures

All procedures for making application for original licensure or certification, for foreign-educated licensure, for endorsement for renewal, for relicensure after a lapse, etc., should be included in detail within rules. This includes reference to various application forms (the actual application forms should not be included in rules), various application fees, and any other supporting documentation required under the application procedures. Although the specific form need not be included in rules, the detail of what the form will require an applicant to report should be specified in rules. For example, listing what will be required regarding names, addresses and phone numbers, names and addresses of colleges attended, previous jurisdictions where licensed, prior professional employment history, disclosure of prior convictions or actions by other jurisdictions' boards or legal entities, malpractice judgment disclosures, etc., will all need to be specified in rules.

### Disciplinary Database

A rule should be developed specifying the obligation of the board to always check the Federation of State Boards of Physical Therapy's database for previous or current disciplinary actions related to each applicant. This should occur with anyone applying for licensure by endorsement or for certification where the applicant was previously regulated in another state. This should also include a requirement that the applicant report all previous states of licensure or certification, not just the one of previous residence.

### Educational Accreditation

The name of the national accrediting agency is not specified in statutes but is more appropriately referenced in rules. The following is suggested for rules inclusion, and may be appropriately included in definitions:

> The board-approved accrediting agency for physical therapist professional education and physical therapist assistant education programs is the Commission on Accreditation of Physical Therapy Education (CAPTE).

### Foreign-Educated Applications

All procedures for foreign-educated physical therapist application should be specified in rules, either in conjunction with the application process for any physical therapist seeking licensure or as a separate area of rules.

The following rule suggestions regarding foreign-educated physical therapist licensure application were previously outlined under the discussion in key area Licensure and Examination and are repeated here due to the specific rule-making suggestions:

### Definition of "Foreign-Educated Applicant"

Either in this section or under definitions, it would be appropriate to define what a "foreign-educated applicant" means. For example:

A "foreign-educated applicant" means a physical therapist who graduated from any physical therapy educational program outside the fifty states, Puerto Rico, District of Columbia, or U.S. territories.

### Definition of "Substantially Equivalent"

Either in this section or under definitions, educational equivalency should be defined. This may be done by requiring a certain number of credit hours in specific areas of both general and professional education curricula. However, this may not guarantee exact equivalency of course content, which may be virtually unachievable from country to country, particularly non-English speaking countries. Again, the more specific states are, the more consistent a board can be with foreign-educated applicants. It would be appropriate to also specify a grade standard, for example, that foreign-educated applicants must have obtained at least a C grade or better in professional education courses. CAPTE's criteria for accrediting foreign educational programs, APTA's *A Normative Model of Physical Therapist Professional Education, Version 97,* and also the Federation's "Course Work Evaluation Tool for Persons Who Received their Physical Therapy Education Outside the United States" may be consulted for additional help in this area.

### English Proficiency Examinations

Rules should specify the exact English proficiency examinations required and under what circumstances they are required. The Federation recommends the following three tests be taken and passed: *Test of English as a Foreign Language (TOEFL), Test of Spoken English (TSE),* and *Test of Written English (TWE).* Also, states may wish to include the passing scores required for each test. The Federation recommends requiring passage of all three tests; the passing score recommendation for each test is:

TOEFL: 560 TSE: 50 TWE 4.5 (See *Appendix F.)*

Some of the following procedures/guidelines for interim permit holders were previously discussed in key area Licensure and Examination, but are repeated here due to rule-making implications:

## Interim Permits

The parameters of supervised clinical experience for the foreign-educated interim permit holder prior to examination should be specified in rules. This should include the length of time (both the minimum and maximum number of weeks or months the supervised clinical experience can occur), the minimum and maximum number of hours worked per week, the options for types of facilities or clinical settings that will be approved (for example, that only broader exposure to general physical therapy, as opposed to narrow specialty care, would be approved by the board) the nature of supervision (direct on-site, for example), the qualifications of a clinical supervisor (for example, the length of time they have been licensed), the reporting requirements and forms used by the clinical supervisor for reporting back to the board, provisions for extension of time or for transfer to another clinical setting if the first supervised clinical experience is not deemed successful, and options for a second supervised clinical experience.

## Failing the Examination

It should be specified, in rules if not in statutes, that once an examination is taken and failed by a foreign-educated applicant, continued clinical practice, even under supervision is not permitted. This same standard should apply to U.S.-educated graduates as well. U.S.-educated physical therapists participate in clinical training as part of their educational curriculum prior to graduation. They then are eligible to take the licensing examination. The reason a supervised clinical training period is required of foreign-educated applicants is the variance in educational inclusion of clinical experience in foreign educational programs, and the importance of exposure to clinical practice in the United States. When the application for licensure is completed by a foreign-educated physical therapist and they are approved for an interim supervised clinical education period, there exists an assumption of competence. If an examination is subsequently failed, that assumption of competence is deemed void and no approval for continued clinical practice should be extended. The U.S. Immigration and Naturalization Service should then be notified of the applicant's status. In case of revocation of an interim permit due to failure of the examination, retesting should be subject to the same provisions as specified in the *Examinations* section of the statutes.

No temporary licenses are proposed under the Model Practice Act.

## Waiving Foreign-Educated Requirements

Under key area *Licensure and Examination: Qualifications for Licensure of Foreign-Educated Physical Therapists,* if a foreign-educated applicant graduated from a CAPTE accredited program, several of the requirements under this section may be waived by the board. Rules may be formulated that address this board option and any further criteria for waiving these requirements.

## Pre-Screening of Foreign-Educated Applicants

The Federation's Foreign Credentialing Commission on Physical Therapy (FCCPT) reviews applicants and grants prescreening certificates. The Federation's *Coursework Evaluation Tool* is used as the standard for assessing educational equivalency. Other pre-screening requirements such as language testing and requirements for a license or authority to practice in the country of education are identical to foreign-educated requirements listed in the Model Practice Act. However, FCCPT is not the only organization authorized to grant pre-screening certificates, but the standards and processes used by other organizations are not known. Jurisdictions maintain their authority and should maintain a process for reviewing all applications for foreign-educated physical therapist. To facilitate and streamline such a process, jurisdictions may wish to adopt a rule requiring an FCCPT certificate for application. Following is suggested rule language:

A Comprehensive Credential Evaluation Certificate for the Physical Therapist from the Foreign Credentialing Commission on Physical Therapy (FCCPT) is required for all applicants who received their education outside the United States to verify that the applicant's education is substantially equivalent to a U.S. degree in physical therapy, that the applicant satisfies the FCCPT's English proficiency requirements, and that the license or authority to practice obtained in the applicant's country of education is unencumbered.

## Approval of Credential Evaluation Agencies

If a jurisdiction's statutes include the requirement that a foreign-educated applicant obtains a credential evaluation from a "board approved credential evaluation agency," rules may be required that specify the criteria for board approval of such agencies. For example, one state included the following criteria in rules:

The Board shall approve an agency to perform credential evaluation of foreign-educated applicants based upon:

1. *The Recommended Guidelines for Reviewing Credentialing Agencies* (amended February 1997) of The Federation of State Boards of Physical Therapy, 509 Wythe Street, Alexandria, VA, 22314, which is incorporated herein by reference and on file with the Secretary of State, and no later editions;
2. The agency agreement to use the *Course Work Evaluation Tool* (amended March 1999) of the Federation of State Boards of Physical Therapy,

509 Wythe Street, Alexandria, VA 22314, which is incorporated herein by reference and on file with the Secretary of State, and no later editions; and

3. The agency agreement to evaluate the specific areas of both general and professional education curriculum as determined by the Board requirements in [reference to another rule specifying specific hour requirements in various components of general and professional education].

### Fees

A section of rules should include all fees and list all types of fees that may be imposed by the board upon those regulated. Penalties for late or lapsed licenses or certificates are also "fees" and should be included in the same rules area as other fees. Rules may state that there will be additional fees associated with computerized testing (fees paid directly to a testing center for use of its facility, equipment, etc.) that are not part of the board fees, but that are acknowledged and authorized. The authority to enact various fees by rule must be stated in statutes, or if specific fee categories with fee ceilings are listed in statutes, then rules must be consistent with the categories authorized in the statutes.

### Examination

Rules specifying the examination process, determining and identifying the passing scores, the reporting of scores, etc, should be developed.

### License and Certificate Renewal

Rules should address licensure and certificate renewal in a timely manner and the information required for renewal. If not previously included in statutes, it may be appropriate here to include a requirement of those regulated to always provide the board with current business and residence mailing addresses. It might be further stated that not having a current address on file with the board is not sufficient reason for failure to renew in a timely manner.

### Reinstatement

A rule should address the process for reinstatement of a lapsed license or certificate as differentiated from a physical therapist reapplying for a license after a lapse of more than 3 years. Refer to previous discussion under the *Licensure and Examination* key area.

### Restricted License or Certificate

The model statute language specifies the existence of restricted licenses and certificates. Rules should be developed giving further clarification to the processes and procedures for such restrictions, for example, the criteria for what circumstances and for whom restricted licenses or certificates could be imposed and the procedures for imposing restrictions, for determining the extent of the restrictions, and for lifting the restrictions. It will be important to include in rules that in addition to disciplinary actions, a restricted license can also be used with physical therapists in professional re-entry programs or physical therapists in substance abuse recovery programs. Where a restricted license is imposed as part of formal discipline, reinstatement to an unrestricted license should not be automatic but should always be associated with an appearance or rehearing of the licensee or certificate holder before the board. The supervision required of someone under such restriction should be addressed in rules.

### Professional Re-Entry

As mentioned, an appropriate use of a restricted license also includes those re-entering the profession after more than a 3-year absence from licensure and practice. Rules may be needed to address the specific needs of re-entry professionals. This should include specifying the procedures for demonstrating competence, possibly by serving an internship under a restricted license.

### Continuing Competence

Any criteria that the board may adopt and use for determining continuing competence requirements associated with relicensure should be clearly outlined in rules. The Federation is developing guidelines for such rules. In addition, states needing assistance may wish to refer to other states that have adopted the Model Practice Act language, including rules related to continuing competence requirements for ongoing licensure.

### National Emergencies

States may wish to include in rules the consideration for discretion under possible national emergencies. For example, in situations such as natural disasters, armed forces reserve call-ups or overseas military duty, the board should be granted flexibility in the area of license or certificate renewal.

### Time-Frame Rules

Some jurisdictions may require what are know as "time-frame rules" that specify the maximum time allowed for certain board procedures. For example, a time-frame rule may require an applicant for a license be granted approval to take the examination within so many days from submission of a completed application. Time-frame rules are designed to keep a board timely and responsive toward those being regulated.

## KEY AREA #5 • LAWFUL PRACTICE

Paragraphs (A) and (C) under the *Lawful Practice* section of statutes may need further clarification in rules:

### Direct Access/Full Authorization to Practice

Paragraph (A) in statutes is the direct access clause. It states: "Physical therapists licensed under this act shall be fully authorized to practice physical therapy as defined herein." The intent is that there be no further qualifications or restrictions to direct access other than licensure. If, for political purposes, states must attach certain restrictions, this would be the place in rules to specify what those restrictions might be. Again, it is recommended that no such restrictions be included, and in fact, paragraph (A) provides no statutory basis for adding other restrictions in rules. Additional restrictions would first require changing the model statute clause to authorize them, and then this area of rules would be the proper place for their inclusion if not addressed specifically enough in statutes. Examples currently seen in a few states include a requirement to refer a patient to a physician within 30 days of initiating direct access treatment and a restriction on direct access practice by a license after a certain time limit, for example, one year after initial licensure. The rationale for inclusion of such restrictions is weak. It has been required in a few states for purposes of political expediency in getting direct access legislation passed.

### Recognized Standards of Ethics

Paragraph (C) under *Lawful Practice* is the requirement to adhere to the recognized standards of ethics of the physical therapy profession. Much has already been said about the need for careful attention in drafting language that links law with ethics, or that adopts ethical standards also as legal standards. This is an area where another operational definition is strongly suggested. It could be included in this area of rules, later under rules associated with *Grounds for Disciplinary Action*, or in definitions. An example would be as follows:

> "The recognized standards of ethics" of the physical therapy profession means the *Code of Ethics* and the accompanying *Guide for Professional Conduct* of the American Physical Therapy Association.

This language may be sufficient to create the link to these ethical standards, but states may wish to seek additional legal counsel on whether this language will suffice, or whether some or all of the language from the *Code of Ethics* and accompanying *Guide* needs to be specifically included in rules. Another requirement may be that a specific date of publication or version of these documents be specified and be on file, for example, with the secretary of state.

Also, it is not recommended that states include references to the *Standards of Ethical Conduct for the Physical Therapist Assistant* and the *Guide for Conduct of the Affiliate Member.* Ultimately, the responsibility for ethical practice rests with the licensed professional physical therapist.

### Standards of Practice

It may be noted that the Model Practice Act does not include a recommendation for "Standards of Practice" in statutes or rules. The concept of standards of practice remains somewhat vague and not well defined. The practice act itself and the rules promulgated thereby, in a regulatory sense, is the standard of practice. Most standards of practice concepts are addressed in the statutes and conforming rules of a practice act. "Guidelines for Physical Therapist Practice," "Practice Parameters" and "Best Practice" are other relatively new concepts that influence standards of practice.

### Wound Management and Medication Storage

Paragraphs (D) and (E) are the optional statute clauses regarding wound debridement and application of topical and aerosol medications. Wound debridement, use of topical medications for iontophoresis or phonophoresis, and application of aerosol medications should be considered entry-level skills not requiring further regulation in rules. Medication storage may need further rule language, even though it has been addressed in the optional model statute language.

## KEY AREA #6 • USE OF TITLES

### "RPT" and "LPT" Prohibited

The only rule suggested under Use of Titles is a rule prohibiting the use of the letters "RPT" and "LPT" by licensed physical therapists. Although these are "protected terms" under the restricted use of titles, they are also archaic terms and add nothing, actually detracting from professionalism, and should be prohibited from use. Consistent use of the "PT" designation is envisioned under this model. An example of rule language may be:

> The proper letter designation of a licensed physical therapist is "PT." "RPT" and "LPT," while protected designations under [cite use of titles section of statutes], are not to be used by a physical therapist or any other person. The "PT" designation

shall be used immediately following the licensee's name or signature. Improper use of designations may result in disciplinary action.

The statutory authority to include this prohibition in rules would be under *Grounds for Disciplinary Action*, paragraph (14), "Making misleading, deceptive, untrue or fraudulent representations in violation of this [chapter, etc.] or in the practice of the profession."

## KEY AREA #7 • PATIENT CARE MANAGEMENT

### On-Site Supervision of Physical Therapist Assistants

States vary considerably regarding on-site or off-site supervision of physical therapist assistants. These requirements should be carefully addressed in both statutes and rules. In states where only on-site supervision exists, then the *Patient Care Management* section needs to be altered slightly or rules need to be altered to specify this restriction, or both. The statute can be altered by simply inserting the word "on-site" before the word "supervision" in paragraph (C.1). This paragraph would then read:

C.1. A physical therapist assistant shall work under a physical therapist's on-site supervision. A physical therapist assistant may document care provided without the co-signature of the supervising physical therapist.

"On-site" supervision is defined in the *Definitions* section of the statutes.

### Physical Therapy Aide Qualifications

Jurisdictions may want to consider a checklist of what skills should be included for onsite training of PT aides, whether the tasks have been observed and performed satisfactorily and the signature and date of the supervising physical therapist reviewing the task list.

### Off-Site Supervision of Physical Therapist Assistants

In states where off-site supervision of physical therapist assistants is permitted, further clarification in rules should specify restrictions or limitations based on the practice setting, the acuity of the patient population, and the types of diagnoses. The method of communication and how often it occurs between the supervising physical therapist and the physical therapist assistant should be included in rules.

### General Supervision of Physical Therapist Assistants

The question of who supervises the physical therapist assistant for each patient should be addressed. Is it the physical therapy department director, the same staff physical therapist always, or the physical therapist working with or responsible for a patient on each date of service? These are questions that licensing boards may wish to address in rules. The concept of a "physical therapist of record" is not a term defined or recommended by the Model Practice Act.

### Documentation

Documentation requirements, in general, should be specified. This area of rules should at least address assistive personnel's authority and extent of involvement in documenting treatment intervention. Model statute language under Patient Care Management recommends that physical therapist assistants be authorized to document in patient charts without requirement for co-signature by the physical therapist. States may wish to refer to APTA documentation guidelines, which may be the most concise model to follow.

## KEY AREA #8 • GROUNDS FOR DISCIPLINARY ACTION

### Substandard Care

Paragraphs (4) and (5) in the model statutes use the term "substandard care." If not included in the rules definitions, an operational definition of this term should be included in this section of the rules. As previously discussed, this Model Practice Act does not include a reference to a specific "standards of care" document. The practice act and rules set legal levels of conduct for practice and have clear ties to ethical standards of conduct for practitioners. The following suggested language might be considered:

"Substandard care" means the failure of a physical therapist or physical therapist assistant to meet the required standards of care as contained in [reference the entire section of statutes for the physical therapy law] and this [reference the entire rules section].

### Unreasonable Fees

A procedure for determining "unreasonable fees" may be a helpful inclusion in rules. Many states have not dealt with, and prefer not to deal with, complaints regarding excessive fees. In regard to regulating the practice of physical therapy, the Model Practice Act addresses greater responsiveness to legitimate public complaints and concerns. Clearly, unreasonable fees represent a legitimate public concern. One approach some states have used when a complaint of this nature is submitted is to survey a number of practitioners in the same geographic area and practice setting for historical information on charges for the procedures in question. This allows the board to have information about average fees and ranges for the same or similar procedures as those being considered. Boards are not in the business of price-fixing or price regulation; this should not be construed in any way as such an activity. Nevertheless, it does afford boards the latitude and means to address a public protection issue. Another option is to appoint a board "complaint resolution" subcommittee to attempt satisfactory resolution of such complaints without formal action of the entire board. Such a committee might comprise a public and a professional member of the board, plus the executive staff of the board.

### Recognized Standards of Ethics

Previous discussion under the *Lawful Practice* key area, in the model statute and *Guidelines for Rules* sections, created the link between ethical guidelines and the statutes. In paragraph (12) under *Grounds for Disciplinary Action* in the model statutes, this tie is again stated. A clear reference to the *Code of Ethics* and *Guide for Professional Conduct* of the American Physical Therapy Association should be established in rules, whether in this section, or previously in the *Lawful Practice* section, or in definitions. (Refer to previous discussion under *Guidelines for Rules: Key Area #5, Lawful Practice* section.)

## KEY AREA #9 • DISCIPLINARY ACTIONS/PROCEDURES

### Administrative Procedures Act

Most states have a uniform Administrative Procedures Act or similar law that governs the disciplinary process and provides consistency in disciplinary action between the various licensing agencies. There either needs to be clear reference in the rules to the Administrative Procedures Act of that state, or the details of all disciplinary procedures need to be fully outlined in rules. Rule language may even be adopted that accepts the Administrative Procedures Act as part of the rules of the physical therapy practice act.

This area of rules usually constitutes a more comprehensive section of various practice acts. Discipline-imposing restrictions on someone's livelihood deserves very careful attention to all legal and procedural details. A few basic principles need to be emphasized as states consider rule development:

### Receiving Complaints

Rules should specify how complaints can be received and may allow for written, verbal, telephone, facsimile, or any other electronic submission of complaints. A complaint form could be used, whether completed by the complainant or by board staff when accepting phone complaints. Overly burdensome requirements that a form must be mailed from the board, completed and returned in all cases by the complainant may place further obstacles and extends the response time in dealing with some complaints.

### Investigations

An investigation process should be in place that provides for timely and thorough investigation of all complaints determined by the board to require investigation. Experienced investigators who understand physical therapy practice, as well as the laws and rules governing that practice, should be employed or contracted to perform necessary investigations. There also may be "time-frame rules" proscribed by states that specify such things as the time from when a complaint is received to when a licensee is notified, and the number of days required to provide notice of an appearance at a hearing.

### Issuing Advisory Letters

An advisory letter is a non-disciplinary communication. It is not to be reported to any disciplinary database. As such, a jurisdiction may not consider it an official "action" of a board, and might choose not to include such a letter in the public file of a licensee or certificate holder. However, further rules may wish to clarify board policy or procedure.

### Hearing Officers or Administrative Law Judges

It is recommended that a process for utilizing hearing officers be employed with all formal hearings. This will guarantee another level of fairness and sense of responsiveness to public concerns. Where only the board and the board's assistant attorney general act in hearing formal cases, there may be a perception of conflict and self-interest. A hearing officer or administrative law judge presides over the case, usually with the board members present to hear testimony and to question witnesses, and then the presiding officer renders an opinion and makes recommendations to the board for the board's final decision.

### Subpoenas

Rules specifying the subpoena process should be developed. Subpoenas may be necessary for compelling witnesses to testify and for examining pertinent documentation. Consideration of whether the board alone can approve a subpoena or if the executive director can be granted this authority should be addressed in rules.

### Hearings

The entire process related to the order of hearings and the role of hearing officers should be specified in rules. Much of this may be in Administrative Procedures Acts, but if not, it should be included in rules.

### Censure

A rule should clarify whether a censure remains as a permanent record in a licensee or certificate holder's file, or if it is removed after a certain period.

### Restricted License or Certificate

Rules should address all aspects of restricted licenses and certificates. Previous discussion under the *Licensure and Examination* key area is again repeated in this section for consideration in rule development:

The model statute language specifies the existence of restricted licenses and certificates. Rules should be developed giving further clarification to the processes and procedures for such restrictions; for example, the criteria for what circumstances and for whom restricted licenses or certificates could be imposed, the procedures for imposing restrictions, for determining the extent of the restrictions, and for lifting the restrictions. It will be important to include in rules that, in addition to disciplinary actions, a restricted license can also be used with physical therapists in professional reentry programs or physical therapists in voluntary substance abuse programs. Where a restricted license is imposed as part of formal discipline, reinstatement of an unrestricted license should not be automatic but should always be associated with an appearance or rehearing of the licensee or certificate holder before the board. The supervision required of someone under such restriction should be addressed in rules.

### Voluntarily Surrendering a License/Certificate

The process for voluntarily surrendering a license or certification when the individual admits guilt should be included in rules.

### Civil Penalties

The procedure for determining the costs of an investigation and hearing and imposing such costs in the form of civil penalties should be clarified in rules.

### Refusal to Issue a License or Certificate

If not addressed in statute, rules should specify the board's authority to refuse to issue or renew a license or certificate when there is a concurrent disciplinary investigation or action involving a licensee or certificate holder. This may be an important legal consideration. For example, if an active investigation alone would be considered grounds for refusing to issue or renew a license, or if an actual action or determination would be required before denial could occur.

### Reapplication of Licensure/Certificate After Revocation/Surrender

Rules should include the process for reapplication for a license or certificate after revocation. A revoked license is not reinstated and is usually revoked with no mention of time frame for potential reapplication. It may be appropriate to consider establishing a minimum amount of time, such as one year, that must pass before a person may reapply. Any reapplication after revocation of a license or certificate should automatically require a rehearing by the board, even if a license or certificate was revoked in another state. Rules should specify what information needs to be included in a potential application, including information from previous disciplinary proceedings. A time frame is usually set in a suspension of a license and, at the end of that period, the license is reinstated. All of these procedural issues need to be addressed in rules. Potential rule language might include:

Following revocation of a licensee or certificate in any jurisdiction, an individual may not reapply for a license or certificate for a period of 2 years.

Reapplication following suspension or revocation of a license or certificate requires a hearing before the Board with a review of the prior disciplinary action and current qualifications of the applicant.

### Emergency Actions

Rules can further clarify criteria that constitute grounds for emergency actions and for enacting summary suspensions.

## KEY AREA #10 • UNLAWFUL PRACTICE

### Cease and Desist Orders and Injunctions

The process for initiating cease and desist orders, as well as administrative procedures for initiating injunctive relief, should be identified in rules. This will allow the board to take action against anyone not regulated by a practice act but who may violate or attempt to violate such an act.

## KEY AREA #11 • CONSUMER ADVOCACY

### Substance Abuse Recovery Program

Rules should outline the process for a licensee opting to participate in a voluntary substance abuse program. Criteria for board authorization of substance abuse programs should be established as well as reporting requirements for licensees who use these services.

### Use of Information

Rules should include policies for information distribution, including use of directories. For example, if a list is not to be used for commercial purposes, then rules should specifically prohibit making lists available for commercial purposes.

### Public Access to Information

Rules should clarify the content, format and extent of information made public by any official action of the board.

### Disclosure

Rules should define what constitutes written disclosure. It should be stated if conspicuous posting is required, if a personal letter is sufficient, and if signed acknowledgment by either party or both parties is required. Rules may also specify the exact language for such disclosure. For example, *Key Area #11* includes model language that, "If a referring practitioner is deriving direct or indirect compensation from the referral to physical therapy the physical therapist shall disclose this information in writing to the patient." Such a disclosure might be specifically required to read:

> Under [cite specific statute requiring disclosure of financial involvement of the referral source] I am required by law to inform you in writing that your referring physician (or specify if different than a physician) derives either direct or indirect compensation related to physical therapy provided in this clinic. You may choose to receive physical therapy in this clinic or, if you elect not to receive physical therapy in this clinic, I will provide you with the names, addresses and telephone numbers of two other physical therapists qualified to provide you with physical therapy.

### Freedom of Choice

There may be guidelines developed on how licensees can support the concept of freedom of choice. For example, a rule may specify, as a matter of guidance, that when a patient is referred to another appropriate provider, at least two provider options must always be given to the patient.

# Appendices

# Appendix A
# The Model Practice Act for Physical Therapy

**MODEL STATUTE LANGUAGE ONLY**

## CONTENTS

### Article 1 • General Provisions



### Article 2 • Board of Physical Therapy



### Article 3 • Licensure and Examination



### Article 4 • Regulation of Physical Therapy

## Physical Therapy Law

[Include proper numerical statute reference, e.g., Chapter # and/or Title #]

### ARTICLE 1 • GENERAL PROVISIONS

#### Legislative Intent

This [chapter, act, section, law] is enacted for the purpose of protecting the public health, safety, and welfare, and of providing for state administrative control, supervision, licensure and regulation of the practice of physical therapy. It is the legislature's intent that only individuals who meet and maintain prescribed standards of competence and conduct may engage in the practice of physical therapy as authorized by this [chapter, etc.]. This [chapter, etc.] shall be liberally construed to promote the public interest and to accomplish the purpose stated herein.
**Bracketed areas in the model language throughout the Model Practice Act indicate optional language each state should adapt to its own needs.*

#### Definitions

A. "Board" means the [specify the state] board of physical therapy.
B. "Physical therapy" means the care and services provided by or under the direction and supervision of a physical therapist who is licensed pursuant to this [chapter, act, section, law].
C. "Physical therapist" means a person who is licensed pursuant to this [chapter, etc.] to practice physical therapy.
D. "Practice of physical therapy" means:
   1. Examining, evaluating and testing individuals with mechanical, physiological and developmental impairments, functional limitations, and disability or other health and movement-related conditions in order

to determine a diagnosis, prognosis, plan of therapeutic intervention, and to assess the ongoing effects of intervention.

2. Alleviating impairments and functional limitations by designing, implementing, and modifying therapeutic interventions that include, but are not limited to therapeutic exercise; functional training in self care and in home, community or work reintegration; manual therapy including soft tissue and joint mobilization and manipulation; therapeutic massage; assistive and adaptive orthotic, prosthetic, protective and supportive devices and equipment; airway clearance techniques; debridement and wound care; physical agents or modalities; mechanical and electrotherapeutic modalities; and patient-related instruction.
3. Reducing the risk of injury, impairment, functional limitation and disability, including the promotion and maintenance of fitness, health and quality of life in all age populations.
4. Engaging in administration, consultation, education and research.

E. Assistive Personnel
   1. "Physical therapist assistant" means a person who meets the requirements of this act for certification and who assists the physical therapist in selected components of physical therapy intervention.
   2. "Physical therapy aide" means a person trained under the direction of a physical therapist who performs designated and supervised routine tasks related to physical therapy.

F. "Restricted license" means a license on which the board places restrictions or conditions, or both, as to scope of practice, place of practice, supervision of practice, duration of licensed status, or type or condition of patient or client to whom the licensee may provide services.

G. "Restricted certificate" means a certificate on which the board has placed any restrictions due to action imposed by the board.

H. "On-site supervision" means the supervising physical therapist is continuously on-site and present in the department or facility where services are provided, is immediately available to the person being supervised and maintains continued involvement in appropriate aspects of each treatment session in which assistive personnel are involved in components of care.

I. "Testing" means standardized methods and techniques used to gather data about the patient, including electrodiagnostic and electrophysiologic tests and measures.

J. "Consultation by means of telecommunication" means that a physical therapist renders professional or expert opinion or advice to another physical therapist or health care provider via telecommunications or computer technology from a distant location. It includes the transfer of data or exchange of educational or related information by means of audio, video or data communications. The physical therapist may use telehealth technology as a vehicle for providing only services that are legally or professionally authorized. The patient's written or verbal consent will be obtained and documented prior to such consultation. All records used or resulting from a consultation by means of telecommunications are part of a patient's records and are subject to applicable confidentiality requirements.

K. "Jurisdiction of the United States" means any state, territory or the District of Columbia that licenses physical therapists.

[Optional Statute or Rule Language] If using only the term "manual therapy" and not using the additional descriptor of manual therapy, i.e. the phrase "including soft tissue and joint mobilization and manipulation" in the "practice of physical therapy" definition:

[L. "Manual therapy" means a broad group of skilled hand movements used by physical therapists to mobilize soft tissues and joints for the purpose of modulating pain, increasing range of motion, reducing or eliminating soft tissue inflammation, inducing relaxation, improving contractile and noncontractile tissue extensibility, or improving pulmonary function.]

## ARTICLE 2 • BOARD OF PHYSICAL THERAPY

### Board of Physical Therapy

A. The board of physical therapy shall consist of [five] members appointed by the governor. [Three] members shall be physical therapists who are residents of this state, possess unrestricted licenses to practice physical therapy in this state and have been practicing in this state for no less than [5] years before their appointments. The governor shall also appoint [two] public members who shall be residents of this state and who are not affiliated with, nor have a financial interest in, any health care profession and who have an interest in consumer rights.

B. Board members serve staggered 4-year terms. Board members shall serve no more than two successive 4-year terms nor for more than 10 consecutive years. By approval of the majority of the board, the service of a member may be extended at the completion of a 4-year term until a new member is appointed or the current member is reappointed.

C. If requested by the board the governor may remove any member of the board for misconduct, incompetence or neglect of duty.

D. Board members are eligible for reimbursement of expenses pursuant to [cite applicable statute relating to reimbursement] to cover necessary expenses for attending each board meeting or for representing the board in an official board-approved activity.

E. A board member who acts within the scope of board duties, without malice and in the reasonable belief that the member's action is warranted by law is immune from civil liability.

### Powers and Duties of the Board

The board shall:

1. Evaluate the qualifications of applicants for licensure and certification.
2. Provide for the national examinations for physical therapists and physical therapist assistants and adopt passing scores for these examinations.
3. Issue licenses, permits, or certificates to persons who meet the requirements of this [chapter, act, section, law].
4. Regulate the practice of physical therapy by interpreting and enforcing this [chapter, etc.].
5. Adopt and revise rules consistent with this [chapter, etc.]. Such rules, when lawfully adopted, shall have the effect of law.
6. Meet at least once each quarter in compliance with the open meeting requirements of [cite applicable statute]. A majority of board members shall constitute a quorum for the transaction of business. The board shall keep an official record of its meetings.
7. Establish mechanisms for assessing continuing competence of licensees.
8. Establish and collect fees for sustaining the necessary operation and expenses of the board.
9. Elect officers from its members necessary for the operations and obligations of the board. Terms of office shall be one year.
10. Provide for the timely orientation and training of new professional and public appointees to the board regarding board licensing and disciplinary procedures, this [chapter, etc.] and board rules, policies and procedures.
11. Maintain a current list of all persons regulated under this chapter, including the person's name, current business and residential address, telephone numbers and license or certificate number.
12. Provide information to the public regarding the complaint process.
13. Employ necessary personnel to carry out the administrative work of the board. Board personnel are eligible to receive compensation pursuant to [cite specific statute].
14. Enter into contracts for services necessary for adequate enforcement of this chapter.
15. Report final disciplinary action taken against a licensee or certificate holder to a national disciplinary database recognized by the board or as required by law.

16. Publish, at least annually, final disciplinary action taken against a licensee or certificate holder.
17. Publish, at least annually, board rulings, opinions, and interpretations of statutes or rules in order to guide persons regulated pursuant to this [chapter, etc.].
18. Participate in or conduct performance audits of the board.

### Disposition of Funds

[No model language is offered under this section heading. See *Discussion* for additional information.]

## ARTICLE 3 • LICENSURE AND EXAMINATION

### Qualifications for Licensure and Certification

A. An applicant for a license as a physical therapist shall:
   1. Be of good moral character.
   2. Have completed the application process.
   3. Be a graduate of a professional physical therapy education program accredited by a national accreditation agency approved by the board.
   4. Have successfully passed the national examination approved by the board.
B. An applicant for a license as a physical therapist who has been educated outside of the United States shall:
   1. Be of good moral character.
   2. Have completed the application process.
   3. Provide satisfactory evidence that the applicant's education is substantially equivalent to the requirements of physical therapists educated in accredited educational programs as determined by the board. If it is determined that a foreign-educated applicant's education is not substantially equivalent the board may require the person to complete additional course work before it proceeds with the application process.
   4. Provide written proof that the applicant's school of physical therapy education is recognized by its own ministry of education.
   5. Provide written proof of authorization to practice as a physical therapist without limitations in the country where the professional education occurred.
   6. Provide proof of legal authorization to reside and seek employment in a jurisdiction of the United States.
   7. Have the applicant's educational credentials evaluated by a board-approved credential evaluation agency.

8. Have passed the board-approved English proficiency examinations if the applicant's native language is not English.
9. Have participated in an interim supervised clinical practice period prior to being approved to take the national examination.
10. Have successfully passed the national examination approved by the board.

C. Notwithstanding the provisions of subsection (B), if the foreign-educated physical therapist applicant is a graduate of an accredited educational program as approved by the board, the board may waive the requirements in subsection (B), paragraphs 3, 4, 7 and 9.

D. An applicant for certification as a physical therapist assistant shall:
1. Be of good moral character.
2. Have completed the application process.
3. Be a graduate of a physical therapist assistant education program accredited by an agency approved by the board.
4. Have successfully passed the national examination approved by the board.

## Application, Statement of Deficiencies, Hearing

A. An applicant for licensure or certification shall file a complete application as required by the board. The applicant shall include application and examination fees as prescribed in [reference the specific statute and/or rules specifying the fees].

B. The board shall notify an applicant of any deficiencies in the application. An applicant who disagrees with the identified deficiencies may request in writing and, upon request, shall be granted a hearing pursuant to [reference the section of the state administrative procedures act where an appeals process is addressed].

## Examination

A. The board shall conduct examinations within the state at least quarterly at a time and place prescribed by the board. The passing score shall be determined by the board.

B. An applicant may take the examination for licensure after the application process has been completed. The national examination shall test entry-level competency related to physical therapy theory, examination and evaluation, diagnosis, prognosis, treatment intervention, prevention, and consultation.

C. An applicant may take the examination for certification after the application process has been completed. The national examination shall test for requisite knowledge and skills in the technical application of physical therapy services.

D. An applicant for licensure or certification who does not pass the examination after the first attempt may retake the examination one additional time without reapplication for licensure or certification within 6 months of the first failure. Before the board may approve an applicant for subsequent testing beyond two attempts, an applicant shall re-apply for licensure or certification and shall demonstrate evidence satisfactory to the board of having successfully completed additional clinical training or course work, or both, as determined by the board.

### Interim Permit

A. If a foreign-educated applicant satisfies the requirements of section [specify the *Qualifications for Licensure and Certification* sections], subsection B, the board shall issue an interim permit to the applicant for the purpose of participating in a supervised clinical practice period prior to the applicant being approved to take the national examination. An applicant who has previously failed the national examination is not eligible for an interim permit until the applicant passes the examination.
B. The board may issue an interim permit for at least 90 days but not more than 6 months.
C. An interim permit holder shall complete, to the satisfaction of the board, a period of clinical practice in a facility approved by the board and under the on-site supervision of a physical therapist who holds an unrestricted license issued pursuant to this [chapter, act, section, law].
D. An interim permit is immediately revoked when the board notifies an interim permit holder that the permit holder has failed the licensing examination.

### Licensure by Endorsement

The board shall issue a license to a physical therapist who has a valid unrestricted license from another jurisdiction of the United States if that person, when granted the license, met all requirements prescribed in section [specify the *Qualifications for Licensure and Certification* section], subsections (A) and (B) and any applicable board rules. [See *Guidelines for Rules, Key Area #4.*]

### Exemptions from Licensure

A. This [chapter, act, section, law] does not restrict a person licensed under any other law of this state from engaging in the profession or practice for which that person is licensed if that person does not represent, imply or claim that he/she is a physical therapist or a provider of physical therapy.

B. The following persons are exempt from the licensure requirements of this [chapter, etc.] when engaged in the following activities:
   1. A person in a professional education program approved by the board who is pursuing a course of study leading to a degree as a physical therapist and that person is satisfying supervised clinical education requirements related to the person's physical therapy education while under on-site supervision of a licensed physical therapist.
   2. A physical therapist who is practicing in the United States Armed Services, United States Public Health Service or Veterans Administration pursuant to federal regulations for state licensure of health care providers.
   3. A physical therapist who is licensed in another jurisdiction of the United States or a foreign-educated physical therapist credentialed in another country of that person is performing physical therapy in connection with teaching or participating in an educational seminar of no more than 60 days in a calendar year.
   4. A physical therapist who is licensed in another jurisdiction of the United States if that person is providing consultation by means of telecommunication to a physical therapist licensed under this [chapter, etc.].

### License or Certificate Renewal, Changes of Name or Address

A. A licensee or certificate holder shall renew the license or certificate pursuant to board rules. A licensee or certificate holder who fails to renew the license or certificate on or before the expiration date shall not practice as a physical therapist or work as a physical therapist assistant in this state.

B. Each licensee and certificate holder is responsible for reporting to the board a name change or change in business or home address within 30 days after the date of change.

### Reinstatement of License or Certificate

A. The board may reinstate a lapsed license or certificate upon payment of a renewal fee and reinstatement fee.

B. If a person's license has lapsed for more than 3 consecutive years that person shall reapply for a license and pay all applicable fees. The person shall also demonstrate to the board's satisfaction competence to practice physical therapy, or shall serve an internship under a restricted license or take remedial courses as determined by the board, or both, at the board's discretion. The board may also require the applicant to take an examination.

[Optional statute language] For states requiring maximum fee ceilings within the statutes.

### [Fees

The board shall establish and collect fees not to exceed:

1. ______________ dollars for an application for an original license or certificate. This fee is nonrefundable.
2. ______________ dollars for an examination for licensure or certification.
3. ______________ dollars for a certificate of renewal of a license or certificate.
4. ______________ dollars for an application for reinstatement of a license or certificate.
5. ______________ dollars for each duplicate license or certificate.]

## ARTICLE 4 • REGULATION OF PHYSICAL THERAPY

### Lawful Practice

A. A physical therapist licensed under this act is fully authorized to practice physical therapy as defined herein.
B. A physical therapist shall refer a patient or client to appropriate health care practitioners if the physical therapist has reasonable cause to believe symptoms or conditions are present that require services beyond the scope of practice or when physical therapy is contraindicated.
C. A physical therapist shall adhere to the recognized standards of ethics of the physical therapy profession and as further established by rule. [Rules should specify ethical conduct or specifically reference the APTA's *Code of Ethics* and *Guide for Professional Conduct* at *Appendix E*.]

[Optional Statute Clauses]

[D. A physical therapist may perform wound management that includes, but is not limited to, sharp debridement, debridement with other agents, dry dressings, wet dressings, topical agents including enzymes, and hydrotherapy.

[E. A physical therapist may purchase, store and administer topical and aerosol medications as part of the practice of physical therapy as defined herein. A physical therapist shall comply with any regulation duly adopted by the [specify the state] Board of Pharmacy (or other regulatory board) specifying protocols for storage of medications.]

### Use of Titles, Restrictions, Classification of Violation

A. A physical therapist shall use the letters "PT" in connection with the physical therapist's name or place of business to denote licensure under this [chapter, act, section, law].

B. A person or business entity, its employees, agents or representatives shall not use in connection with that person's name or the name or activity of the business, the words "physical therapy," "physical therapist," "physiotherapy," "physiotherapist" or "registered physical therapist," the letters "PT," "LPT," "RPT," or any other words, abbreviations or insignia indicating or implying directly or indirectly that physical therapy is provided or supplied, including the billing of services labeled as physical therapy, unless such services are provided by or under the direction of a physical therapist licensed pursuant to this [chapter, etc.]. A person or entity that violates this subsection is guilty of a [cite specific legal sanction].
C. A physical therapist assistant shall use the letters "PTA" in connection with that person's name to denote certification hereunder.
D. A person shall not use the title "physical therapist assistant," the letters "PTA," or any other words, abbreviations or insignia in connection with that person's name to indicate or imply, directly or indirectly, that the person is a physical therapist assistant unless that person is certified as a physical therapist assistant pursuant to this [chapter, etc.]. A person who violates this subsection is guilty of a [cite specific legal sanction].

### Patient Care Management

A. A physical therapist is responsible for managing all aspects of the physical therapy care of each patient. The physical therapist shall provide:
   1. The initial written evaluation for each patient;
   2. Periodic written re-evaluation of each patient;
   3. A written discharge plan for the patient and the patient's response to treatment at discharge.
B. A physical therapist shall assure the qualifications of all assistive personnel to perform specific designated tasks through written documentation of the assistive personnel's education or training.
C. For each date of service, a physical therapist shall provide all therapeutic interventions that require the expertise of a physical therapist and shall determine the use of assistive personnel that provides delivery of service that is safe, effective, and efficient for each patient.
   1. A physical therapist assistant shall work under a physical therapist's supervision. A physical therapist assistant may document care provided without the co-signature of the supervising physical therapist. [Any further limitations on supervision of the physical therapist assistant should be specified here and/or clarified in rules.]
   2. A physical therapist may use physical therapy aides for designated routine tasks. A physical therapy aide shall work under the on-site supervision of a physical therapist who is continuously on-site and

present in the facility. This may extend to an off-site setting only when the physical therapy aide is accompanying and working directly with a physical therapist assistant with a specific patient. [Any further limitations on the use of physical therapy aides should be specified here and/or clarified in rules.]

D. A physical therapist may concurrently utilize no more than any combination of [specify the number] assistive personnel. In addition to [specify the number] assistive personnel, a physical therapist may supervise any combination of [specify the number] additional persons who are physical therapist students, physical therapist assistant students or physical therapists under restricted license or interim permit.

E. A physical therapist's responsibility for patient care management shall include oversight of all documentation for services rendered to each patient, including awareness of fees charged or reimbursement methodology used. A physical therapist shall also be aware of what constitutes unreasonable or fraudulent fees.

### Grounds for Disciplinary Action

The following are grounds for disciplinary action:

1. Violating any provision of this [chapter, act, section, law], board rules or a written order of the board.
2. Practicing or offering to practice beyond the scope of the practice of physical therapy.
3. Obtaining or attempting to obtain a license or certificate by fraud or misrepresentation.
4. Engaging in the performance of substandard care by a physical therapist due to a deliberate or negligent act or failure to act regardless of whether actual injury to the patient is established.
5. Engaging in the performance of substandard care by a physical therapist assistant, including exceeding the authority to perform components of intervention selected by the supervising licensee regardless of whether actual injury to the patient is established.
6. Failing to supervise assistive personnel in accordance with this [chapter, etc.] and board rules.
7. Having been convicted of a felony in the courts of this state or any other state, territory or country. Conviction, as used in this paragraph, shall include a finding or verdict of guilt, an admission of guilt, or a plea of *nolo contendere.*
8. Practicing as a physical therapist or working as a physical therapist assistant when physical or mental abilities are impaired by the use of controlled substances or other habit-forming drugs, chemicals or alcohol.

9. Having had a license or certificate revoked or suspended, other disciplinary action taken, or an application for licensure or certification refused, revoked or suspended by the proper authorities of another state, territory or country.
10. Engaging in sexual misconduct. For the purpose of this paragraph sexual misconduct includes:
    (a) Engaging in or soliciting sexual relationships, whether consensual or non-consensual, while a physical therapist or physical therapist assistant/patient relationship exists.
    (b) Making sexual advances, requesting sexual favors or engaging in other verbal conduct or physical contact of a sexual nature with patients or clients.
    (c) Intentionally viewing a completely or partially disrobed patient in the course of treatment if the viewing is not related to patient diagnosis or treatment under current practice standards.
11. Directly or indirectly requesting, receiving or participating in the dividing, transferring, assigning, rebating or refunding of an unearned fee, or profiting by means of a credit or other valuable consideration such as an unearned commission, discount, or gratuity in connection with the furnishing of physical therapy services. This does not prohibit the members of any regularly and properly organized business entity recognized by law and comprising physical therapists from dividing fees received for professional services among themselves as they determine necessary to defray their joint operating expense.
12. Failing to adhere to the recognized standards of ethics of the physical therapy profession.
13. Charging unreasonable or fraudulent fees for services performed or not performed.
14. Making misleading, deceptive, untrue or fraudulent representations in violation of this [chapter, etc.] or in the practice of the profession.
15. Having been adjudged mentally incompetent by a court of competent jurisdiction.
16. Aiding or abetting a person who is not licensed or certified in this state and who directly or indirectly performs activities requiring a license or certificate.
17. Failing to report to the board any act or omission of a licensee, certificate holder, applicant or any other person who violates the provisions of this [chapter, etc.].
18. Interfering with an investigation or disciplinary proceeding by willful misrepresentation of facts or by the use of threats or harassment against any patient or witness to prevent them from providing evidence in a disciplinary proceeding or any legal action.

19. Failing to maintain patient confidentiality without prior written consent of the patient or unless otherwise required by law.
20. Failing to maintain adequate patient records. For the purposes of this paragraph, "adequate patient records" means legible records that contain at a minimum sufficient information to identify the patient, an evaluation of objective findings, a diagnosis, the plan of care, the treatment record and a discharge plan.
21. Promoting an unnecessary device, treatment intervention or service for the financial gain of the practitioner or of a third party.
22. Providing treatment intervention unwarranted by the condition of the patient, or continuing treatment beyond the point of reasonable benefit.
23. Participating in underutilization or overutilization of physical therapy services for personal or institutional financial gain, or participation in services that are in any way linked to the financial gain of a referral source.

## Investigative Powers, Emergency Action, Hearing Officers

A. To enforce this [chapter, act section, law] the board is authorized to:
   1. Receive complaints filed against licensees or certificate holders and conduct a timely investigation.
   2. Conduct an investigation at any time and on its own initiative without receipt of a written complaint if the board has reason to believe that there may be a violation of this [chapter, etc.].
   3. Issue subpoenas to compel the attendance of any witness or the production of any documentation relative to a case.
   4. Take emergency action ordering the summary suspension of a license or certificate or the restriction of the licensee's practice or certificate holder's employment pending proceedings by the board.
   5. Appoint hearing officers authorized to conduct hearings. Hearing officers shall prepare and submit to the board findings of fact, conclusions of law and an order that shall be reviewed and voted on by the board.
   6. Require a licensee to be examined in order to determine the licensee's mental, physical or professional competence.

B. If the board finds that the information received in a complaint or an investigation is not of sufficient seriousness to merit disciplinary action against a licensee or certificate holder it may take the following actions:
   1. Dismiss the complaint if the board believes the information or complaint is without merit.
   2. Issue a confidential advisory letter to the licensee or certificate holder. An advisory letter is non-disciplinary and notifies a licensee or cer-

tificate holder that, while there is insufficient evidence to support disciplinary action, the board believes that the licensee or certificate holder should modify or eliminate certain conduct or practices.

### Hearings

[No model statute language is offered under this section heading. See *Discussion* for additional information.]

### Disciplinary Actions/Penalties

Upon proof that any grounds prescribed in section [cite section on Grounds for Disciplinary Action] have been violated, the board may take the following disciplinary actions singly or in combination:

1. Issue a censure.
2. Restrict a license or certificate. The board may require a licensee or certificate holder to report regularly to the board on matters related to the grounds for the restricted license or certificate.
3. Suspend a license or certificate for a period prescribed by the board.
4. Revoke a license or certificate.
5. Refuse to issue or renew a license or certificate.
6. Impose a civil penalty of at least ____________ but not more than ____________. [Include minimum and maximum dollar amounts of civil penalties.] In addition the board may assess and collect the reasonable costs incurred in a disciplinary hearing when action is taken against a person's license or certificate.
7. Accept a voluntary surrendering of a license or certificate.

### Procedural Due Process

Actions of the Board shall be taken subject to the right of notice, hearing and adjudication and the right of appeal in accordance with [specify the state] law relating to administrative law and procedure. [Or specify the state statute that addresses appeals or review of board decisions.]

### Unlawful Practice, Classification, Civil Penalties, Injunctive Relief

A. It is unlawful for any person to practice or in any manner to represent, imply or claim to practice physical therapy or use any word or designation that implies that the person is a physical therapist unless that person is licensed pursuant to this [chapter, act, section, law]. A person who engages in an activity requiring a license pursuant to this [chapter, etc.] or uses any word, title, letters, or any description of services that incorporates one or more of the terms, designations or abbreviations in violation of section [cite specific *Use of Titles* section] that implies that the person is licensed to engage in the practice of physical therapy is guilty of a [cite specific legal sanction, e.g., class 1 misdemeanor.]

B. The board may investigate any person to the extent necessary to determine if the person is engaged in the unlawful practice of physical therapy. If an investigation indicates that a person may be practicing physical therapy unlawfully, the board shall inform the person of the alleged violation. The board may refer the matter for prosecution regardless of whether the person ceases the unlawful practice of physical therapy.

C. The board, through the [Office of the Attorney General or the appropriate county attorney], may apply for injunctive relief in any court of competent jurisdiction to enjoin any person from committing any act in violation of this [chapter, etc.]. Injunction proceedings are in addition to, and not in lieu of, all penalties and other remedies prescribed in this [chapter, etc.]. [It may be the Justice Department, a county attorney, or other appropriate agency other than or in addition to the office of the Attorney General. Language should reflect those options.]

D. A person who aids or requires another person to directly or indirectly violate this [chapter, etc.] or board rules, who permits a license to be used by another person, or who acts with the intent to violate or evade this [chapter, etc.] or board rules is subject to a civil penalty of not more than [$ amount of violation] for the first violation and not more than [$ amount of violation] for each subsequent violation. [At least one thousand dollars and five thousand dollars, respectively, are suggested.]

[Optional Statute]

[E. The board shall transmit all monies it collects from civil penalties pursuant to this [chapter, etc.] to the [specify the disposition of these funds if different from other funds].]

### Reporting Violations, Immunity

A. Any person, including but not limited to a licensee, corporation, insurance company, health care organization or health care facility and state or local governmental agencies shall report to the board any conviction, determination or finding that a licensee has committed an act that constitutes a violation of section [cite section on *Grounds for Disciplinary Action*].

B. A person is immune from civil liability, whether direct or derivative, for providing information in good faith to the board pursuant to paragraph (A) of this section.

C. The board shall not disclose the identity of a person who provides information unless such information is essential to proceedings conducted pursuant to sections [cite the *Investigative Powers and Hearings* sections] or unless required by a court of law.

### Substance Abuse Recovery Program

In lieu of a disciplinary proceeding prescribed by this [chapter, act, section, law], the board may permit a licensee or certificate holder to actively participate in a board-approved substance abuse recovery program if:

A. The board has evidence that the licensee or certificate holder is impaired.
B. The licensee or certificate holder has not been convicted of a felony relating to a controlled substance in a court of law of the United States or any other territory or country.
C. The licensee or certificate holder enters into a written agreement with the board for a restricted license or certificate and complies with all the terms of the agreement, including making satisfactory progress in the program and adhering to any limitations on the licensee's practice or certificate holder's work imposed by the board to protect the public. Failure to enter into such an agreement shall activate an immediate investigation and disciplinary proceeding by the board.
D. As part of the agreement established between the licensee or certificate holder and the board, the licensee or certificate holder signs a waiver allowing the substance abuse program to release information to the board if the licensee or certificate holder does not comply with the requirements of this section or is unable to practice or work with reasonable skill or safety.

### Rights of Consumers

A. The public shall have access to the following information:
   1. A list of licensees and interim permit holders that includes place of practice, license or interim permit number, date of license or interim permit expiration and status of license.
   2. A list of physical therapist assistants certified in the state, including place of employment, certification number, and date of certificate expiration.
   3. A list of official actions taken by the board.
B. The home address and telephone numbers of physical therapists and physical therapist assistants are not public records and shall be kept confidential by the board unless they are the only addresses and telephone numbers of record.
C. If a referring practitioner is deriving direct or indirect compensation from the referral to physical therapy the physical therapist shall disclose this information in writing to the patient prior to the initial evaluation.

D. A physical therapist shall disclose in writing to a patient any financial interest in products that the physical therapist endorses and recommends to the patient at the time of such endorsement or recommendation.
E. A physical therapist shall inform each patient that the patient has freedom of choice in services and products.
F. Information relating to the physical therapist-patient relationship is confidential and shall not be communicated to a third party who is not involved in that patient's care without the prior written consent of the patient. A physical therapist shall divulge to the board information it requires in connection with any investigation, public hearing or other proceedings. The physical therapist-patient privilege does not extend to cases in which the physical therapist has a duty to report information as required by law.
G. Any person may submit a complaint regarding any licensee, certificate holder, or any other person potentially in violation of this [chapter, act, section, law]. Confidentiality shall be maintained subject to law.
H. The board shall keep all information relating to the receiving and investigation of complaints filed against licensees or certificate holders confidential until the information becomes public record or as required by law. Patient records, including clinical records, files, any other report or oral statement relating to diagnostic findings or treatment of patients, any information from which a patient or his family might be identified, or information received and records or reports kept by the board as a result of an investigation made pursuant to this chapter shall not be available to the public and shall be kept confidential by the board.
I. Each licensee shall display a copy of the licensee's license or current renewal verification in a location accessible to public view at the licensee's place of practice.

### Temporary Provisions

[No model statute language is offered under this section heading. See *Discussion* for additional information.]

# Appendix B
# Model Definition of Physical Therapy

**APTA Board of Directors • March 1997**
Reprinted With Permission

Physical therapy, which is the care and services provided by or under the direction and supervision of a physical therapist, includes:

1. Examining (history, systems review, and tests and measures) individuals with impairments, functional limitations, and disability or other health-related conditions in order to determine a diagnosis, prognosis, and intervention; tests and measures may include the following:
   - Aerobic capacity or endurance
   - Anthropometric characteristics
   - Arousal, mentation and cognition
   - Assistive and adaptive devices
   - Community or work (job/school/play) integration/reintegration
   - Cranial nerve integrity
   - Environmental, home and work (job/school/play) barriers
   - Ergonomics or body mechanics
   - Gait, locomotion and balance
   - Integumentary integrity
   - Joint integrity and mobility
   - Motor function
   - Muscle performance
   - Neuromotor development and sensory integration
   - Orthotic, protective and supportive devices
   - Pain
   - Posture
   - Prosthetic requirements
   - Range of motion

- Reflex integrity
- Self-care and home-management
- Sensory integrity
- Ventilation, respiration and circulation

2. Alleviating impairment, functional limitation, and disability by designing, implementing and modifying therapeutic interventions that may include the following:
   - Coordination, communication and documentation
   - Patient-related instruction
   - Therapeutic exercise (including aerobic conditioning)
   - Functional training in self-care and home-management (including activities of daily living and instrumental activities of daily living)
   - Functional training in community or work (job/school/play) integration/reintegration activities (including instrumental activities of daily living, work hardening, and work conditioning)
   - Manual therapy techniques, including mobilization and manipulation
   - Prescription, application, and as appropriate, fabrication of assistive, adaptive, orthotic, protective, supportive and prosthetic devices and equipment
   - Airway clearance techniques
   - Wound management
   - Electrotherapeutic modalities
   - Physical agents and mechanical modalities
3. Preventing impairments, functional limitations, disability and injury including the promotion and maintenance of fitness, health and quality of life in all age populations.
4. Engaging in consultation, education and research.

# Appendix C Position Paper on Physical Therapist Assistant Regulation

FEDERATION OF STATE BOARDS OF PHYSICAL THERAPY

APPROVED BY THE BOARDS OF DIRECTORS • OCTOBER 1998

## THE IMPORTANCE OF REGULATING PHYSICAL THERAPIST ASSISTANTS

It is the position of the Federation of State Boards of Physical Therapy that physical therapist assistants should be regulated in each jurisdiction. The purpose of regulation is to protect the safety and welfare of the public. Physical therapists remain legally and professionally responsible for all physical therapy services including decisions for the appropriate use of assistive personnel. However, physical therapist assistants working under the supervision of physical therapists may perform many components of physical therapy treatment, and in the majority of states supervision of physical therapist assistants is not necessarily "on-site." A physical therapist assistant may be in a patient's home or in the clinic alone. Even with "on-site" supervision, the assistant may be with a patient on another floor in a building or behind a drawn curtain or closed door. Thus, where a greater potential for harm to the public exists, even with physical therapist supervision, regulation of the physical therapist assistant is advisable.

There are instances in states where physical therapist assistants are not regulated and a patient has withdrawn a complaint against an assistant once they learned that any action could only be taken against the supervising physical therapist. Without regulation, a physical therapist assistant has little accountability for making an error in clinical or behavioral judgment that may harm a patient. While a job may be at stake, a physical therapist assistant can easily move and work in another location. Without regulation there is no mechanism to notify other states of any action taken against an assistant since assistants who are not regulated are not subject to any Federation disciplinary database.

In 1997, 92 disciplinary actions against physical therapists were reported to the Federation of State Boards of Physical Therapy Disciplinary Database. Thirty-one disciplinary actions were reported against physical therapist assistants. As of December 31, 1997, there were 104,115 licensed physical therapists and 26,650 physical therapist assistants reported to the database.[1] In spite of the fact that they must work under supervision, there were more disciplinary actions taken per PTA than per PT.

FIGURE 1

**1997 Disciplinary Data Showing More Disciplines per PTA than per PT**

| | |
|---|---|
| PT Disciplines | 92 |
| PTA Disciplines | 31 |
| Total PTs | 104,115 |
| Total PTAs | 26,650 |
| Ratio of PT Disciplines to 1000 PTs | 0.8836 |
| Ratio of PT Disciplines to 1000 PTAs | 0.1163 |

The question then arises: What level of regulation is needed in order to enhance public protection? There are three options available in most states: licensure, certification or registration. Typically, the intent has been that licensure is most restrictive, followed by certification and finally registration. Unfortunately these terms have not been consistently defined or applied in various states. Most states require that the least restrictive or burdensome regulation that provides sufficient protection to the public be used. The Commonwealth of Virginia describes this:

> Regulations of any type constitute restraints on the exercise of free choice. Government should only exercise its power to regulate when it is found that regulation is clearly necessary for the preservation of the health, safety, and welfare of the public. Each provision of every regulation must have as its sole objective the protection of the public, must constitute the least burdensome method of achieving that purpose, and must be no more restrictive than the minimally acceptable standards of care to be provided to the public.[2]

## DEFINITIONS OF TERMS

Each of these regulatory terms may be defined as follows.

*Registration:* Registration, which is the least restrictive form of regulation, "should be considered when there is a low probability that the practitioner will inflict serious harm on the public."[3] In the purest form of registration, an applicant does not have to demonstrate any special qualifications. All that is required is that an individual registers his or her name, address and perhaps some relevant background information. The most basic form of registration carries neither warranty of competence nor any assurance that the registrant has met any predetermined standards, such as level of education or experience.[4]

*Certification:* Statutory certification implies a greater risk of harm to the public. It offers title protection.[5] Requirements at this level of regulation often include a specified level of education and passing entry competency examination. Statutory certification also allows a state board to discipline the certified individual if they violate established legislative and regulatory standards.

*Licensure:* Licensure implies the highest risk of harm to the public. It also implies a protection of scope of practice. Licensure usually requires an entry-level competency examination, educational requirements and the ability of a state board to discipline the licensee if they don't meet the established legislative and regulatory standards.

*Non-governmental certification:* To add confusion to the terminology, many private agencies offer non-governmental certification. It is important to maintain a distinction between non-governmental and statutory certification. Non-governmental certification is strictly voluntary. Non-governmental certification developed in the early 1900s, as physicians wanted to establish specialties.[6] Today many disciplines that have not warranted licensure or governmental certification have non-governmental certification. They include certified athletic trainers and personal trainers. Personal trainers have many private certifications they can choose from with varying requirements and focus for each one. However, none of these non-governmental certifications can prevent anyone who is not certified from calling himself or herself a personal trainer. This paper will consider only governmental certification.

In summary, each of the governmental regulatory terms can be defined to include the following distinctions.

***Registration • Much less potential danger to the public***

1. No independent scope of practice
2. May or may not have examination
3. May or may not have education requirements

4. No title protection
5. Usually voluntary

*Certification • Less potential danger to the public (i.e. may be under a form of supervision)*

1. Does not necessarily have an independent scope of practice or practice protection
2. Entry level examination required
3. Graduation from an approved education program
4. Ability for a board to discipline and revoke certification
5. Title protection
6. Mandatory in order to use the title

*Licensure • Requires the highest level of protection due to potential danger to the public*

1. Independent scope of practice with practice protection
2. Entry level examination required
3. Graduation from an approved education program
4. Ability for a board to discipline and revoke license
5. Title protection
6. Mandatory

FIGURE 2

**Differences Among Three Categories of Regulation**

| | Registration | Certification | Licensure |
|---|---|---|---|
| Potential for harm to the public | *Little* | *Moderate* | *High* |
| Scope pf practice protection | | | x |
| Mandatory | | *Maybe* | x |
| Ability of a board to discipline | | x | x |
| Title protection | | x | x |
| Entry-level examination | | x | x |
| Educational requirements | | x | x |

## APPROPRIATE REGULATION

The least restrictive form of regulation that will still afford public protection determines the appropriate level of regulation. When considering the regulation of assistants, the following should be mandatory requirements of the regulation: 1) minimal educational requirements, 2) entry competency examination, 3) title protection and 4) ability to discipline the individual and ultimate authority to revoke the regulatory certificate or license. All of these are needed to assure protection of the public. Registration does not meet these requirements. Registration as defined herein is not appropriate for regulation of physical therapist assistants.

Following the principle of the least restrictive form of regulation that affords public protection, it follows that governmental certification, as defined here, is the most appropriate form of regulation for the physical therapist assistant. Certification allows title protection, educational requirements, entry-level examination and disciplinary action. It does not necessarily afford scope of practice protection. However since physical therapist assistants do not have a unique body of knowledge nor an independent scope of practice, but are defined and regulated within the physical therapy practice act, this is not an issue. This would be an issue only with a certified profession with an independent scope. Because it is prohibited in state practice acts for anyone to perform physical therapy unless they are a physical therapist or under the supervision of a physical therapist, scope of practice protection is not necessary for physical therapist assistants. The scope of practice of the physical therapist is already protected and extends to any acts under the physical therapist's supervision.

It is recognized that not all states follow the "ideal" definitions of the regulatory terms. In fact, in a few states governmental certification is not available. Non-governmental certification would be optional and not afford disciplinary provisions or title protection. Certification would not be the appropriate form of regulation in such a state and the state may need to require licensure of its physical therapist assistants. Therefore:

It is the position of the Federation of State Boards of Physical Therapy that the least restrictive form of regulation available within a state should be used for physical therapist assistants that allows for 1) minimal educational requirements, 2) entry competency examination, 3) title protection, and 4) the board's power to discipline. This can usually be accomplished by statutory certification. When this is the case, regulation by licensure should be reserved for the physical therapist.

## Endnotes

[1] Federation of State Boards of Physical Therapy Disciplinary Database.

[2] Code of Virginia, 1950, 1993 Cumulative Supplement, The Mitchie Company, *Law Publishers*, Charlottesville, Virginia: 3.

[3] Kara Schmitt and Benjamin Shimberg, *Demystifying Occupational and Professional Regulation: Answers to Questions You May Have Been Afraid To Ask*, Council on Licensure, Enforcement and Regulation, 1996, p. 21.

[4] *Ibid*, p. 21.

[5] *Ibid*, p. 21–22.

[6] *Ibid*, p. 22–23.

# Appendix D
# FSBPT Model Language Changes for Licensure of Physical Therapist Assistants

*Appendix C* outlines the rationale for the Model Practice Act's recommendation that physical therapist assistants be regulated by state certification. As stated in the position statement on physical therapist assistant regulation, there may be times when state certification is not an option, or a state chooses to license rather than certify physical therapist assistants. In those instances, changes in the model statute language are not as simple as deleting references to certification or replacing those references with a reference to licensure.

*Appendix D* provides a sequential review of the Model Practice Act's key areas and shows the changes that should be made in the model statute language to accommodate licensing rather than certifying physical therapist assistants. Changes demonstrated in this appendix are formatted with the legislative ~~strike out~~ and LARGE CAP additions to demonstrate how the changes in the original language should be made.

If questions arise regarding these specific language recommendations please contact the FSBPT's Vice President of Professional Standards or a member of the Federation's Legislative Committee.

## KEY AREA #2 • DEFINITIONS

E. Assistive Personnel
   1. "Physical therapist assistant" means a person who meets the requirements of this act for ~~certification~~ LICENSURE AS A PHYSICAL THERAPIST ASSISTANT and who assists the physical therapist in selected components of physical therapy intervention.

F. "Restricted PHYSICAL THERAPIST license" means a license on which the board places restrictions or conditions, or both, as to scope of practice, place of practice, supervision of practice, duration of licensed status, or type or condition of patient or client to whom the licensee may provide services.

G. "Restricted PHYSICAL THERAPIST ASSISTANT LICENSE" ~~certificate~~ means a ~~certificate~~ LICENSE on which the board has placed any restrictions due to action imposed by the board.

## KEY AREA #3 • POWERS AND DUTIES OF THE BOARD

The board shall:

1. Evaluate the qualifications of applicants for licensure~~ and certification~~.
3. Issue licenses OR permits~~, or certificates~~ to persons who meet the requirements of this [chapter, act, section, law].
7. Establish mechanisms for assessing continuing competence of ~~licensees~~ PHYSICAL THERAPISTS.
11. Maintain a current list of all persons regulated under this chapter, including the person's name, current business and residential address, telephone numbers and license ~~or certificate~~ number.
15. Report final disciplinary action taken against a licensee ~~or certificate holder~~ to a national disciplinary database recognized by the board.
16. Publish, at least annually, final disciplinary action taken against a licensee ~~or certificate holder~~.

## KEY AREA #4 • LICENSURE AND EXAMINATION

### Qualifications for Licensure ~~and Certification~~

D. An applicant for ~~certification~~ LICENSURE as a physical therapist assistant shall:

### Application, Statement of Deficiencies, Hearing

A. An applicant for licensure ~~or certification~~ shall file a completed application as required by the board. The applicant shall include application and examination fees as prescribed in [reference the specific statute and/or rules specifying the fees].

### Examination

B. An applicant may take the examination for PHYSICAL THERAPIST licensure after the application process has been completed. The national examination shall test entry-level competency related to physical therapy theory, examination and evaluation, diagnosis, prognosis, treatment intervention, prevention, and consultation.
C. An applicant may take the examination for ~~certification~~ PHYSICAL THERAPIST ASSISTANT LICENSURE after the application process has been completed. The national examination shall test for requisite knowledge and skills in the technical application of physical therapy services.
D. An applicant for licensure ~~or certification~~ who does not pass the examination after the first attempt may re-take the examination one additional time without re-application for licensure ~~or certification~~ within 6 months after the first failure. Before the board may approve an applicant for subsequent testing beyond two attempts, an applicant shall re-apply for licensure ~~or certification~~ and shall demonstrate evidence satisfactory to the board of having successfully completed additional clinical training or course work, or both, as determined by the board.

### License ~~or Certificate~~ Renewal, Changes of Name or Address

A. A licensee ~~or certificate holder~~ shall renew the license ~~or certificate~~ pursuant to board rules. A licensee ~~or certificate holder~~ who fails to renew the license ~~or certificate~~ on or before its expiration date shall not practice as a physical therapist or work as a physical therapist assistant in this state.
B. Each licensee ~~or certificate holder~~ is responsible for reporting to the board a name change and changes in business and home address within 30 days after the change.

### Reinstatement of License ~~or Certificate~~

A. The board may reinstate a lapsed license ~~or certificate~~ on payment of a renewal fee and reinstatement fee.
B. If a ~~person's~~ PHYSICAL THERAPIST'S license has lapsed for more than 3 consecutive years ~~that person~~ THE PHYSICAL THERAPIST shall reapply for a license and pay all applicable fees. The ~~person~~ PHYSICAL THERAPIST shall also demonstrate to the board's satisfaction competency in the practice of physical therapy, or shall serve an internship under a restricted license or take remedial courses as determined by the board, or both, at the board's discretion. The board may also require the applicant to take an examination.

[Optional statute language] For states requiring maximum fee ceilings within the statutes.

### [Fees

[The board shall establish and collect fees not to exceed:

1. __________ dollars for an application for an original license ~~or certificate~~. This fee is nonrefundable.
2. __________ dollars for an examination for licensure ~~or certificate~~.
3. __________ dollars for a certificate of renewal of a license ~~or certificate~~.
4. __________ dollars for an application for reinstatement of a license ~~or certificate~~.
5. __________ dollars for each duplicate license ~~or certificate~~.]

## KEY AREA #6 • USE OF TITLES

### Use of Titles, Restrictions, Classification of Violation

C. A physical therapist assistant shall use the letters "PTA" in connection with that person's name to denote ~~certification~~ LICENSURE hereunder.

D. A person shall not use the title "physical therapist assistant," the letters "PTA," or any other words, abbreviations or insignia in connection with that person's name to indicate or imply, directly or indirectly, that the person is a physical therapist assistant unless that person is ~~certified~~ LICENSED as a physical therapist assistant pursuant to this [chapter, etc.]. A person who violates this subsection is guilty of a [cite specific legal sanction].

## KEY AREA #8 • GROUNDS FOR DISCIPLINARY ACTION

### Grounds for Disciplinary Action

The following are grounds for disciplinary action:

3. Obtaining or attempting to obtain a license or certificate by fraud or misrepresentation.
5. Engaging in the performance of substandard care by a physical therapist assistant, including exceeding the authority to perform tasks selected and delegated by the supervising ~~licensee~~ PHYSICAL THERAPIST regardless of whether actual injury to the patient is established.
9. Having had a license or certificate revoked or suspended, other disciplinary action taken, or an application for licensure or certification refused, revoked or suspended by the proper authorities of another

state, territory or country. [*Note:* This is one statutory paragraph that should be left unmodified, since it addresses forms of regulation in other states that may include licensure or certification.]

16. Aiding or abetting a person who is not licensed ~~or certified~~ in this state and who directly or indirectly performs activities requiring a license ~~or certificate~~.
17. Failing to report to the board any act or omission of a licensee, ~~certificate holder~~, applicant or any other person who violates the provisions of this [chapter, etc.].

## KEY AREA #9 • DISCIPLINARY ACTIONS/PROCEDURES

### Investigative Powers, Emergency Action, Hearing Officers

A. To enforce this [chapter, act section, law] the board may:
   1. Receive complaints filed against licensees or certificate holders and conduct a timely investigation.
   4. Take emergency action ordering the summary suspension of a license or certificate or the restriction of the ~~licensee's~~ A PHYSICAL THERAPIST'S practice or ~~certificate holder's~~ A PHYSICAL THERAPIST ASSISTANT'S employment pending proceedings by the board.
   6. Require a ~~licensee~~ PHYSICAL THERAPIST to be examined in order to determine the ~~licensee's~~ PHYSICAL THERAPIST'S mental, physical or professional competence.

B. If the board finds that the information received in a complaint or an investigation is not of sufficient seriousness to merit direct action against the licensee ~~or certificate holder~~ it may take either of the following actions:
   2. Issue a confidential advisory letter to the licensee ~~or certificate holder~~. An advisory letter is non-disciplinary and notifies a licensee ~~or certificate holder~~ that, while there is insufficient evidence to support disciplinary action, the board believes that the licensee ~~or certificate holder~~ should modify or eliminate certain conduct or practices.

### Disciplinary Actions, Penalties

On proof that any grounds prescribed in section [cite section on *Grounds for Disciplinary Action*] have been violated, the board may take the following disciplinary actions singly or in combination:

2. Restrict a license ~~or certificate~~. The board may require a licensee ~~or certificate holder~~ to report regularly to the board on matters related to the grounds for the restricted license ~~or certificate~~.
3. Suspend a license ~~or certificate~~ for a period prescribed by the board.

4. Revoke a license ~~or certificate~~.
5. Refuse to issue or renew a license ~~or certificate~~.
6. Impose a civil penalty of at least __________ but not more than __________. [Include minimum and maximum dollar amounts of civil penalties.] In addition the board may assess and collect the reasonable costs incurred in a disciplinary hearing when action is taken against a person's license ~~or certificate~~.
7. Accept a voluntary surrendering of a license ~~or certificate~~.

## KEY AREA #10 • UNLAWFUL PRACTICE

### Unlawful Practice, Classification, Civil Penalties, Injunctive Relief

A. It is unlawful for any person to practice or in any manner to claim to practice physical therapy or claim any word or designation that implies that the person is a physical therapist unless that person is licensed AS A PHYSICAL THERAPIST pursuant to this [chapter, act, section, law]. A person who engages in an activity requiring a PHYSICAL THERAPIST license pursuant to this [chapter, etc.] or uses any word, title, letters, or any description of services that incorporates one or more of the terms, designations or abbreviations in violation of section [cite specific *Use of Titles* section] that implies that the person is licensed to engage in the practice of physical therapy is guilty of a [cite specific legal sanction, e.g., class 1 misdemeanor].

## KEY AREA #11 • CONSUMER ADVOCACY

### Substance Abuse Recovery Program

In lieu of a disciplinary proceeding prescribed by this [chapter, act, section, law], the board may permit a licensee ~~or certificate holder~~ to actively participate in a board-approved substance abuse recovery program if:

1. The board has evidence that the licensee ~~or certificate holder~~ is impaired.
2. The licensee ~~or certificate holder~~ has not been convicted of a felony relating to a controlled substance in a court of law of the United States or any other territory or country.
3. The licensee ~~or certificate holder's~~ enters into a written agreement with the board for a restricted license ~~or certificate~~ and complies with all the terms of the agreement, including making satisfactory progress in the program and adhering to any limitations on the ~~licensee's~~ PHYSICAL THERAPIST'S practice or ~~certificate holder's~~ THE PHYSICAL THERAPIST ASSISTANT'S work imposed by the board to protect the public. Failure to enter into such an agreement shall activate an immediate investigation and disciplinary proceeding by the board.

4. As part of the agreement established between the licensee ~~or certificate holder~~ and the board, the licensee ~~or certificate holder~~ signs a waiver allowing the substance abuse program to release information to the board if the licensee ~~or certificate holder~~ does not comply with the requirements of this section or is unable to practice or work with reasonable skill or safety.

## Rights of Consumers

A. The public shall have access to the following information:
   1. A list of ~~licensees~~ PHYSICAL THERAPISTS and interim permit holders that includes place of practice, license or interim permit number, date of license or interim permit expiration and status of license.
   2. A list of physical therapist assistants ~~certified~~ LICENSED in the state, including place of employment, ~~certification~~ LICENSE number and date of ~~certificate~~ LICENSE expiration.

G. Any person may submit a complaint regarding any licensee, ~~certificate holder~~, or any other person potentially in violation of this [chapter, act, section, law]. Confidentiality shall be maintained subject to law.

H. The board shall keep all information relating to the receiving and investigation of complaints filed against licensees ~~or certificate holders~~ confidential until the information becomes public record or as required by law.

# Appendix E
# Code of Ethics and Guide for Professional Conduct

Reprinted With Permission

## PREAMBLE

This *Code of Ethics* sets forth ethical principles for the physical therapy profession. Members of this profession are responsible for maintaining and promoting ethical practice. This *Code of Ethics,* adopted by the American Physical Therapy Association, shall be binding on physical therapists who are members of the Association.

***Principle 1*** • Physical therapists respect the rights and dignity of all individuals.

***Principle 2*** • Physical therapists comply with the laws and regulations governing the practice of physical therapy.

***Principle 3*** • Physical therapists accept responsibility for the exercise of sound judgment.

***Principle 4*** • Physical therapists maintain and promote high standards for physical therapy practice, education, and research.

***Principle 5*** • Physical therapists seek remuneration for their services that is deserved and reasonable.

***Principle 6*** • Physical therapists provide accurate information to the consumer about the profession and about those services they provide.

***Principle 7*** • Physical therapists accept the responsibility to protect the public and the profession from unethical, incompetent, or illegal acts.

***Principle 8*** • Physical therapists participate in efforts to address the health needs of the public.

Adopted by the House of Delegates, June 1981 Amended June 1987, June 1991

## GUIDE FOR PROFESSIONAL CONDUCT

### Purpose

This *Guide for Professional Conduct (Guide)* is intended to serve physical therapists who are members of the American Physical Therapy Association (Association) in interpreting the *Code of Ethics (Code)* and matters of professional conduct. The *Guide* provides guidelines by which physical therapists may determine the propriety of their conduct. The *Code* and the *Guide* apply to all physical therapists who are Association members. These guidelines are subject to changes as the dynamics of the profession change and as new patterns of health care delivery are developed and accepted by the professional community and the public. This *Guide* is subject to monitoring and timely revision by the Ethics and Judicial Committee of the Association.

### Interpreting Ethical Principles

The interpretations expressed in this *Guide* are not to be considered all inclusive of situations that could evolve under a specific principle of the *Code* but reflect the opinions, decisions, and advice of the Ethics and Judicial Committee. Although the statements of ethical principles apply universally, specific circumstances determine their appropriate application. Input related to current interpretations, or situations requiring interpretation, is encouraged from Association members.

### Principle 1

Physical therapists respect the rights and dignity of all individuals.

*1.1 Attitudes of Physical Therapists*

A. Physical therapists shall recognize that each individual is different from all other individuals and shall respect and be responsive to those differences.
B. Physical therapists are to be guided at all times by concern for the physical, psychological, and socioeconomic welfare of those individuals entrusted to their care.
C. Physical therapists shall not engage in conduct that constitutes harassment or abuse of, or discrimination against, colleagues, associates, or others.

*1.2 Confidential Information*

A. Information relating to the physical therapist/patient relationship is confidential and may not be communicated to a third party not involved in that patient's care without the prior written consent of the patient, subject to applicable law.

B. Information derived from component-sponsored peer review shall be held confidential by the reviewer unless written permission to release the information is obtained from the physical therapist who was reviewed.
C. Information derived from the working relationships of physical therapists shall be held confidential by all parties.
D. Information may be disclosed to appropriate authorities when it is necessary to protect the welfare of an individual or the community. Such disclosure shall be in accordance with applicable law.

*1.3 Patient Relations*

Physical therapists shall not engage in any sexual relationship or activity, whether consensual or nonconsensual, with any patient while a physical therapist/patient relationship exists.

*1.4 Informed Consent*

Physical therapists shall obtain patient informed consent before treatment, to include disclosure of: (i) the nature of the proposed intervention, (ii) material risks of harm or complications, (iii) reasonable alternatives to the proposed intervention, and (iv) goals of treatment.

## Principle 2

Physical therapists comply with the laws and regulations governing the practice of physical therapy.

*2.1 Professional Practice*

Physical therapists shall provide consultation, evaluation, treatment, and preventive care in accordance with the laws and regulations of the jurisdiction(s) in which they practice.

## Principle 3

Physical therapists accept responsibility for the exercise of sound judgment.

*3.1 Acceptance of Responsibility*

A. Upon accepting a patient/client for provision of physical therapy services, physical therapists shall assume the responsibility for examining, evaluating, and diagnosing that individual; prognosis and intervention; re-examination and modification of the plan of care; and maintaining adequate records of the case including progress reports. Physical therapists establish the plan of care and provide and/or supervise the appropriate intervention.

B. If the diagnostic process reveals findings that are outside the scope of the physical therapist's knowledge, experience, or expertise, the physical therapist shall so inform the patient/client and refer to an appropriate practitioner.
C. Regardless of practice setting, physical therapists shall maintain the ability to make independent judgments.
D. The physical therapist shall not provide physical therapy services to a patient while under the influence of a substance that impairs his or her ability to do so safely.
E. When the patient is referred from another practitioner, the physical therapist shall communicate the findings of the examination, the diagnosis, the proposed intervention, and re-examination findings (as indicated) to the referring practitioner and any other appropriate individuals involved in the patient's care, while maintaining standards of confidentiality.

*3.2 Delegation of Responsibility*

A. Physical therapists shall not delegate to a less qualified person any activity that requires the unique skill, knowledge, and judgment of the physical therapist.
B. The primary responsibility for physical therapy care rendered by supportive personnel rests with the supervising physical therapist. Adequate supervision requires, at a minimum, that a supervising physical therapist perform the following activities:
   1. Designate or establish channels of written and oral communication.
   2. Interpret available information concerning the individual under care.
   3. Examine, evaluate, and determine a diagnosis.
   4. Develop plan of care, including short- and long-term goals.
   5. Select and delegate appropriate tasks of plan of care.
   6. Assess competence of supportive personnel to perform assigned tasks.
   7. Direct and supervise supportive personnel in delegated tasks.
   8. Identify and document precautions, special problems, contraindications, goals, anticipated progress, and plans for re-evaluation.
   9. Re-evaluate, adjust plan of care when necessary, perform final evaluation, and establish follow-up plan.

*3.3 Provision of Services*

A. Physical therapists shall recognize the individual's freedom of choice in selection of physical therapy services.
B. Physical therapists' professional practices and their adherence to ethical principles of the Association shall take preference over business prac-

tices. Provisions of services for personal financial gain rather than for the need of the individual receiving the services are unethical.

C. When physical therapists judge that an individual will no longer benefit from their services, they shall so inform the individual receiving the services. Physical therapists shall avoid overutilization of their services.

D. In the event of elective termination of a physical therapist/patient relationship by the physical therapist, the therapist should take steps to transfer the care of the patient, as appropriate, to another provider.

E. Physical therapists shall recognize that third-party payer contracts may limit, in one form or another, provision of physical therapy services. Physical therapists shall inform patients of any known limitations. Third-party limitations do not absolve the physical therapist from adherence to ethical principles. Physical therapists shall avoid underutilization of their services.

*3.4 Practice Arrangements*

A. Participation in a business, partnership, corporation, or other entity does not exempt the physical therapist, whether employer, partner, or stockholder, either individually or collectively, from the obligation of promoting and maintaining the ethical principles of the Association.

B. Physical therapists shall advise their employer(s) of any employer practice that causes a physical therapist to be in conflict with the ethical principles of the Association. Physical therapist employees shall attempt to rectify aspects of their employment that are in conflict with the ethical principles of the Association.

**Principle 4**

Physical therapists maintain and promote high standards for physical therapy practice, education, and research.

*4.1 Continued Education*

A. Physical therapists shall participate in educational activities that enhance their basic knowledge and provide new knowledge.

B. Whenever physical therapists provide continuing education, they shall ensure that course content, objectives, and responsibilities of the instructional faculty are accurately reflected in the promotion of the course.

*4.2 Review and Self-Assessment*

A. Physical therapists shall provide for utilization review of their services.

B. Physical therapists shall demonstrate their commitment to quality assurance by peer review and self-assessment.

*4.3 Research*

A. Physical therapists shall support research activities that contribute knowledge for improved patient care.
B. Physical therapists engaged in research shall ensure:
   1. The consent of subjects
   2. Confidentiality of the data on individual subjects and the personal identities of the subjects
   3. Well-being of all subjects in compliance with facility regulations and laws of the jurisdiction in which the research is conducted
   4. The absence of fraud and plagiarism
   5. Full disclosure of support received
   6. Appropriate acknowledgment of individuals making a contribution to the research
   7. That animal subjects used in research are treated humanely and in compliance with facility regulations and laws of the jurisdiction in which the research experimentation is conducted
C. Physical therapists shall report to appropriate authorities any acts in the conduct or presentation of research that appear unethical or illegal.

*4.4 Education*

A. Physical therapists shall support high-quality education in academic and clinical settings.
B. Physical therapists functioning in the educational role are responsible to the students, the academic institutions, and the clinical settings for promoting ethical conduct in educational activities. Whenever possible, the educator shall ensure:
   1. The rights of students in the academic and clinical settings
   2. Appropriate confidentiality of personal information
   3. Professional conduct toward the student during the academic and clinical educational processes
   4. Assignment to clinical settings prepared to give the student a learning experience
C. Clinical educators are responsible for reporting to the academic program student conduct that appears to be unethical or illegal.

**Principle 5**

Physical therapists seek remuneration for their services that is deserved and reasonable.

*5.1 Fiscally Sound Remuneration*

A. Physical therapists shall never place their own financial interest above the welfare of individuals under their care.

B. Fees for physical therapy services should be reasonable for the service performed, considering the setting in which it is provided, practice costs in the geographic area, judgment of other organizations, and other relevant factors.
C. Physical therapists should attempt to ensure that providers, agencies, or other employers adopt physical therapy fee schedules that are reasonable and that encourage access to necessary services.

*5.2 Business Practices/Fee Arrangements*

A. Physical therapists shall not:
   1. Directly or indirectly request, receive, or participate in the dividing, transferring, assigning, or rebating of an unearned fee
   2. Profit by means of a credit or other valuable consideration, such as an unearned commission, discount, or gratuity in connection with the furnishing of physical therapy services
B. Unless laws impose restrictions to the contrary, physical therapists who provide physical therapy services in a business entity may pool fees and monies received. Physical therapists may divide or apportion these fees and monies in accordance with the business agreement.
C. Physical therapists may enter into agreements with organizations to provide physical therapy services if such agreements do not violate the ethical principles of the Association.

*5.3 Endorsement of Equipment or Services*

A. Physical therapists shall not use influence on individuals under their care or their families for utilization of equipment or services based on the direct or indirect financial interest of the physical therapist in such equipment or services. Realizing that these individuals will normally rely on the physical therapists' advice, their best interest must always be maintained, as must their right of free choice relating to the use of any equipment or service. Although it cannot be considered unethical for physical therapists to own or have a financial interest in equipment companies or services, they must act in accordance with law and make full disclosure of their interest whenever such companies or services become the source of equipment or services for individuals under their care.
B. Physical therapists may be remunerated for endorsement or advertisement of equipment or services to the lay public, physical therapists, or other health professionals provided they disclose any financial interest in the production, sale, or distribution of said equipment or services.
C. In endorsing or adverting equipment or services, physical therapists shall use sound professional judgment and shall not give the appearance of Association endorsement.

*5.4 Gifts and Other Considerations*

A. Physical therapists shall not accept nor offer gifts or other considerations with obligatory conditions attached.
B. Physical therapists shall not accept nor offer gifts or other considerations that affect or give an objective appearance of affecting their professional judgment.

**Principle 6**

Physical therapists provide accurate information to the consumer about the profession and about those services they provide.

*6.1 Information About the Profession*

Physical therapists shall endeavor to educate the public to an awareness of the physical therapy profession through such means as publication of articles and participation in seminars, lectures, and civic programs.

*6.2 Information About Services*

A. Information given to the public shall emphasize that individual problems cannot be treated without individualized evaluation and plans/programs of care.
B. Physical therapists may advertise their services to the public.
C. Physical therapists shall not use, or participate in the use of, any form of communication containing a false, plagiarized, fraudulent, misleading, deceptive, unfair, or sensational statement or claim.
D. A paid advertisement shall be identified as such unless it is apparent from the context that it is a paid advertisement.

**Principle 7**

Physical therapists accept the responsibility to protect the public and the profession from unethical, incompetent, or illegal acts.

*7.1 Consumer Protection*

A. Physical therapists shall report any conduct that appears to be unethical, incompetent, or illegal.
B. Physical therapists may not participate in any arrangements in which patients are exploited due to the referring sources enhancing their personal incomes as a result of referring for, prescribing, or recommending physical therapy.
C. Physical therapists shall be obligated to safeguard the public from underutilization or overutilization of physical therapy services.

*7.2 Disclosure*

The physical therapist shall disclose to the patient if the referring practitioner derives compensation from the provision of physical therapy. The physical therapist shall ensure that the individual has freedom of choice in selecting a provider of physical therapy.

## Principle 8

Physical therapists participate in efforts to address the health needs of the public.

*8.1 Pro Bono Service*

Physical therapists should render pro bono publico (reduced or no fee) services to patients lacking the ability to pay for services, as each physical therapist's practice permits.

Issued by Ethics and Judicial Committee, American Physical Therapy Association, October 1981. Last Amended January 1999.

# Appendix F
# FSBPT Guidelines on English Proficiency Test Standards

FEDERATION OF STATE BOARDS OF PHYSICAL THERAPY

## ENGLISH LANGUAGE PROFICIENCY

It is recommended that all three of the following passing scores on the respective examinations be requirements for licensure for all candidates who have not graduated from a U.S. program accredited by CAPTE.

Test of English as a Foreign Language (TOEFL): 560
Test of Written English (TWE): 4.5
Test of Spoken English (TSE): 50

Individuals who meet both of the following conditions may be exempt from this requirement for language proficiency testing:

1. The native language of the country of origin is English.
2. Graduated from a PT program that was conducted in English.

## BACKGROUND INFORMATION

English language proficiency is critical for competent performance at the entry level of practice. Common passing scores among jurisdictions is consistent with the FSBPT goal of reasonable uniformity of standards, which facilitates mobility of qualified physical therapists. All three examinations should be required because each examination measures different language proficiency skills:

TOEFL: Listening Comprehension
Structure and Written Comprehension
Vocabulary and Reading Comprehension
TWE: Written Language Ability
TSE: Oral Language Ability

APPENDIX III

# American Physical Therapy Association

**Organizational Chart**

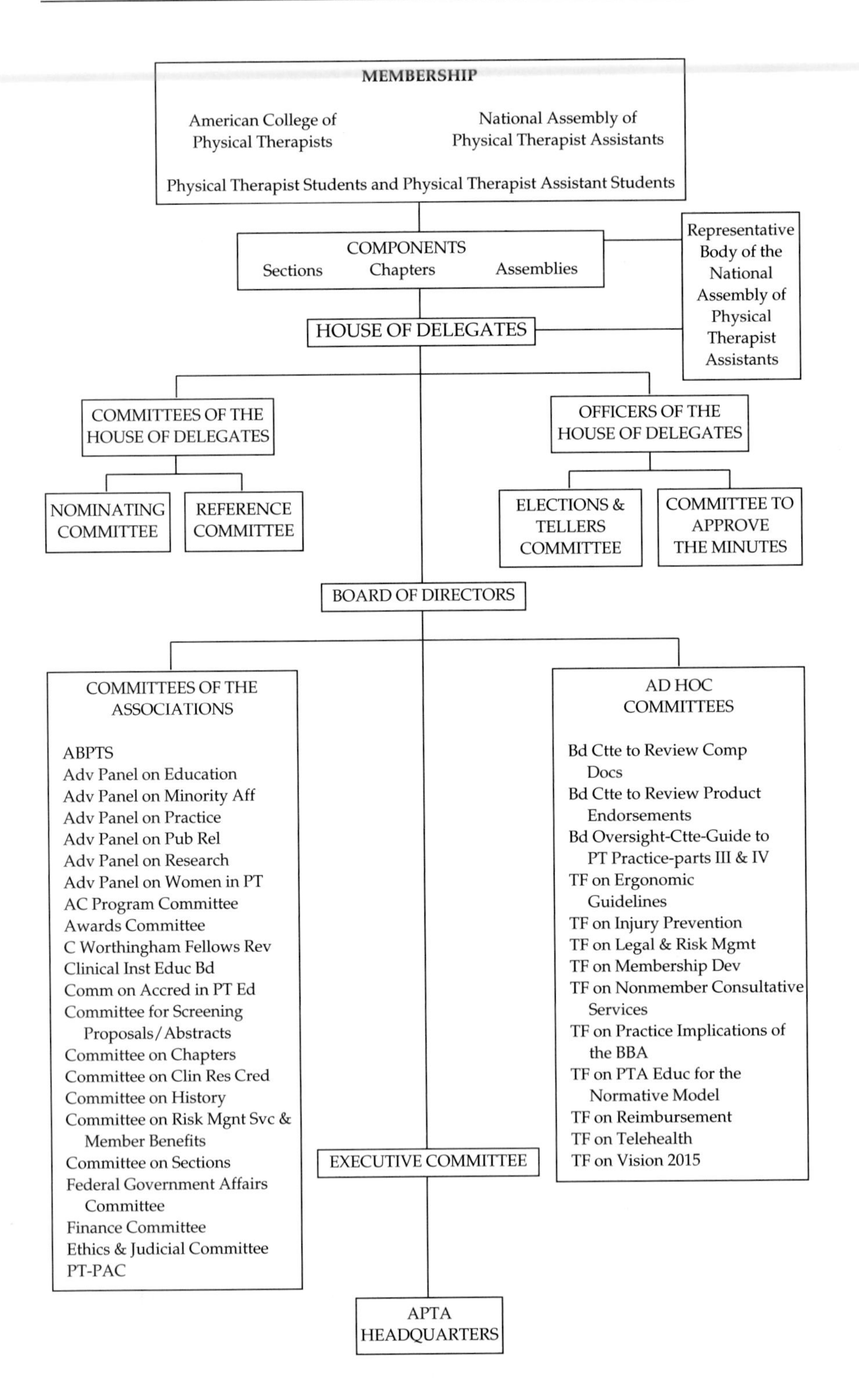
MEMBERSHIP
American College of Physical Therapists
National Assembly of Physical Therapist Assistants
Physical Therapist Students and Physical Therapist Assistant Students
COMPONENTS
Sections
Chapters
Assemblies
Representative Body of the National Assembly of Physical Therapist Assistants
HOUSE OF DELEGATES
COMMITTEES OF THE HOUSE OF DELEGATES
OFFICERS OF THE HOUSE OF DELEGATES
NOMINATING COMMITTEE
REFERENCE COMMITTEE
ELECTIONS & TELLERS COMMITTEE
COMMITTEE TO APPROVE THE MINUTES
BOARD OF DIRECTORS
COMMITTEES OF THE ASSOCIATIONS
ABPTS
Adv Panel on Education
Adv Panel on Minority Aff
Adv Panel on Practice
Adv Panel on Pub Rel
Adv Panel on Research
Adv Panel on Women in PT
AC Program Committee
Awards Committee
C Worthingham Fellows Rev
Clinical Inst Educ Bd
Comm on Accred in PT Ed
Committee for Screening Proposals/Abstracts
Committee on Chapters
Committee on Clin Res Cred
Committee on History
Committee on Risk Mgnt Svc & Member Benefits
Committee on Sections
Federal Government Affairs Committee
Finance Committee
Ethics & Judicial Committee
PT-PAC
AD HOC COMMITTEES
Bd Ctte to Review Comp Docs
Bd Ctte to Review Product Endorsements
Bd Oversight-Ctte-Guide to PT Practice-parts III & IV
TF on Ergonomic Guidelines
TF on Injury Prevention
TF on Legal & Risk Mgmt
TF on Membership Dev
TF on Nonmember Consultative Services
TF on Practice Implications of the BBA
TF on PTA Educ for the Normative Model
TF on Reimbursement
TF on Telehealth
TF on Vision 2015
EXECUTIVE COMMITTEE
APTA HEADQUARTERS

# Index

**B**

## C

**Q**



**R**